The
Treatment of Haemophilia A and B and
von Willebrand's Disease

The Treatment of Haemophilia A and B and von Willebrand's Disease

EDITED BY

ROSEMARY BIGGS

BSc, PhD, MD, MRCP, MA.

Director, Oxford Haemophilia Centre.
Lecturer in Haematology
University of Oxford

BLACKWELL SCIENTIFIC PUBLICATIONS
OXFORD LONDON EDINBURGH MELBOURNE

© 1978 Blackwell Scientific Publications
Osney Mead, Oxford, OX2 0EL
8 John Street, London, WC1N 2ES
9 Forrest Road, Edinburgh, EH1 2QH
P.O. Box 9, North Balwyn, Victoria, Australia

All rights reserved. No part of this
publication may be reproduced, stored in a
retrieval system, or transmitted, in any
form or by any means, electronic,
mechanical, photocopying, recording or
otherwise, without the prior permission
of the copyright owner.

First published 1978

British Library Cataloguing in
Publication Data

The treatment of Haemophilia A and B and von Willebrand's disease.
1. Haemophilia
I. Biggs, Rosemary
616. 1'57   RC642
ISBN: 0-632-00216-6

Distributed in the U.S.A. by
J. B. Lippincott Company, Philadelphia
and in Canada by
J. B. Lippincott Company of Canada Ltd, Toronto

Printed in Great Britain by
Burgess & Son Ltd, Abingdon, Oxon
and bound by
Kemp Hall Bindery Ltd, Oxford

Contents

Preface   x

1 Blood Coagulation and Haemostasis   1
  R. G. MACFARLANE
  Blood coagulation 2
  Platelet aggregation and adhesion 9
  Vascular and tissue function in haemostasis 10
  The haemostatic mechanism as a whole 11
  The consequences of haemostatic failure 12
  The clinical picture in haemophilia, Christmas disease and von Willebrand's disease 19
     Haemophilia A 19
     Christmas disease (haemophilia B) 25
     Von Willebrand's disease 26
  References 27

2 Factor VIII   29
  D. E. G. AUSTEN
  Introduction and nomenclature 29
  Measurement of factor VIII 30
  Factor VIII in the body 31
  Factor VIII synthesis *in vivo* 33
  The purification of factor VIII 34
  The stability of factor VIII 36
  Buffers for factor VIII 37
  Animal factor VIII 37
  The chemical structure of factor VIII 39
  Molecular weights, sub-units and the segregation of factor VIII activity 41
  Sub-units of factor-VIII-related antigen and ristocetin co-factor 45
     Molecular weight of factor VIII in polyacrylamide gels 46
     Reaggregation of factor VIII 47
  Antibodies to factor VIII 47
  Chemical conclusions about factor VIII 49
  References 51

3 The Laboratory and Clinical Diagnosis of Patients with Coagulation Defects   58
  ROSEMARY BIGGS
  Clinical History and diagnosis 59

Chapter 3 continued
    Laboratory diagnosis   63
        Assay of factor VIII   65
        Errors in measuring factor VIII   70
        Standards of normality for factor VIII   70
        Assay of factor IX   71
        The diagnosis of patients having anti-factor VIII antibodies   73
            The kinetics of factor VIII and antibody interaction   74
            The measurement of antifactor VIII antibodies   77
        The diagnosis of carriers of haemophilia using the level of factor VIII as criterion   79
            The absorption of antibody by factor VIII   80
        Factor-VIII-related antigen and detection of carriers of haemophilia   82
    Clinical syndromes   84
        Von Willebrand's disease   84
        Factor IX deficiency   84
        Factor I (fibrinogen) deficiency   85
        Factor II (prothrombin) deficiency   85
        Deficiency of factors V, VII and X   86
        Defects in the contract phase of clotting (factors XI and XII)   86
        Factor XIII deficiency   86
        Abnormalities of coagulation due to the presence of inhibitors   86
    Concluding remarks   87
    References   87

4 The Amount of Blood Required Annually to make Concentrates to Treat Patients with Haemophilia A & B   **89**
ROSEMARY BIGGS

The number of patients with haemophilia A in the population   90
The amount of factor VIII expressed as units of activity required on average by each haemophiliac   93
    The number of doses given per year to haemophilia A patients in Oxford   94
    The average units of factor VIII given per infusion   98
The types of therapeutic material available to treat haemophilia A patients   98
    Fresh frozen plasma   100
    Cryoprecipitate   101
    Intermediate purity NHS factor VIII   102
    Commercial human factor VIII   103
    Animal factor VIII   103
The total amount of factor VIII required annually for all haemophilia A patients in the United Kingdom   104
What is the best form in which the factor VIII should be presented?   104
Is it possible to provide the factor VIII from a wholly voluntary blood transfusion service?   105
The treatment of patients with factor IX deficiency   106
References   107

5 Plasma Concentrations of Factor VIII and Factor IX and Treatment of Patients who do not have Antibodies directed against these Factors   **110**
ROSEMARY BIGGS

The patient's response to treatment in relation to plasma volume and weight   110

Contents

Chapter 5 continued
    The response of haemophilia A patients to treatment 112
    The response of haemophilia B patients to treatment 115
    The half-life of factors VIII and IX following infusion to patients who lack these factors 115
    Whole blood or plasma as source of factor VIII or IX 120
    Concentrated preparations from human plasma as source of factor VIII 121
        Animal factor VIII in the treatment of haemophilia A 123
    Calculation of the dose of factor VIII for haemophilic patients 124
    The response of factor IX deficient patients to factor IX 124
    Conclusion 125
    References 125

6 The Control of Haemostasis in Haemophilic Patients   127
ROSEMARY BIGGS AND C. R. RIZZA

    Spontaneous bleeding into soft tissues, muscles and joints 128
    Spontaneous bleeding into specific sites other than joints 130
        Deep muscle haematomata 131
        Other types of spontaneous bleeding 132
    Treatment of the spontaneous type of bleeding in patients who have Christmas disease 132
    The administration of factor VIII or factor IX to the patient 132
    Home therapy and prophylaxis 134
    The dental care of patients having haemophilia or Christmas disease 135
        Dental extraction in haemophilia A patients 135
        Dental extraction in haemophilia B patients 138
        A suggested regime for dental extraction in haemophilic patients 139
    The control of haemorrhage following major surgery 142
        The factor VIII treatment of haemophilia A patients who require surgery 143
        The factor IX treatment of Christmas disease patients who require surgery 146
    Conclusion 151
    References 151

7 Home Therapy   153
C. R. RIZZA, ROSEMARY BIGGS AND ROSEMARY SPOONER

    The criteria for admitting patients to the home therapy programme 154
    The introduction of a patient to home therapy 156
    The dosage of factors VIII and IX for home therapy 159
    Observations on Oxford home therapy patients 159
    The amounts and types of material used for home therapy at the Oxford Haemophilia Centre 162
    Home therapy for haemophilia B patients 165
    Home therapy for special occasions 166
    Complications of treatment 166
    The assessments of benefits of treatment 167
        A year in the life of a haemophilic boy 167
        Comments by haemophilic patients and their parents on the benefits of home therapy 169

8 Von Willebrand's Disease   172
C. R. RIZZA

   Nature of the disease   172
   Clinical features   172
The defect in von Willebrand's disease   173
The work of the Oxford Haemophilia Centre
   Bleeding time   173
   Factor VIII deficiency   174
   Capillary and platelet defects   174
   Adhesion of platelets to glass beads   174
   Aggregation of platelets in the presence of ristocetin   174
   Factor-VIII-related antigen   175
   Transfusion studies in von Willebrand's disease   175
The diagnosis of von Willebrand's disease   176
The Management of patients with von Willebrand's disease   178
   Epistaxis   178
   Dental extraction   178
   Menorrhagia   179
   Major surgery   179
References   179

9 Complications of Treatment   181
ROSEMARY BIGGS

Transmission of diseases contained in the fractions   181
   Hepatitis   181
   The diagnosis of hepatitis   183
   The susceptibility of patients to infection with hepatitis   184
   The need for future observations for the prevention of hepatitis   187
   An attempt to analyse the source of hepatitis in patients during 1974 in Oxford   187
   Other diseases transmitted by whole blood or other fractions   188
   Pyrogenic and other adverse reactions to infusion therapy   189
Thrombosis and the administration of clotting factor concentrates   190
The occurrence of antibodies directed against factor VIII or factor IX   193
   Antibodies to factor IX   194
   The treatment of patients who have factor VIII antibodies   195
      The treatment of patients with low titre antibodies or those whose antibodies have temporarily disappeared   195
   The natural history of factor VIII antibodies   198
   The circumstances which influence the decision to treat a patient having factor VII antibody   198
      The use of bovine or porcine factor VIII for patients having factor VIII antibodies   199
      The use of cyclocapron in patient having factor VIII antibodies   199
      Factor IX and the treatment of patients having factor VIII antibodies   200
      Immunosuppressing drugs and the treatment of patients who have factor VIII antibodies   200
      References   200

10 Organisation of Haemophilia Treatment   203
ROSEMARY BIGGS

    The Haemophilia Centre (Historical) 205
    The organisation of a Haemophilia Centre 206
        Haemophilia Centres 206
        Associate Haemophilia Centres 207
        Reference Centres 207
    The work of the Oxford Haemophilia Centre 210
        Diagnosis and laboratory testing 210
        Treatment and general advice 211
            Home therapy 215
            Consultation 216
    Conclusion 217
    References 218

11 Haemophilia, Medical Science and Society   219
ROSEMARY BIGGS AND C. R. RIZZA

    Academic research and the treatment of patients 219
        Chemical studies of the structure of factor VIII 221
        Why do haemophilic patients bleed in the way that they do? 222
            Inhibitors in haemophilia 222
            Aspirin and haemophilia 223
            Haemophilia and von Willebrand's disease 223
            Platelets and haemophilia 223
    Limitation of haemophilia by genetic counselling 224
    Factor VIII and the blood transfusion service 226
    How much factor VIII is enough? 229
    The treatment of haemophilic patients in society 229
    How can the effectiveness of the medical services be judged? 231
    Conclusion 234
    References 234

Index

Preface

The present book was started as a Second Edition of *The Treatment of Haemophilia and other Coagulation Disorders* (Blackwell Scientific Publications 1966). This first book described in detail, almost case by case, the experience gained in Oxford in treating patients having haemophilia and related conditions. Before 1966 the treatment of haemophilic patients was a worrying cooperative enterprise involving conferences between many different specialists. Surgical procedures had to be modified on account of the patient's haemostatic defect and local aids to haemostasis such as dental splints were developed. Each case presented a problem in assuring haemostasis with the very limited supply of factor VIII then available. In 1966 many patients having relatively mild haemarthroses were treated by rest and immobilisation without factor VIII infusion. Had factor VIII been used for these patients none would have been available for patients who had more serious bleeding. In fact patients also had to wait for months or even years for operations until enough factor VIII could be stockpiled for their post-operative care.

Cooperation between doctors of different specialities is still important in planning the treatment of haemophilic patients, but the much greater availability of therapeutic materials has, in most cases, removed the need to use special surgical procedures. This book contains no chapters on special surgical and dental procedures simply because many of such special procedures are out-dated by the more certain and effective haemostatic control. In the case of orthopaedic management in Oxford this subject has been developed separately by Duthie and his colleagues (*The Management of Musculo-skeletal Problems in the Haemophilias*, Blackwell Scientific Publications 1972). The present book is thus written by staff at the Oxford Haemophilia Centre. We should like to thank all of the doctors, nurses, physiotherapists, social workers and others who have helped us, over the years, to develop the system of treatment now used.

The greater availability of therapeutic material has also meant that even the most minor episodes of bleeding are now treated by infusion therapy and this has opened up a new set of problems in the management of haemophilia. It is now possible to plan for patients having haemophilia to live nearly normal lives. The frequent treatments needed to ensure safety in all circumstances has prompted the development of a new approach to the treatment of haemophilia in the patients' homes. In addition, the large amounts of therapeutic material now available raise questions about the cost of this treatment, the supply of plasma and the social implications of the medical services now used by haemophilic patients. Thus the present book has a very different emphasis from the previous book (*The Treatment of Haemophilia and other Coagulation Disorders*). The present book is written for haematologists and physicians and surgeons who care for haemophilic patients. Much of the approach is rather academic. A number of difficult problems are discussed in detail: for example, the standardization of the factor VIII assay, the absorption of factor VIII antibody by factor VIII, the chemistry of factor VIII and the kinetics of interaction of factor VIII and antibody. These are problems which have interested us and we hope the discussion about them will be helpful or stimulating to other specialists. In the more clinical chapters a rather authoritarian approach has been adopted. We have simply described what we do without too much talk about what others do or might have done.

The book is not written for patients but many patients and their parents undertake much responsibility for therapy in their own homes. In this new situation patients may find this book helpful for reference. Patients may also be interested in the social and economic problems raised by haemophilia treatment. If patients do consult this book they should bear in mind the biased point of view that we present. In medicine there are often many ways of achieving essentially the same results. If the treatment that a patient receives does not correspond exactly with that described in this book the treatment is not necessarily wrong. It may also happen that advances in science may outdate the treatment regimes that we now advocate in the same way that recent advances have outdated the policies that we put forward in 1966.

We have made no attempt to cover all of the literature about the treatment of haemophilia which has accumulated in the last 10 years. The book is deliberately biased to emphasize the experience gained in Oxford. This does not mean that we do not appreciate the valuable observations of others. We do appreciate the literature and many papers not quoted here have influenced our points of view. A full discussion of the literature would, we feel, have confused what we hope is a simple description of our own practice and our own opinions.

The data in some of the tables used in chapters other than chapter 7 was collected, sifted and calculated by Miss Rosemary Spooner. The diagrams were drawn by Mr Roger Matchett and Mr Raymond Borrett.

Much of the therapeutic material used to treat patients was prepared in the Oxford Plasma Fractionation Laboratory by Dr E. Bidwell and her staff from plasma collected by the Oxford Regional Blood Transfusion Service. We should like to thank all of those concerned for their continued and ever increasing efforts over the years to supply the needs of haemophilic patients.

The Oxford Haemophilia Centre has also received much help and encouragement from the Oxford Area and Oxford Regional Health Authorities and from the DHSS. All of those with whom we have had dealings over the years have done their utmost to see that haemophilic patients receive optimum therapy. The DHSS gave kind permission for an extensive quotation from their circular HC (76)4 which appears between pages 206 and 210.

We should like to thank Dr J.J.Sixma who provided data used in Table 5.1.

We should like to acknowledge permission to publish data or short quotations in the text as follows:

1 To *Nature* **253**, page 55 (1975) for figures 2.3 and 2.5.
2 To *The British Journal of Haematology* as follows:
   27, page 89 (1974) for figures 2.2 and 2.4.
   22, page 735 (1972) for figure 3.4.
   24, page 65 (1973) for tables 3.7, 9.4, 9.5 and figure 3.5.
   30, page 44 (1975) for figure 3.6.
   28, page 35 (1974) for figure 8.3.
   35, page 483 (1977) for tables 9.1, 9.2 and 9.3.
We also thank Dr Peter Kernoff for permission to use figure 3.4.
3 To *Thrombosis and Haemostasis* **35**, 274 (1976) for table 3.8.
4 Figures 5.1, 5.2, 5.3, and 8.1 are taken from *The Treatment of Haemophilia and other Coagulation Disorders* by Biggs R. and Macfarlane R.G., Blackwell Scientific Publications 1966.
5 Short quotations as follows:
   To Mr Hermans, Dr K.Brinkhous and Excerpta Medica for a quotation from *A Handbook of Haemophilia* on page 153.
   To Professor Max Perutz and the Editor of *New Scientist,* London; a weekly review of science and technology, for a quotation from an article entitled 'Haemoglobin the molecular lung' on page 221.
   Professor Sir Peter Medawar and his publishers, Methuen, for a short quotation from *The Art of the Soluble* on page 219.
   Mr Robert Massie and Mrs Suzanne Massie and Irving and Hudson N.Y. 10533, publishers, for short quotations on page 153 and page 218.

Chapter 1. Blood Coagulation and Haemostasis

R. G. MACFARLANE

The clinical problems presented by patients with haemophilia and similar conditions are essentially the results of abnormal bleeding, and they can only be dealt with on a rational basis if the causes of such bleeding are known and understood. But an understanding of the abnormal implies knowledge of the normal, and there is still no clear picture of the pattern of events which constitute the normal haemostatic mechanism. In a first approach to this subject, it might be supposed that the factors involved in haemorrhage and haemostasis are relatively simple since they are basically mechanical ones of the sort confronting the plumber or engineer in everyday life. But biological systems are immensely complicated in relation to man-made contrivances, and even the apparently well-known physical principles of flow and adhesion have unexpected complexities when applied at the scale of blood capillaries and platelets. As long ago as 1810, Jones wrote 'we can no longer consider the suppression of haemorrhage as a simple or mechanical effect, but a process performed by the concurrent and successive operations of many causes'. These causes are still obscure more than a century and a half later.

As a first approach to the problem of haemostasis, it is necessary to consider the circumstances which determine bleeding. Loss of whole blood can only occur if the wall of a blood vessel is damaged or permeable to an extent which allows the escape of cells and plasma, and if the fluid pressure within the vessel exceeds that outside it. The rate of blood loss is determined by the size and number of the vessels injured, and the pressure at which blood is supplied to them, and the haemostatic response differs greatly both in nature and effectiveness in different types of injury. For example, incised wounds of large arteries usually cause bleeding which is not controlled by natural haemostasis and may be fatal unless artificial aids such as tourniquets or ligatures are used, whereas crush injuries of similar vessels may bleed surprisingly little. Bleeding from veins is very variable, since the pressure within them may be so low that an accumulation of blood in the surrounding tissues, or elevation of the injured part may stop the flow. Bleeding from smaller vessels depends, of course, on the number injured and on the volume of blood they carry, that is, on the degree of hyperaemia or ischaemia of the tissue concerned. It is particularly in the case of these smaller vessels—arterioles, venules and capillaries—that the normal haemostatic mechanism is so effective. Though literally millions of such vessels may be severed as a result of an abrasion or contusion, bleeding usually ceases spontaneously within a few minutes. It is only when this mechanism fails to operate, as in haemophilia, that its importance in normal life becomes apparent.

At the mechanical level, the normal cessation of bleeding can be analysed fairly simply. The escape of blood will cease (a) if there is no longer a pressure difference between the lumen and the exterior of the damaged vessel and (b) if the hole in the vessel wall or the lumen itself becomes blocked by solid or extremely viscous material. These two situations can be brought about by different factors. Equalisation of pressure can be produced by a rise in external pressure (e.g. by haematoma formation) or by a fall in the blood pressure in the vessel, which, in turn may be due to a general reduction in blood supply (e.g. in shock or fainting) or to an active constriction of the damaged vessel above the point of injury, or to the opening up of shunts with diversion of blood through alternative pathways. Blocking of the vessel or wound opening can occur through the formation of a solid mass, usually derived from the blood itself and composed of fibrin, and aggregated platelets and cells. Blocking can also occur by the active constriction of the vessel at the site of injury, or the 'elastic recoil' of the surrounding tissues. It may also be due to the mutual adhesion of endothelial surfaces at the site of injury, though this is probably only significant in the case of very small vessels. The sequence in which these factors operate, and their relative importance varies greatly according to the site and nature of the injury. The physiological mechanism which controls their operation is extremely complex, and there is a curious interdependence underlying apparently unrelated events which probably stems from the evolution of injury reactions from a primitive and simpler pattern. The apparently separate functions of platelet adhesion, fibrin formation and vascular contraction or dilatation are all interconnected at one or more points in their operational pathways. But, for the sake of clarity they will be briefly described as separate entities before the integrated mechanism of haemostasis is considered as a whole.

Blood coagulation

The importance of the coagulation of the blood as a haemostatic factor has been recognised for centuries, and it is strongly emphasised by the disastrous clinical consequences of any serious fault in the clotting mechanism. The relatively sudden transformation of fluid blood into solid gel is a striking phenomenon which has apparently obvious haemostatic consequences. It is, of course, due to the conversion of the soluble protein fibrinogen into insoluble strands of fibrin. These entangle the cells of the blood and give the clot a degree of solidity which is surprising when one considers that the fibrin so formed represents only about 0·15% of the total mass of clot.

Fibrinogen is the most unstable of the plasma proteins as regards precipitation by heat or salt, and has a normal concentration of 200–400 mg per 100 ml of plasma. It has a high molecular weight (about 340,000) and its molecule is a nodular rod composed of three pairs of polypeptide chains. The conversion of soluble fibrinogen to solid fibrin follows the action of thrombin. Thrombin is a highly specific proteolytic enzyme that splits off certain peptide fragments (fibrinopeptides) from each fibrinogen molecule. The fibrinopeptides are negatively charged, and the loss of these charges from the remaining portions of the fibrinogen results in a loss of mutual repulsion between the molecules and a consequent tendency to aggregation. At this stage the original fibrinogen has become 'fibrin monomer' and under physiological conditions the monomer polymerises by end-to-end and side-to-side alignment of its molecules to form fibres. The initial bonding is relatively weak and can be reversed by urea. Normal plasma, however, contains a specific factor, known as 'fibrin stabilizing factor' (factor XIII) which, when activated by thrombin, becomes a transglutaminase that forms stronger, co-valent bonds within the fibrin structure.

Thrombin does not exist in the normal circulating blood in detectable amounts, otherwise significant intravascular coagulation would occur. It is derived from an inert precursor, prothrombin, which is thus a proenzyme or zymogen. Most of the very considerable confusion and complexity of blood clotting theories during the past 50 years has centred on the problems of the physiological activation of prothrombin.

For many years it was supposed that normal haemostatic clotting was due to the release from damaged tissue blood cells or platelets of a factor capable of converting prothrombin to thrombin. This view was based on the fact that the addition to blood of extracts of certain tissues such as brain or lung caused clotting in about 15 seconds, the reaction requiring the presence of ionised calcium. Many attempts were made to isolate and identify this tissue factor, which was variously called 'thromboplastin' or 'thrombokinase'. Beyond the fact that certain phospholipids, including ethanolamine phosphatide, form one component, and that a labile factor, probably a protein, is another component, little definite information has been obtained.

The introduction by Quick in 1935 of the 'prothrombin time' test led to a series of discoveries and the recognition that prothrombin activation is far more complex than supposed. If only four factors are concerned in clotting, prothrombin, thromboplastin, fibrinogen and calcium, then, in a system in which the last three are present 'in excess' the clotting time should be proportional to the prothrombin concentration. But experience with the clinical application of this 'prothrombin time test' revealed many anomalies, which were explained by the unsuspected existence of other plasma clotting factors concerned in the activation of prothrombin in the presence of tissue thromboplastin. The first of these to be discovered was named 'factor V' by Owren (1947), and this was followed by factor VII (the term factor VI having been used in another context) and, some time later by factor X. The factors concerned in the clotting of blood by tissue factor are listed in Figure 1.1.

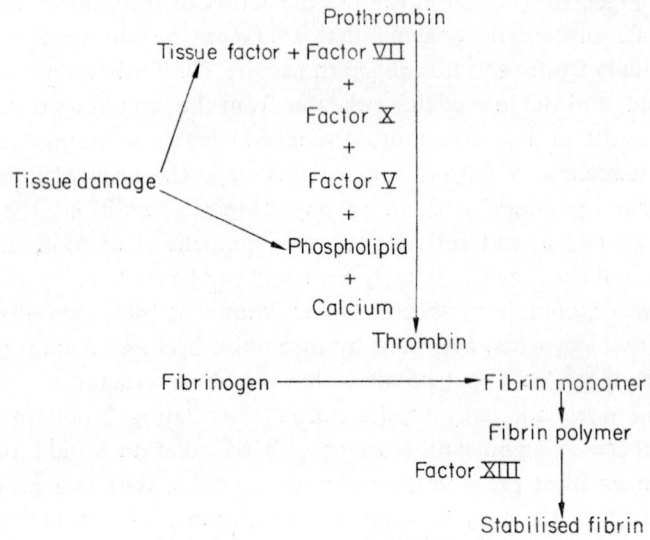

Figure 1.1. The factors concerned with the clotting of blood by the products of tissue damage (usually referred to as 'tissue thromboplastin'), which constitute the 'extrinsic system' or prothrombin activation.

The increased understanding of the action of tissue thromboplastin in the clotting mechanism did not explain several important aspects of the physiological mechanism. It did not explain, for example, why patients with haemophilia have defective clotting, because haemophilic blood clots apparently quite normally when tissue thromboplastin (even if derived from haemophilic tissue) is added to it. It could be inferred therefore that all the factors concerned with the 'extrinsic system' of clotting are normal, and that the action of tissue thromboplastin is not enough for normal haemostasis, since, if it were, haemophilic patients would not bleed abnormally.

Attention was therefore turned to another phenomenon, which had been emphasised by Lister in 1863, the initiation of clotting by contact of the blood with a 'foreign' surface. Following contact with glass, metals, fabrics and a wide variety of substances other than normal vascular endothelium, the blood will clot firmly and quite suddenly after an interval of a few minutes. The significance of this fact had been under-estimated by comparison with the more immediate effect of tissue extracts, but it can be shown that, though its onset occurs later, contact activation produces a generation of thrombin which is just as rapid as that produced by the addition of thromboplastin. In haemophilia and other clinically important clotting defects, the fault lies in the mechanism which connects the surface-contact reaction with prothrombin conversion.

Table 1.1. The roman numerical nomenclature of blood clotting factors, together with some common synonyms.

Factor	Synonyms
I	Fibrinogen
II	Prothrombin
III	Thromboplastin; tissue extract
IV	Calcium
V	Accelerator globulin; proaccelerin; labile factor
VI	This number is not now used
VII	Proconvertin; stable factor: auto-prothrombin I
VIII	Antihaemophilic factor; antihaemophilic globulin; platelet co-factor I; antihaemophilic factor A
IX	Plasma thromboplastin component (PTC); Christmas factor; platelet co-factor II; auto-prothrombin II; antihaemophilic factor B
X	Stuart-Prower factor
XI	Plasma thromboplastin antecedent (PTA)
XII	Hageman factor
XIII	Fibrin stabilising factor

The idea that surface-contact leads to the production in the blood itself of a 'plasma-thromboplastin' resulted in the development of the 'thromboplastin generation test' by Biggs and Douglas (1953). As in the case of the prothrombin time test, its clinical application revealed the existence of new factors. Considerable confusion resulted from the application, by different groups of workers, of different names to the same factors, and this was not resolved until the matter was taken in hand by an International Committee which introduced the Roman Numeral system of nomenclature. This system is now in general use, and it is listed, together with some of the better known synonyms, in Table 1.1. The result of this work in different centres showed that at least 6 plasma factors together

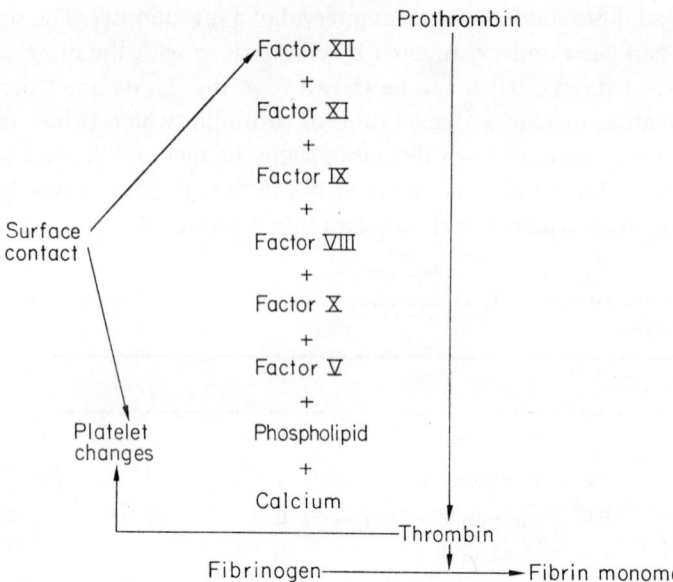

Figure 1.2. The factors concerned with the activation of prothrombin following surface contact, constituting the 'intrinsic system'. It is probable that contact activates factor XII (Hageman factor).

with the platelets and calcium are concerned with the activation of prothrombin by the contact-activated or intrinsic system, as shown in Figure 1.2.

The contact-sensitive component in this system is factor XII which is activated, possibly by an unfolding of its molecule, as a result of its adsorption to any 'foreign' surface. The chemical or physical property which determines surface activation has not yet been defined, but certain surfaces, such as silicones, oils, waxes and some plastics are inert and are used in practice to coat containers or apparatus in which blood clotting is to be avoided. Of the other factors concerned, factor VIII is also known as antihaemophilic factor (AHF) or antihaemophilic globulin (AHG), and factor IX as Christmas factor, and it is the natural and hereditary deficiency of one or other of these factors which causes haemophilia and Christmas disease respectively. But natural deficiencies may occur of any of the plasma factors shown in Figure 1.2, though their incidence is less than that of haemophilia, and, in general, their effects are less severe (see Table 1.2).

The identification of the components of a mechanism does not explain how it works. There are many possible interactions between the thirteen clotting factors, but experimental evidence favoured a sequential reaction between pairs and also defined the order in which they were involved. There was also evidence that some, at least, of the stages were enzymatic. For example, thrombin is an enzyme. It is

Table 1.2. The recognised coagulation defects, their probable mode of inheritance, probable incidence and some acquired defects.

Deficient factor	Congenital defect — Probable inheritance	Probable incidence per million of population	Acquired defect
I	Autosomal recessive	0·1	Defibrination syndrome; liver disease
II	?	0·1	Coumarin anti-coagulants; vitamin K deficiency; liver disease
III IV	No deficiency causing coagulation defect		
V	Autosomal recessive	0·1	Defibrination syndrome
VII	Autosomal recessive	0·1	Liver disease; Coumarin anti-coagulants; vitamin K deficiency
VIII	Sex-linked recessive	40–60	Defibrination syndrome; circulating anticoagulants
IX	Sex-linked recessive	4–6	Coumarin anti-coagulants; vitamin K deficiency; liver disease
X	Autosomal recessive	0·1	
XI	Autosomal dominant	1	
XII	Autosomal recessive	0·1	
XIII	Autosomal recessive	0·1	

derived from prothrombin by an enzymatic splitting of the prothrombin molecule. Factor X, like prothrombin, can be activated enzymatically, the product being itself an enzyme and concerned with prothrombin activation. Factor XII develops esterase activity on surface contact, and this in turn can induce an esterase activity in factor XI.

On the basis of this and other evidence it was proposed as a general hypothesis (Macfarlane, 1964) that all the plasma clotting factors, except calcium and fibrinogen, were proenzymes. Each could be activated to yield an enzyme that could activate the next proenzyme in the sequence. The intrinsic clotting system began with the contact activation of factor XII and proceeded in sequence through factors XI, IX, VIII, X, V and II (prothrombin) to yield thrombin. The extrinsic system began with the release from damaged cells of 'tissue factor' which activated factor VII and thence factors X, V, and II. Thus, from factor X onwards the two systems shared a common path. It was suggested that the active derivative of a clotting factor should be indicated by the letter 'a' after the Roman numeral. Thrombin, for example, would be IIa. It was pointed out that such an enzyme cascade would function as a biochemical amplifier and thus explain how the minute stimulus of surface contact finally promotes the large effect of fibrin formation. The known concentrations of the clotting factors supported the idea of amplification. The clotting of about 250 mgm of fibrinogen involves about 15 mgm of prothrombin, 1·6 mgm of factor X and 0·17 mgm of factor VIII.

Though subsequent work has supported the principle of the cascade hypothesis, it is now seen to have been too simple in its original form. Factor V is probably not a proenzyme but a co-factor with phospholipid and calcium that catalyses the activation of prothrombin by Xa. It seems likely that factor VII also has a similar function as a co-factor between tissue factor and its activation of factor X, and that factor VIII takes part with (not after) IXa in the intrinsic activation of factor X. Thrombin has other actions besides its effect on fibrinogen. It apparently 'activates' factor VIII; it causes aggregation of the platelets and the release from them of phospholipids that catalyse earlier stages of its own generation, and it also activates factor XIII (fibrin stabilising factor). A diagram setting out this current scheme of interactions is shown in Figure 1.3.

The diagram does not show the inhibitors that destroy each activated clotting factor within a short time. The average life span of a thrombin molecule, for

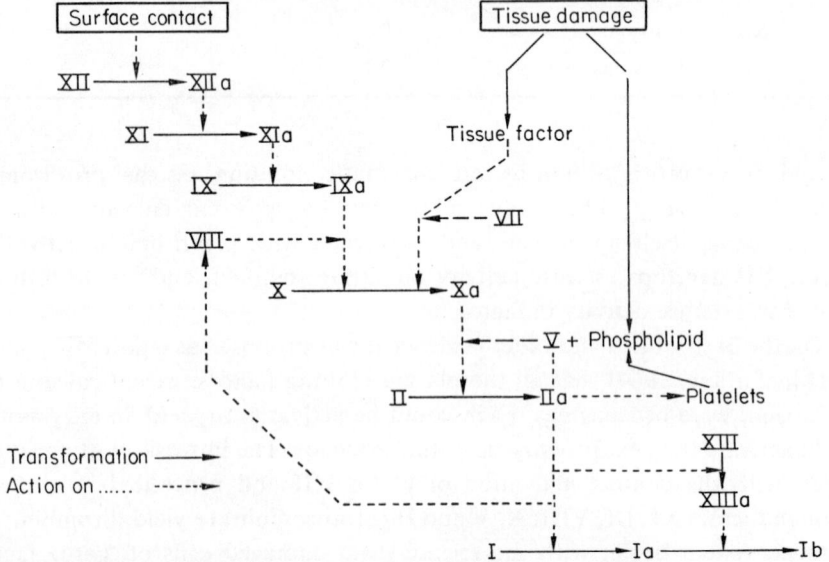

Figure 1.3. A blood coagulation scheme based on existing evidence, and including the autocatalytic effects of thrombin. Ia = fibrin and Ib = stabilised fibrin.

example, is about 24 seconds in normal plasma and it is probable that other active factors are equally short lived. This destruction is essential to limit the activation of this powerful and auto-catalytic clotting system to a site of injury, and to prevent the spread of an otherwise disastrous thrombosis. It is only at such local sites that activation can outstrip inactivation and promote haemostasis, and it is the loss of power in one of the early stages of the amplification system that causes the haemostatic failure in haemophilia and similar conditions.

Platelet aggregation and adhesion

Fibrin formation is not the only way in which solid material can form in wound areas and damaged vessels and obstruct bleeding. Wharton-Jones (1851) described the formation of a 'grey granulous substance' at the site of injuries to vessels in the frog's web, which he considered was composed of colourless corpuscles. Hayem (1882) investigated the structure of the mass which forms at the site of an incision in veins in dogs. He called this mass the 'clou hémostatique' and showed that it was mainly composed of 'hematoblasts' or platelets. From that time, the phenomenon of platelet adhesion to damaged surfaces and to each other has been intensively studied, not only on account of its haemostatic importance but also because it is an important factor in thrombosis.

Platelets are complex and sensitive structures capable of metabolic and synthetic activity and of rapid morphological change. They contain several known enzyme systems and pharmacologically active substances such as adenosine triphosphate, 5-hydroxytryptamine, histamine and adrenaline. They also contain a phospholipoprotein (platelet factor 3) which is active in the clotting mechanism, a lipoprotein (platelet factor 4) which antagonises heparin, and a contractile protein (thrombosthenin).

The most striking reaction of the platelets is their immediate adhesion to 'foreign' surfaces, in particular to collagen that may be exposed by damage to the vascular endothelium. This adhesion is selective, since platelets show no tendency to adhere to normal endothelial or blood cells, and its mechanism is obscure. But adherent platelets themselves become adhesive for other platelets and this phenomenon (platelet cohesion or aggregation) has been much studied and is partially explained. Surface contact can trigger a series of platelet changes known as the 'release reaction'. In this, ATP is broken down to ADP, which is released at the platelet surface and, since ADP itself can cause platelet cohesion and the release of further ADP, a chain reaction ensues. Aggregation by ADP requires the presence of ionised calcium and of a plasma factor which may be identical with fibrinogen. Morphologically, platelets clumped by ADP retain their individual outlines and granules, and after a few minutes the clumps lose their cohesion and the platelets redisperse.

During physiological haemostasis it is probably thrombin that adds a significant stability and permanence to clumping by ADP. Platelets exposed to thrombin are not only aggregated, they tend to lose their outlines and become welded into a uniform mass. They also lose their visible granules, probably by extrusion, and some of these contain the phospholipid that accelerates further thrombin generation. Adrenaline and 5-hydroxytryptamine are also released, and these have vaso-constrictor activity and promote further platelet aggregation. During these release reactions individual platelets extend long pseudopodia, and where these are adherent to newly-formed fibrin the subsequent contraction of the pseudopodia causes a shortening of the fibres and retraction of the clot. The contractile protein, thrombosthenin, and the breakdown of ATP probably supply the power for this physical change which results in a mechanically stronger clot.

Whatever the cause of platelet adhesion and aggregation, the effect is the building up of solid masses at the site of injury. If the injury is very slight, such as experimental injuries produced in small arterioles by microelectrodes or needles, the 'white bodies' formed by aggregating platelets are unstable, and repeatedly break down after reaching a certain size, usually less than that required to block the vessel. Electron microscopy of these masses shows no detectable fibrin formation. Experimental transection of an arteriole usually leads to the formation of a 'haemostatic plug' and here layers of fibrin are usually visible in addition to platelet masses. Such haemostatic plugs are stable, and do not tend to break down once they have formed. It is possible that the forces of platelet adhesion alone are insufficient to withstand the blood pressure, and that the action of thrombin, which seems to cause an irreversible platelet fusion, and the re-inforcing effect of fibrin layers are required to form a haemostatically efficient mass.

Defective haemostasis may arise from a numerical reduction in platelet numbers, or a functional deficiency which prevents their aggregation, or to a deficiency of their phospholipid component which leads in turn to defective clotting.

Vascular and tissue function in haemostasis

Vascular constriction is a response to injury which has been recognised by surgeons for centuries. Constriction may be observed experimentally, and it is produced not only by direct trauma or transection of a vessel, but by nervous or chemical stimulation, or the presence of shed blood or agglutinated platelets. The constriction may be complete, so that the blood flow is stopped; even when it is incomplete the effect may be to channel the blood supply through alternative vascular pathways, so that the injured area becomes relatively ischaemic and the other haemostatic mechanisms have a better chance to become effective. Constriction in the smaller vessels is usually short-lived, and passes off after 5–10 minutes, perhaps being followed by dilatation. In larger arteries and veins it may persist as a powerful spasm for longer periods. It is usually supposed that active constriction can only occur in those vessels which possess definite coats of smooth muscle. This would preclude active contraction by capillaries, but there is a good deal of evidence suggesting that capillaries have the power to constrict, and recent electron microscopical observations suggest that capillary endothelium may contain contractile elements.

The stimulus responsible for the vaso-constriction of even muscular vessels following injury has not yet been identified. It is possible that there is a direct effect of trauma on the muscle cells or their innervation, and there is also evidence that the shed blood contains or develops vaso-active substances. The relation to platelet aggregation has already been mentioned, and an obvious association would be the local action of vaso-constrictor substances from the platelets during the changes which take place during clotting. Vascular abnormalities can be a cause of abnormal bleeding, but they are rare. In haemorrhagic telangiectasia the greatly dilated capillaries which form the lesions can be a source of severe and prolonged bleeding, despite the normal functioning of the clotting and platelet components of the haemostatic mechanism in this condition. Vascular or perivascular connective tissue also seems to be involved in haemostasis, since certain collagen or elastic tissue defects such as Ehlers Danlos syndrome are associated with abnormal bleeding. It may be that the lack of firm support for the vessels, or their undue friability may predispose the rupture following a degree of trauma which would not cause bleeding in the normal subject, or it may be that the tissues themselves may not promote the haemostatic response of the platelets or blood.

The haemostatic mechanism as a whole

It is clear that no simple nor single picture can be given of the operation of these factors in curtailing the bleeding from injured vessels. The order in which they come into effect, and their importance relative to each other will be determined by the nature and severity of the injury. In the smaller vessels, the formation of the platelet plug and vaso-constriction are probably the earliest and most important events. Fibrin formation is less essential, and even if clotting is defective minor injuries involving only small vessels may not bleed abnormally, whereas platelet or vascular defects may cause prolonged bleeding from injuries

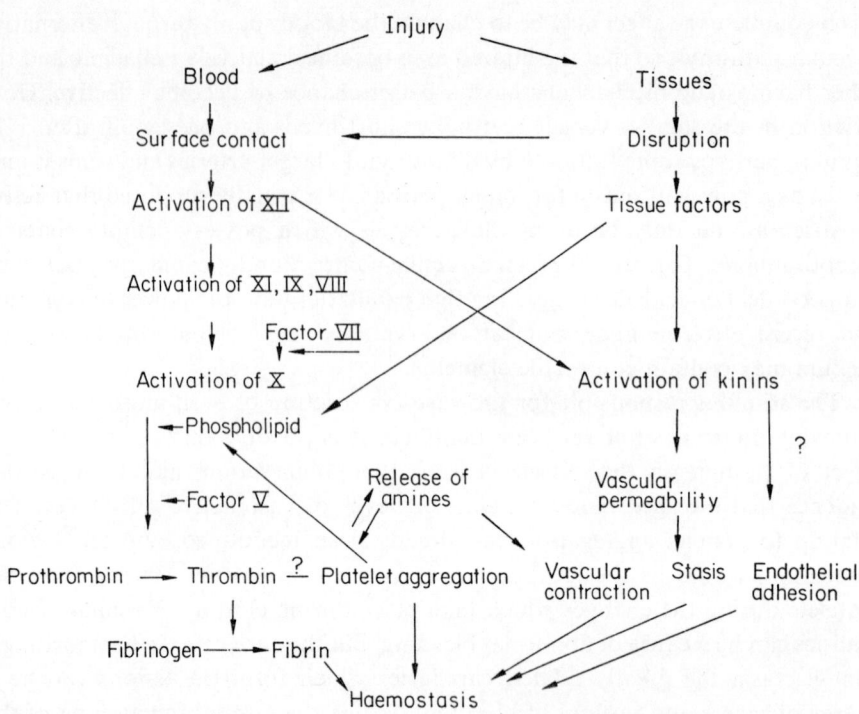

Figure 1.4. A diagram illustrating the factors probably concerned with haemostasis, and their inter-relation.

of this type. This is illustrated by the results of the 'bleeding-time test' which is normal in cases of haemophilia, but greatly prolonged in thrombocytopenic purpura and von Willebrand's disease. In more extensive wounds, normal clotting function seems to be essential for normal haemostasis. In the case of severed arteries, contraction is an important factor, and if it does not occur the other haemostatic factors will be unlikely to arrest the bleeding unaided. The whole mechanism is complicated by the cross links and 'feedback' effects which are illustrated diagrammatically in Figure 1.4

The consequences of haemostatic failure

The effect of severe deficiencies in the haemostatic mechanism is, of course, the occurrence of prolonged bleeding. But it is not easy to predict the clinical severity of a haemorrhagic state from laboratory studies of clotting and platelet function. It is likely that a deficiency in any one component may be compensated to some degree by the normal operation of the others and that relatively mild defects affecting more than one of the main haemostatic functions will cause relatively severe bleeding. For example, total afibrinogenaemia in which no fibrin formation can occur causes less disability than haemophilia in which fibrin formation is merely delayed. The explanation may be that thrombin formation and hence platelet function are normal in afibrinogenaemia, but thrombin formation is much reduced in haemophilia so that platelet aggregation as well as fibrin formation may be reduced.

In some patients severe thrombocytopenia is not associated with bleeding of the purpuric type, in others even moderate reductions in the platelets are correlated with episodes of abnormal bleeding. The explanation may be that vascular damage or dysfunction is superimposed on the thrombocytopenia in the latter cases. In von Willebrand's disease a vascular or platelet abnormality is combined with a deficiency of factor VIII. Treatment of either of these two defects separately may be clinically effective.

In general, the sort of bleeding produced by platelet or vascular defects which we often refer to as capillary bleeding differs from that due to defective clotting. Thrombocytopenic purpura is characteristic of the former group and it is essentially due to an increased vascular fragility combined with prolonged bleeding from small, superficial injuries such as needle pricks. Bleeding into the intact skin or mucous membranes in the form of petechiae or more extensive ecchymoses may follow the slightest trauma such as the constriction of tight clothes, or it may occur apparently spontaneously. Free haemorrhage may occur, also apparently spontaneously, from the mucous membranes particularly of the nose, and uterine tract. Deep tissue haemorrhages are rare, and bleeding into the joints hardly ever occurs, but cerebral haemorrhage is not so uncommon and is responsible for most of the deaths in this condition. The clotting mechanism in thrombocytopenic purpura is normal as regards the plasma factors, but the numerical deficiency of the platelets may reduce the efficiency of prothrombin conversion, presumably because of a reduction in the available platelet factor. It is possible that this interference with clotting may contribute to abnormal bleeding, particularly since the infusion of stored platelets or phospholipid has been reported to improve haemostasis.

The findings in thrombocytopenic purpura are essentially a prolonged bleeding time, positive tourniquet test and a reduced platelet count. The prothrombin consumption test may be abnormal, and clot retraction reduced, but other tests of clotting function are usually normal. It is beyond the scope of this book to discuss the aetiology or treatment of the purpuras, which can be subdivided into a number of entities in which antibodies, auto-antibodies, toxins, drugs and chemicals which may damage platelets or vascular endothelium, have been implicated. The conditions have been mentioned here as an example of a **type of** haemostatic failure distinct from clotting defects, and because

Table 1.3. Laboratory tests used in the diagnosis of patients with coagulation defects.

Deficient factor	Tests likely to give positive information	Tests which may be unhelpful
I	Clotting time; kaolin cephalin clotting time; one-stage prothrombin time; assay of fibrinogen	Prothrombin consumption; T.G.T.
II	Assay of prothrombin; one-stage prothrombin time	One-stage prothrombin time; T.G.T.
V	Clotting time; one-stage prothrombin time; assay of factor V	Thrombotest and P & P techniques; T.G.T.
VII	One-stage prothrombin time; assay of factor VII	Clotting time; P.C.I.; T.G.T.; kaolin cephalin clotting time
VIII Severely affected patients	Clotting time; kaolin cephalin clotting time; P.C.I.; assay of factor VIII	One-stage prothrombin time
VIII Mildly affected patients	Assay of factor VIII	Clotting time; T.G.T.; P.C.I.; kaolin cephalin clotting time
IX Severely affected patients	Clotting time; kaolin cephalin clotting time; P.C.I.; assay of factor IX	One-stage prothrombin time
IX Mildly affected patients	Assay of factor IX	Clotting time; T.G.T.; P.C.I.; kaolin cephalin clotting time
X	Clotting time; kaolin cephalin clotting time; one-stage prothrombin time; T.G.T.; assay of factor X	P.C.I.
XI XII	Clotting time; kaolin cephalin clotting time; tests of surface contact; assays of factors XI and XII	One-stage prothrombin time; T.G.T.
XIII	Solubility of plasma clots in 30% urea and 1% monochloracetic acid	All tests of clotting function

occasionally the two types may occur in the same patient leading to diagnostic troubles, or one type may be mistaken for the other by an unwary or inexperienced doctor.

The uncomplicated coagulation defects present quite a different clinical picture. Petechial haemorrhages and ecchymoses in the skin are very uncommon, though subcutaneous bruising is frequently seen after minor trauma. Spontaneous bleeding from apparently intact mucous membranes is also uncommon. On the other hand, deep tissue haemorrhages into almost any part of the body, and particularly into muscles and joints, are a frequent and major cause of trouble, and lead to pain and perhaps lasting disability. These haemorrhages usually result from trauma. Though minor scratches and needle pricks do not bleed abnormally, cuts, wounds or abrasions of the skin or mucous membranes will lead to persistent bleeding which cannot be controlled by the ordinary haemostatic measures usually effective in normal people. Gastro-intestinal bleeding is not very common and, when it occurs, is usually associated with ulceration. Haematuria also occurs, and is difficult to explain on the basis of a clotting defect alone, unless it is assumed that renal bleeding takes place from time to time in normal people but is checked by clotting before it becomes clinically obvious.

The essential abnormality in this group of conditions is the deficiency or inactivity of one or more of the factors required for normal clotting, or the presence of an inhibitor which prevents their action. Often no other demonstrable abnormality can be found; platelets and platelet function are normal, and there is no indication in most cases of any abnormality of the vessels or tissues which would predispose to excessive bleeding after injury.

The majority of the clotting defects arise as hereditary and congenital conditions, with well marked genetic characters. Of those which are acquired, some may be due to the development of antibodies which inhibit certain normal clotting factors, some are due to the action of toxins, drugs and chemicals, or the effect of deficiency states or disease processes. The action of the coumarin drugs and of Vitamin K deficiency on the production of factors IX, X, VII and II by the liver is the most familiar example of the effect, but any severe liver disease may result in a reduction in these factors, and sometimes of fibrinogen. A summary of the more important laboratory tests used to differentiate the various clotting defects is set out in Table 1.3.

From a correlation of the observed blood levels of these different factors with the clinical history of patients in whom they are deficient, and with the clinical effects of replacement therapy, it is possible to estimate the minimum levels required for haemostatic efficiency. Many such observations are available in the case of factor VIII deficiency, and a general correlation between different levels of this factor and the liability to abnormal bleeding is set out in Table 1.4. It will

Table 1.4. The relation of observed blood levels of factor VIII to the severity of the clinical manifestations of defective haemostasis.

Blood level of factor VIII (per cent of normal)	Level of haemostatic efficiency
50–100	Normal
25–50	Tendency to excessive bleeding after major trauma. Often not diagnosed.
5–25	Severe bleeding after minor trauma or surgical operations
1–5	Gross bleeding after minor injuries. Some haemarthroses and 'spontaneous' bleeding
0	Severe haemophilia. Haemarthroses and crippling. Deep tissue haemorrhages

be seen that this liability is proportional both to the degree of factor VIII deficiency and also to the degree of trauma, so that even mild trauma may produce serious bleeding in a patient with very low factor VIII levels, but not in patients with 10–20% of factor VIII. The latter patients, however, might have seriously abnormal bleeding after such trauma as a major surgical operation. From this table it can be seen that, in general, if the factor VIII level is over 25% the patient can lead a normal life without serious risk of bleeding, but if it is below 25% then abnormal bleeding may be troublesome or dangerous. A level of 25% might therefore be called the 'minimum haemostatic level' for factor VIII. The treatment of patients with various coagulation defects depends on information about the recovery of the relevant clotting factor in the circulation and the half life of the infused activity. In addition experience with treating patients provides information about the level of a given factor required for haemostasis. The experience with haemophilic patients is dealt with in the ensuing chapters and such information as is available about other defects is presented in Table 1.5.

Purely vascular or tissue abnormalities are uncommon causes of serious bleeding, and their clinical manifestations may not be very informative. Essentially, their diagnosis depends on the recognition of structural abnormalities, which may be missed unless they are looked for specifically. In haemorrhagic telangiectasia there are recurrent episodes of profuse and apparently spontaneous epistaxis, gastro-intestinal bleeding, haematuria, or haemoptysis. Telangiectasia is inherited as a simple dominant, but it is not congenital in the sense that the haemorrhagic lesions seldom develop until adult or middle life.

Table 1.5. Data from which to estimate the treatment required by patients having various coagulation defects.

Defect	Recovery of infused activity % of expectation	Half-life of infused activity hours	Haemostatically effective concentration % normal	Therapeutic materials
I	50	120	10–25	Preparations containing fibrinogen including plasma
II	50	80–120	40	Concentrates containing factors II, VII, IX & X or II, IX and X
V	50	24	10–15	Fresh frozen plasma
VII	65	2–5	5–10	Concentrates containing factors II, VII, IX & X or factor VII
VIII Haemophilia A	50–100	10–20	Spontaneous bleeding (a) 10–20 Trauma (b) 50–100	Factor VIII concentrates including cryoprecipitate
VIII von Willebrand's disease	100+	48–72	?	Factor VIII concentrates including cryoprecipitate
IX	25–50	8–24	Spontaneous bleeding (a) 10–20 Surgery (b) 50–100	Concentrates containing factors II, VII, IX and X or II, IX and X
X	50–100	60–70	10–40	Concentrates containing factors II, VII, IX and X or II, IX and X
XI	80–100	60–70	?	Fresh frozen plasma
XII	—	—	—	No treatment needed
XIII	50–100	144	1–2	Fresh frozen plasma or concentrates containing factor XIII

A positive family history and the existence of telangiectasia of the lips, the mucous membranes of the mouth or nose, or in the skin of the fingers make the diagnosis relatively simple, but in some cases the condition is sporadic or acquired and the vascular lesions may only occur in the remote interior leading to much instrumental inspection and often to fruitless surgery. All tests of haemostatic function are usually normal in telangiectasia, but the 'bleeding time' from a lesion pricked by a needle is prolonged and the blood loss usually so profuse that this method of investigation is not recommended unless firm pressure can be applied to the site. It is probable that the widely dilated vessels which constitute the lesions are structurally abnormal and incapable of contraction or possibly of promoting platelet adhesion. Their superficial situation and prominence makes them very liable to damage.

A different and even rarer type of tissue defect is the Ehlers Danlos syndrome. In this condition there is a rather ill-defined tendency to extensive bruising and haematoma formation, and sometimes to epistaxis, haematuria or gastrointestinal bleeding. The most characteristic symptom is the slow and incomplete healing of wounds or operation sites, with a recurrent breakdown of the scar tissue and renewed bleeding. The condition is inherited as an autosomal defect, leading to an abnormality of connective tissue, particularly collagen. The bleeding time, particularly when measured by the Ivy or saline methods may be prolonged but other tests of haemostatic function are normal. On examination the relevant abnormalities are an excessive extensibility of the joints, particularly of the fingers or elbows, which can be bent back to an extreme degree, or a remarkable lax inelasticity of the skin which may hang in folds or pouches over the knees and elbows, and the presence of stretched scars indicating the failure of old injuries to heal and contract properly. There are several clinical varieties of this rare conditon, depending on the relative degrees to which the skin, joints, and other connective tissue structures are involved. All grades of severity occur, varying from a loose or 'double' jointedness of which the patient may be rather proud, to horrifying loss of cohesion resembling lathyrism in chicks in which the connective tissues disintegrate at the slightest trauma. It is probable that the haemorrhagic tendency in Ehlers Danlos syndrome is due to the mechanical weakness of the vessels and their supporting tissues.

A complete review of factor XIII deficiency is given by Favre-Gilly *et al* (1974). The most usual clinical features are inheritance of an autosomal recessive type; bleeding from the umbilical cord; bleeding from skin injuries; bruising and failure to form normal scar tissue. Bleeding from mucous membranes and epistaxis occur, haemarthroses are often seen but intramuscular haematomata are rare. Intracranial bleeding is particularly common. Usually the excessive bleeding is preceded by recollected trauma. The 'spontaneous' type of bleeding so usual with haemophilia is not seen.

The clinical picture in haemophilia, Christmas disease and von Willebrand's disease

In the previous sections the main factors supposed to be concerned with haemostasis have been considered from a rather theoretical point of view, and the effect of the breakdown of each of them has been illustrated by clinical conditions arbitrarily chosen because they conformed to theory. But in actual practice we have to diagnose and treat patients as they come, and often they do not present simple defects or clinical pictures which can be entirely explained on the basis of theory. The three most important hereditary haemorrhagic diseases in terms of incidence and severity are haemophilia, Christmas disease and von Willebrand's disease, and a description of our experience in the treatment of these is the main purpose of this book. The clinical picture of a 'typical' case of these conditions is fairly clear cut, though there are rather wide variations between families and individuals. Most of the clinical manifestations are explicable on the type of haemostatic failure to be expected from laboratory findings, but there are some which are not easily explicable. It is possible that there are many other factors physiological or extraneous, which influence the efficiency of haemostasis to some degree in one direction or the other, or damage or protect the vessels. In the normal individual these secondary factors have little significance because there is a large margin of safety preventing excessive bleeding as a result of the wear and tear of ordinary modern life. But in the patient with defective haemostasis with little or no safety margin the operation of one of these secondary factors may determine whether or not disastrous haemorrhage takes place. This phenomenon may result in a mis-interpretation or over-emphasis of the function of a secondary factor and it is probably responsible for the beneficial clinical results claimed for a wide variety of remedies which have no demonstrable effect on laboratory findings.

It is also probably responsible for a periodic improvement or worsening of the haemorrhagic condition in time cycles of weeks or months to which some patients seem to be subject, and may explain non-specific effects attributed produced by changes in diet, exercise and so on.

HAEMOPHILIA A

During the past 150 years, the term 'haemophilia' has gradually become more restricted. At first, any type of constitutional haemorrhagic condition might be called haemophilia, but the work of Bulloch & Fildes (1911) established the existence of a sex-linked recessively inherited disorder which affected males and was transmitted by apparently normal females. It was to this condition that they restricted the term haemophilia. The discovery and characterisation of factors VIII and IX has shown that the condition defined by Bulloch & Fildes can be divided into two separate entities. In one of these, representing the majority of cases, the condition is a hereditary deficiency of factor VIII. The other entity is a deficiency of factor IX, with a similar sex-linked recessive inheritance, and a similar clinical picture and symptomatology. Both conditions breed true, and are due to separate defective genes located on the X chromosome, factor VIII deficiency being about 10 times commoner (in this country) than factor IX deficiency. The term 'haemophilia A' has been retained here to describe factor VIII deficiency while factor IX deficiency has been called haemophilia B or Christmas disease, after the surname of the first patient with this condition identified in this country. Their mode of inheritance is illustrated in Figure 1.5;

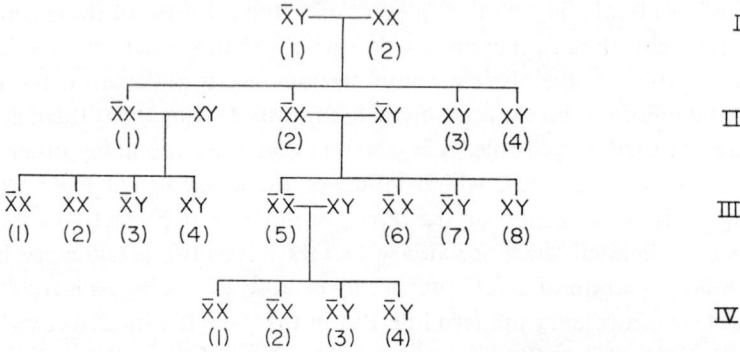

Figure 1.5. The inheritance of haemophilia. The defect is carried by the X chromosome and is shown as $\bar{X}$. In Generation I, an affected male ($\bar{X}Y$) marries a normal female (XX). Two possible genotypes are shown in Generation II, (1) and (2) being heterozygous (carrier) females, (3) and (4) being normal males. In Generation III, the children of a female carrier and a normal male are carriers or normal if females (1) and (2), affected or normal if males (3) and (4). II (2) a carrier is shown as marrying a haemophilic male; in such a case homozygous (affected) female children might occur (III (5)), with offspring as shown in Generation IV.

it should be noted that all the daughters of an affected male are potential carriers, a fact which used sometimes to be overlooked, but his sons are normal. The children of (heterozygous) female carriers have an equal chance of being normal or affected if males, or normal or carriers if females. The marriage of an affected male with a female carrier has occurred on rare occasions, and in such a case affected (homozygous) females have been produced with all the symptoms of haemophilia. Haemophilia occurs in animals, both dogs and horses having been studied experimentally. The genetic, laboratory, and clinical pictures seem to be exactly similar to haemophilia in humans.

The incidence of haemophilia in this country is not known with precision, but it is thought to be about 6 per 100,000 of the population giving at least 3,000

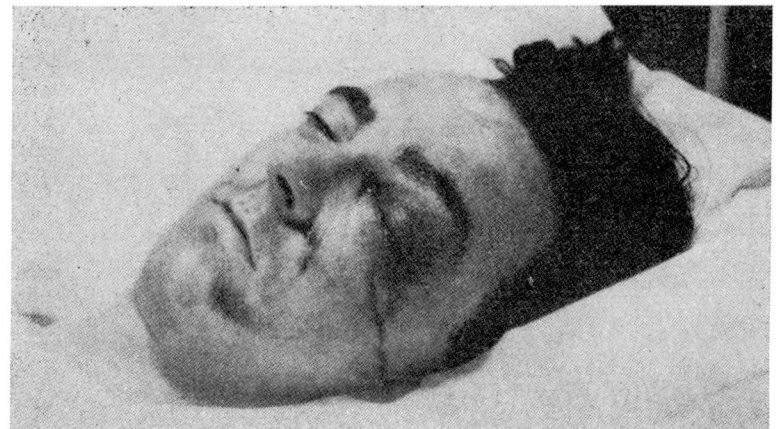

(*a*) Haematoma of the orbit.

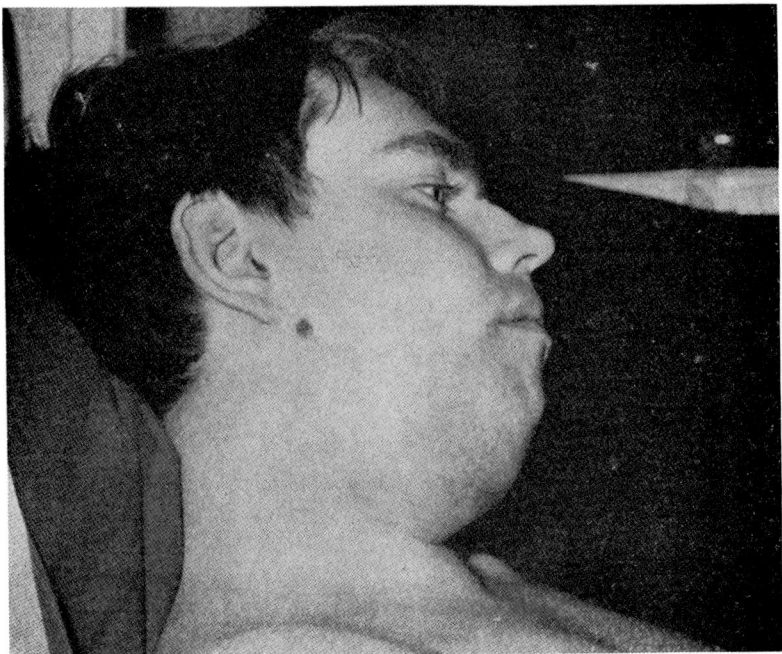

(*b*) Haematoma of the floor of the mouth causing difficulty in swallowing.

Figure 1.6. Haemorrhagic manifestation in haemophilic patients.

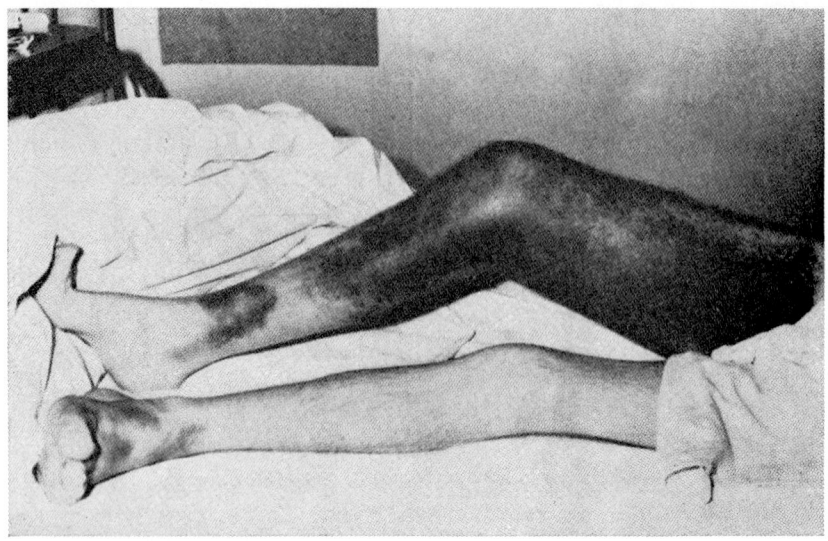

(c) Haematoma of the whole leg following a minor injury.

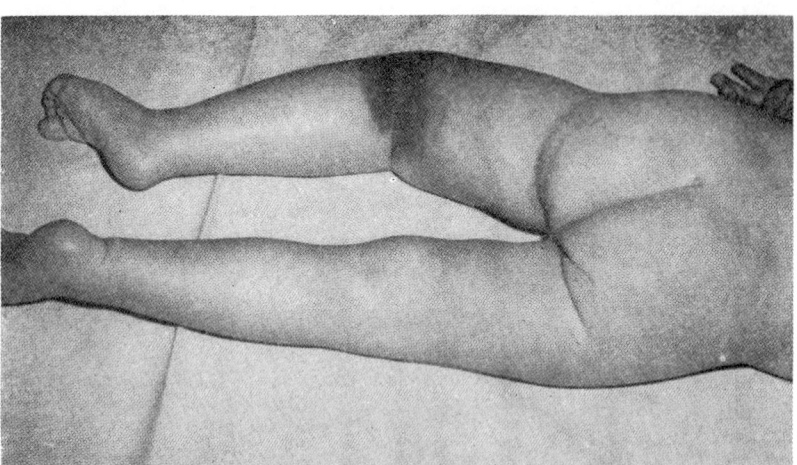

(d) Haematoma of the back of the knee.

Figure 1.6. Haemorrhagic manifestation in haemophilic patients.

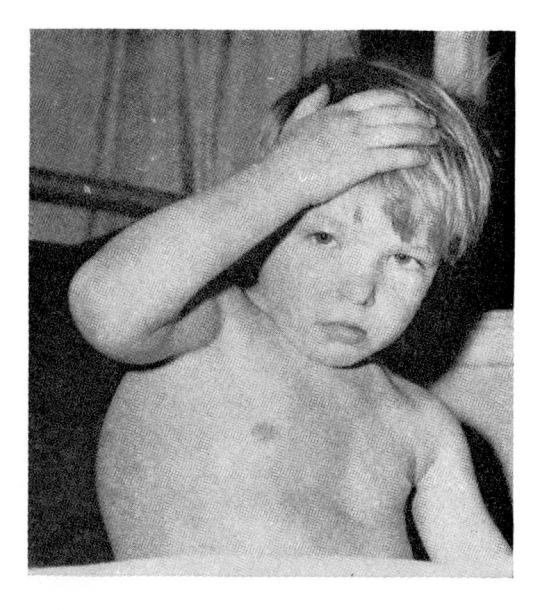

(e) A massive haematoma of the back; apparently spontaneous.

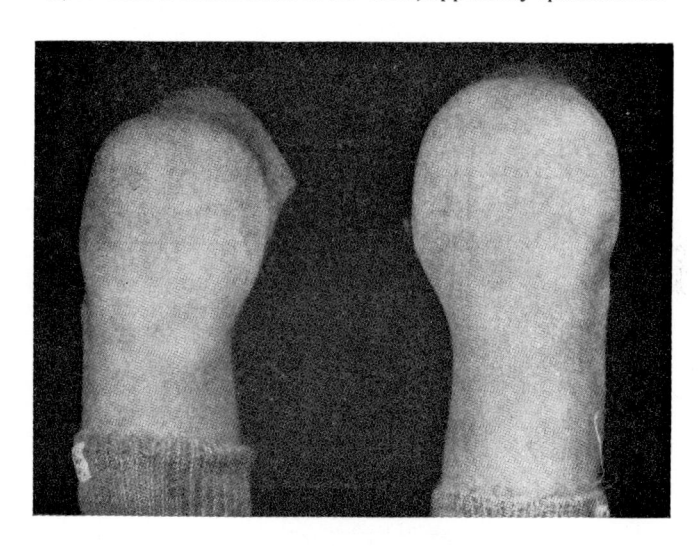

(f) Haemarthroses of the knees.

Figure 1.6. Haemorrhagic manifestation in haemophilic patients.

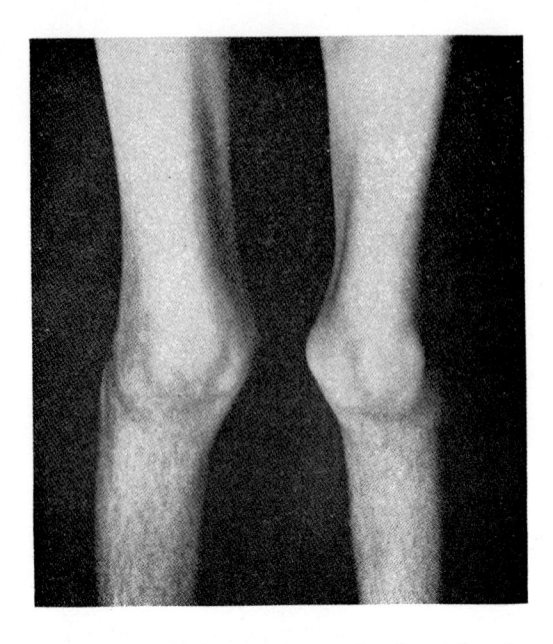

(*a*) Knees affected by multiple haemorrhages, showing deformity and wasting.

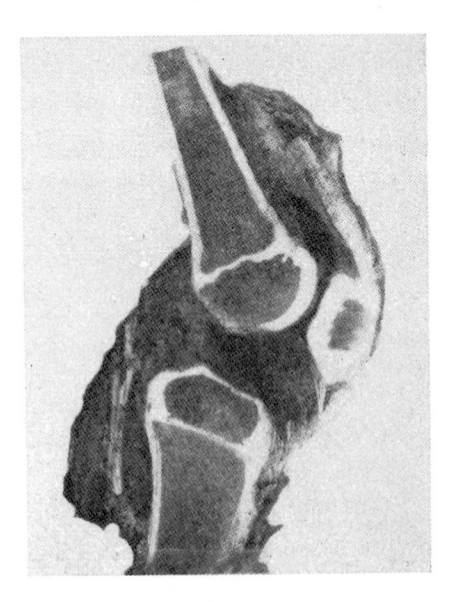

(*b*) Post mortem specimen of a knee joint affected by haemarthroses.

Figure 1.7. Late results of haemophilic haemorrhages.

Figure 1.7. Late results of haemophilic haemorrhages.

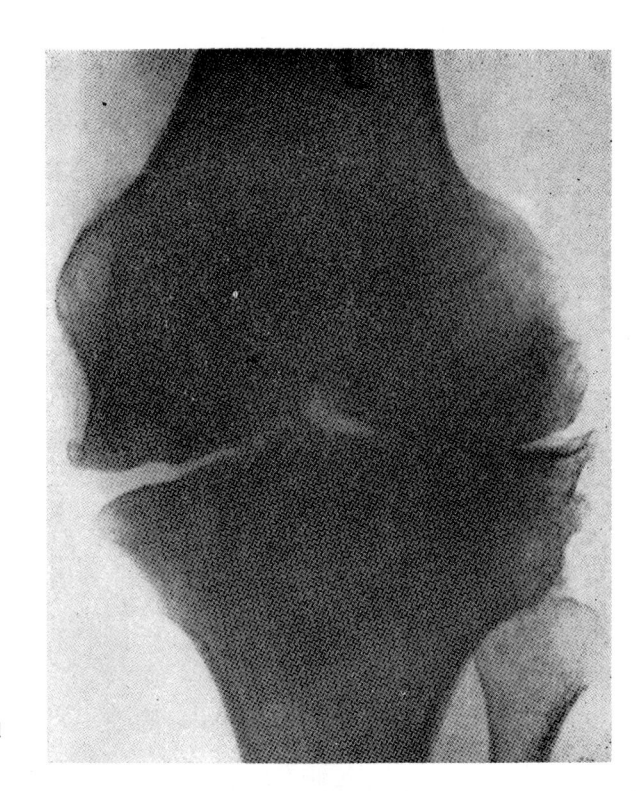

(c) X-ray of a knee affected by multiple haemarthroses.

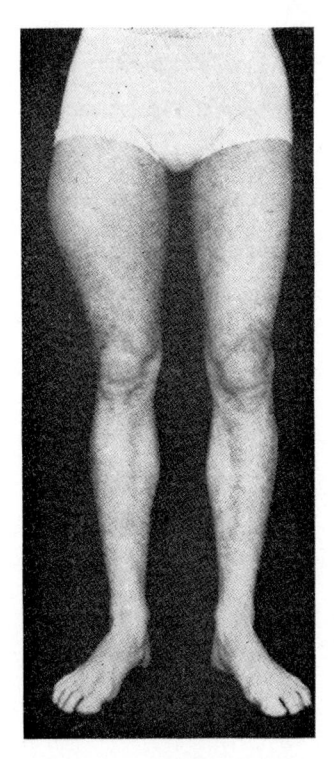

(d) Chronic cyst of the thigh following an unresolved haemorrhage.

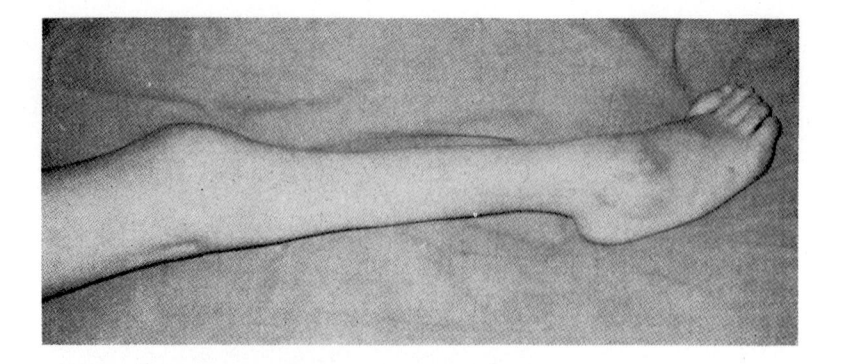

(e) Equinous deformity of the foot following contraction of the calf muscles.

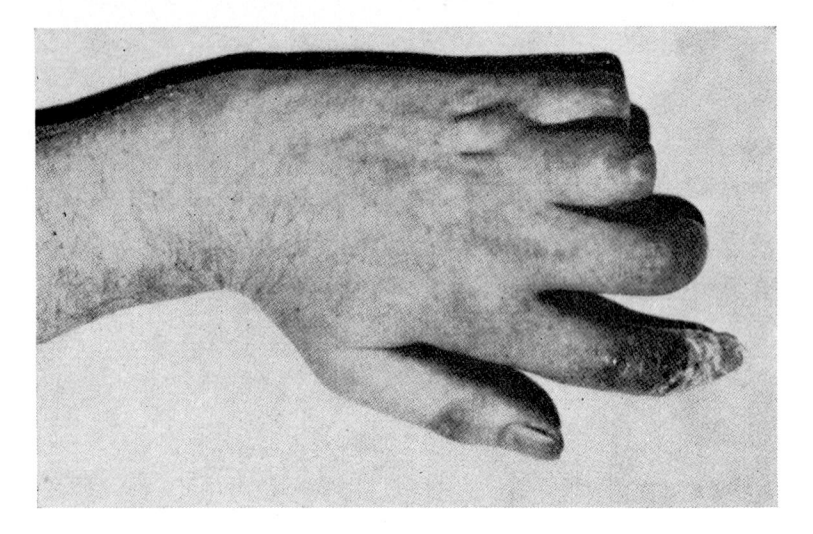

(f) Gangrene of the finger following Volkmann's ischaemic contracture.

Figure 1.7. Late results of haemophiliac haemorrhages.

affected males. There may be many more undetected and mildly affected individuals who have escaped serious injury or surgery and are unaware of anything more than a slight tendency to bleed or bruise more than normal. About two-thirds of our patients have a positive family history of the sex-linked recessive type, in about one-third there is no family history, but in some of these cases there is insufficient evidence or so few males in the pedigree that it cannot be determined that the condition has arisen *de novo* as a mutation in the patient or his mother. Where the family history is positive, it is usually found that the condition is of about the same clinical grade and with similar factor VIII levels in the blood, in the different affected members. Haemophilic relatives of a severely affected patient are thus likely to be severely affected, whereas a mild haemophilic with factor VIII levels about 5% will tend to have relatives with similar levels, perhaps without symptoms.

The first manifestations of haemophilia appear in early childhood, but not, curiously enough, during the neo-natal period. Haemophilic babies very seldom present with the bleeding from the cord and umbilicus, melaena, haematemesis, intracranial bleeding, or bruising characteristic of haemorrhagic disease of the new-born which is due to Vitamin K deficiency. In fact, for the first 6–9 months even severely haemophilic babies may be apparently normal. The reason for this temporary immunity is not known. It is possible that, during the birth trauma the baby's blood contains sufficient factor VIII derived from the mother to give protection, and that during its cradle life it is protected from trauma sufficiently to prevent bleeding. However, as soon as he begins to crawl and walk and suffer the inevitable knocks and twists associated with the process, haemorrhagic troubles begin.

Extensive bruising is usually an early sign of trouble and also the painful swellings produced by deep tissue haematomata which may occur anywhere in the body. These tissue haemorrhages may compress muscles, nerves or blood vessels in the limbs and may lead to ischaemia, paralysis, contractures and permanent crippling. In certain sites tissue haemorrhages can be of immediate danger, particularly in the tongue or throat, and in the tissues of the neck and mediastinum, where they may cause asphyxia and need immediate treatment for relief of the obstruction and control of bleeding. It is a characteristic of haemophilic bleeding into the tissues that the blood, remaining fluid as it does, tracks widely through the tissue spaces and along fascial planes. It is not unusual for subcutaneous bleeding to affect a whole limb as a result of some minor injury, or even half the body (see Figure 1.6). The tissues are not so much separated as infiltrated, in contrast to 'normal' haematoma formation where a solid blood clot is formed, separating the tissues, and which can be evacuated through an incision. Incision of an acute haemophilic haematoma seldom achieves anything except the infliction of further injury, since no localised collection of blood is found, only a sort of oedema in which the fluid is blood. The blood is, however, quite rapidly re-absorbed if the patient's blood level of factor VIII is raised by suitable means. Haemorrhages in the abdomen may give rise to diagnostic difficulties. Right-sided abdominal pain, with tenderness and swelling in the right iliac fossa, some rise of temperature and a moderate leucocytosis which would indicate acute appendicitis in the normal person, in a haemophilic patient is more likely to be due to retro-peritoneal bleeding, initiated, perhaps, by some appendicular inflammation but certainly not justifying an operation. A most curious and serious result of deep tissue bleeding, particularly in the thigh, is the gradual formation of a blood cyst, which may slowly grow to vast proportions, eroding bone, invading the pelvis, and ultimately bursting or becoming infected. It may be that these cysts begin as sub-periosteal haematomata, and some of those presenting in the thigh may have arisen in the para-vertebral region in the abdomen. These blood cysts have been mistaken for sacromata in the past, and, being aware of this, we have made the tragic error of supposing the swelling in the leg of a haemophilic boy was haemorrhagic in origin though it proved, after amputation, to be a sarcoma. The effects of haemorrhage can simulate many infective and neoplastic conditions, and though bleeding should be considered as the most likely cause of trouble in any known haemophilic patient, the more obvious diagnosis applicable in a normal person must always be carefully considered too. Without question, the most characteristic bleeding in haemophilia is into the joints giving rise to recurrent haemarthroses with swelling and pain during the acute phase, and increasing crippling and deformity as a late result of repeated episodes. Haemarthroses begin to occur from the age of 3 or 4 years onwards. In mild haemophilia they may not occur at all, or so infrequently that no permanent damage is done, but in more severe cases they constitute the most distressing and incapacitating feature of the disease. The first episodes are usually the result of definite trauma, but each haemorrhage causes damage that predisposes to further bleeding. The joint structures are weakened or destroyed, and the muscles related to it become atrophic or fibrosed so that the joint itself becomes intrinsically less stable, and less supported by normal muscle. There may be increased vascularisation of the damaged synovial membranes and eroded cartilages, so that the joint is not only more liable to be damaged, it also becomes more liable to bleeding. In the end the joint may become completely fixed by fibrous or even bony union, or worst of all, flail-like and incapable of weight-bearing or control. No joints are exempt from this process, but the knees, elbows, ankles, wrists, shoulders and hips are affected most frequently in that order.

Bleeding into the nervous system is a special problem in haemophilia. Peripheral nerves are likely to be involved in deep tissue haemorrhages with their resultant pressure and later fibrosis, particularly in the limbs, and early treatment is needed if permanent damage is to be avoided. Haemorrhage into or around the spinal cord, which occurs usually as the result of trauma, may cause paraplegia, and the immediate relief of the compression by major surgery or by more conservative means requires careful consideration in each individual case. Intercranial bleeding is also a greater hazard in the haemophilic patient than in the normal subject, to judge by its frequency. Again trauma is usually the cause, but in several cases even comparatively slight head injury has resulted in the occurrence of diffuse intercerebral bleeding and signs of compression. No definite clot is found in such cases, but decompression relieves the symptoms (in conjunction with treatment with factor VIII).

Serious gastro-intestinal bleeding is not very common, and when it occurs repeatedly is usually due to a definite lesion such as a gastric or duodenal ulcer, or colitis. It is a general rule, in fact, that lesions which cause some bleeding in normal people will cause serious and prolonged bleeding in the haemophilic patient. These causes of gastro-intestinal bleeding should therefore be treated in the same way as would be adopted in the non-haemophilic patient, if necessary by surgery with the use of specific factor VIII treatment. A special complication of intestinal bleeding in haemophilia is the formation of a haematoma in the wall of the gut, which may cause obstruction or even intersusception.

Haematuria is common in haemophilia. It occurs, usually without warning or obvious cause, and continues more or less steadily for days or even weeks, and sometimes ceasing abruptly and starting again without obvious cause. The bleeding is usually renal in origin. The amount of blood lost is usually far less than would be judged by simple inspection of the urine, because even a 1 in 100 dilution of blood in a large volume looks almost like pure blood. It is difficult, on the theories of haemostasis already discussed, to account for this apparently spontaneous bleeding. It must be assumed either that the renal vessels are abnormal in haemophilia, or that some intermittent and very slight bleeding occurs in normal people and is stopped by the normal clotting mechanism before the urine is significantly coloured.

Figures 1.6 and 1.7 (following p. 20) show the effects of haemorrhage in haemophilic patients to whom inadequate treatment was given too late. Some of the lesions illustrated (Figure 1.6, Figure 1.7a, c, d, e and f) have caused permanent deformity and will cause life-long disability to the patient. These lesions are now practically all preventable. The key to prevention lies in adequate replacement therapy given as soon after the onset of bleeding as possible. There is now no shortage of therapeutic material in the United Kingdom and the next stage in mastering the disease concerns planning the use of therapeutic materials, the setting up of organisations best suited to deliver the material to the patient and educating the patients and their medical advisors in the new approach.

Overt bleeding is probably the symptom most often associated in the lay mind with the condition of haemophilia. While it is true that in the past patients have bled to death from cuts or superficial injuries, or following minor operations such as tooth extraction or an unwisely performed tonsillectomy, blood transfusion and modern methods of treatment have greatly reduced the hazards of actual blood loss. In fact, haemorrhage of this sort, though alarming for the patient and his relatives is less likely to cause serious danger than an accumulation of blood in the tissues. Small injuries of the skin, such as pin-pricks, scratches or small shaving cuts do not bleed unduly as a rule, but small injuries to the mucous membranes of the mouth or nose, or larger wounds to the skin may bleed persistently. Often there is a 'latent period' of several hours after injury before the onset of this persistent bleeding, a fact which is not easy to explain. It may be that vascular spasm is an important factor in the early stages of haemostasis, and that this is normal in haemophilia, but that the firm clot required to prevent the recurrence of bleeding when these vessels relax is not formed by haemophilic blood. Another explanation might be that platelet aggregates form normally in haemophilia, but are less stable because of the lack of adequate thrombin and fibrin formation and thus tend to break up or loosen some time after their formation.

Without effective treatment bleeding can continue for days or weeks from even slight injuries, such as a small cut on the finger or an abrasion of the tongue. The ordinary remedies usually effective in normal people such as the application of dressings, bandages, or styptics are incapable of arresting this haemophilic blood flow which seeps through dressings like water. Pressure firm enough to arrest the circulation will, of course, stop the bleeding, but as soon as it is relaxed the haemorrhage will restart, and if it is applied for more than a few minutes the tissues become devitalised with consequent sloughing and an extension of the wound. Cauterisation, chemical or thermal, is only temporarily effective for the same reasons, and when the inevitable slough separates the patient bleeds from an area larger than before. There is naturally a temptation to close the wound by sutures, strapping or plugging, but this is actually worse than useless because it simply prevents the escape of blood without stopping the bleeding, and haematoma formation is inevitable. In the mouth, this may have disastrous consequences, and patients have died of asphyxia caused by haematoma formation in the throat following the suturing of bleeding tooth sockets.

The local treatment of surface bleeding can be often quite effective if the haemostatic principles are considered and used intelligently. The main defect in haemophilia is the failure to form a tough, adherent clot at the mouths of the damaged vessels. The local application of an agent which will correct this defect would be effective if the blood with which it is mixed remained *in situ* in the wound. This is unlikely to happen during actual bleeding, since the wound is constantly bathed with fresh, non-clotting blood. But the combination of local pressure and a haemostatic such as Russell's Viper Venom or human thrombin is often successful in dealing with bleeding tooth sockets, or cuts, or epistaxis. Pressure can be applied to the dressing soaked in the haemostatic for long enough to allow the blood to clot firmly, and the pressure can then be relaxed (leaving the dressing in place) without restarting the bleeding. It is an advantage to use an absorbable dressing such as oxidised cellulose, gelatine sponge or fibrin foam which avoids the trauma inevitably inflicted in changing cotton dressings.

More serious injuries require specific factor VIII treatment, and under cover of its administration wounds are dealt with just as they would be in the normal individual; obvious bleeding points are ligatured, and sutures inserted where required. Factor VIII treatment will, of course, need to be continued until healing is complete. Though healthy granulation tissue does not bleed with low factor VIII levels, it is particularly liable to trauma, and infection may erode vessels in the area. Not until epithelisation is complete or skin grafting has been carried out successfully is the patient free from risk of bleeding should the factor VIII level of his blood fall below 20–30% of normal even temporarily. During the healing period protection of the injured area from trauma is therefore a very important part of the treatment.

Throughout his life the haemophilic patient lives on the brink of haemorrhagic disasters of the sort described. The severely affected patient if untreated becomes progressively crippled by repeated haemarthroses and muscle haemorrhages and is often in great pain. Either because he learns to live more effectively with his disability, or because his haemostatic mechanism improves or compensates for its defect in some unknown way, the liability to bleed seems to diminish in some patients as they reach middle or old age, despite the lack of any observable improvement in their clotting defect. It is difficult to give figures for the expectation of life for severely affected haemophilic patients. In 1943, it was assessed at 18 years for haemophilics in Denmark, and this was probably considerably longer than the expectation for similar patients at the beginning of the century. In this country and at the present time the expectation must have considerably improved again. The mean age at death of 56 patients recorded by the Registrar General for the years 1959–62 was between 36 and 37. For 62 deaths recorded between 1969 and 1974 it was 42·3 (Biggs & Spooner, 1977).

CHRISTMAS DISEASE (HAEMOPHILIA B)

Hereditary factor IX deficiency resembles haemophilia A in almost every genetic and clinical aspect. The symptomatology and natural history are practically indistinguishable from haemophilia, except that there is a greater tendency for the heterozygous female carriers to suffer from abnormal bleeding.

The main practical importance in distinguishing the two conditions is the necessity for applying the correct specific treatment, if it is required. Patients with Christmas disease will not respond to factor VIII concentrates, nor will haemophilic patients respond to factor IX, though they will both respond to whole blood or plasma transfusion to the limited extent to which this can be effective. It is possible that the reported success of serum transfusion in cases of 'haemophilia' in the past was due to its use in cases of Christmas disease, then unrecognised. Christmas disease has an incidence of about 1 to every 10 cases of haemophilia in this country, but it is relatively commoner in others because of a rather localised geographical distribution. There are many cases in Switzerland, for example, and it is of interest that the famous bleeders of Tenna, regarded by Bullock and Fildes as a classical haemophilic family, actually suffer from Christmas disease.

VON WILLEBRAND'S DISEASE

The condition now known as von Willebrand's disease has been rather slow to emerge as a clinical entity, and it has been described under a number of different names of which 'pseudohaemophilia', 'hemogenia', 'capillary thrombopathy', 'hereditary angiostaxis' are a selection. Its demarcation from Glantzman's disease and thrombasthenia seems to be established, since in these conditions abnormal platelet function as regards clot retraction or clotting is found, whereas the platelets in von Willebrand's disease are normal in these respects. The condition is inherited as a simple dominant, either sex being affected, and the defect passed directly from the affected parent to his or her children. The main pathological finding is a greatly prolonged bleeding time, and an increased rate of bleeding from the needle punctures used in this investigation. On capillary microscopy patients have been found to have abnormally large and sometimes tortuous skin capillaries which bleed profusely on being pricked and show no sign of contraction. There may be some morphological similarity, therefore, to the capillary defect in telangiectasia, though there is no localisation of abnormal vessels into visible lesions, and the defect is distributed diffusely over the vessels of the skin and mucous membranes. These vessels do not seem to be unduly fragile, since the tourniquet test is usually negative. The platelet count is normal, and all the usual tests of platelet function such as aggregation during normal clotting or on the addition of ADP, ability to promote clot retraction, and thromboplastin generation are normal. It has been shown, however, that adhesion to a particular sort of glass is less than normal, and it is said that platelet adhesion *in vivo* is reduced, but this may be a defect of the tissues to which the platelets normally adhere, or of some factor in the blood which promotes adhesion to damaged tissues rather than a defect of the platelet themselves.

Several 'factors' have been found to be absent from the plasma of patients having von Willebrand's disease. One of these is factor-VIII-related antigen (see Chapter 2). This is a substance which forms a precipitate with rabbit anti-factor VIII antibodies. This factor-VIII-related protein is present in normal plasma, haemophilic plasma, stored normal plasma and normal serum. It is heat resistant. Another 'factor' is one which promotes the adhesion of platelets to glass while another promotes the aggregation of platelets in the presence of ristocetin. These properties may be associated with the same or different plasma proteins and all or some are absent or reduced in patients having von Willebrand's disease. In many cases of von Willebrand's disease, there is a deficiency of factor VIII. In most of such cases the factor VIII level is in the range of 5% to 20% thus resembling mild haemophilia, and it remains fairly constant in any one individual investigated from time to time. More rarely the factor VIII may be lower than 5% and, conversely, in some cases with quite severe haemorrhagic symptoms, it may be normal. When it occurs as a feature of von Willebrand's disease, this factor VIII deficiency is inherited not as a sex-linked X-born defect as in haemophilia, but as an autosomal dominant. One must conclude, therefore, that at least two different genes are concerned with the control of factor VIII levels in the blood. When patients having von Willebrand's disease are treated with crude fractions containing factor VIII, such as cryoprecipitate and Cohn fraction I, the factor VIII level rises and the level is maintained for longer than in haemophiliacs. It seems that the fractions used contain some substance which induces the patient to make some factor VIII. This factor VIII promoting protein may or may not be identical with one or other of the 'factors' which affect platelet function referred to above.

The type of bleeding in von Willebrand's disease is usually quite different from that of haemophilia. The main sites of haemorrhage are the mucous membranes, giving rise to epistaxis, menorrhagia and gastro-intestinal bleeding. Some cases of abdominal operations have given relatively little trouble, but any trauma to the mouth, throat, or nose can produce serious and persistent bleeding. Haemarthroses and deep tissue haemorrhages occur occasionally in the most severely affected patients. Superficial bruising occurs, and persistent bleeding from small cuts or abrasions of the skin. It seems, therefore, as if the haemorrhagic tendency particularly affects the surfaces of the body lined or covered with epithelium. Though these patients do not suffer the severe physical crippling which occurs in haemophilia, their liability to spontaneous or easily induced bleeding is a constant anxiety, and many have died of haemorrhage.

References

BIGGS, R. & DOUGLAS A.S. (1953) The thromboplastin generation test. *Journal of Clinical Pathology*, **6**, 23.

BIGGS R. & SPOONER R. (1977) Haemophilia treatment in the United Kingdom from 1969 to 1974. *British Journal of Haematology.* In press.

BULLOCH W. & FILDES P. (1911) *Haemophilia: Treasury of Human Inheritance,* Parts V & VI. Eugenic Laboratory Memoirs XII, Dulan and Company, London.

FAVRE-FILLY J., PRADER J.P., THOUVEREZ J.P. & BELLEVILLE J. (1974) *Le Facteur Stabilisant de la Fibrine (FSF) et son Deficit Congenital.* Imprimerie des Beaux-Arts, Lyon.

HAYES G. (1882) Sur le mécanisme de l'arrêt des hémorrhagies. *Compte rendus hebdomadaires de séances de l'Académie des Sciences,* **95,** 18.

JONES A.F.D. (1810) *A treatise on the process employed by nature in suppressing its haemorrhage of divided and punctured arteries and the use of the ligature.* Longman, Hurse, Rees, Orine and Brown, London.

MACFARLANE R.G. (1964) An enzyme cascade in the blood clotting mechanism and its function as a biochemical amplifier. *Nature (London),* **202,** 498.

OWREN P.A. (1947) The coagulation of blood. Investigations on a new clotting factor. *Acta Medical Scandinavica,* Suppl. 194.

QUICK A.J. (1935) The prothrombin in hemophillia and obstructive jaundice. *Journal of Biological Chemistry,* **109,** LXXIII.

WHARTON JONES T. (1851) *Guy's Hospital Rept.* **7,** 1.

Chapter 2. Factor VIII

D. E. G. AUSTEN

Introduction and nomenclature

Factor VIII activity is present in normal human blood plasma and is wholly or partially absent in plasma from patients with haemophilia or von Willebrand's disease. It is essential for normal blood clotting and haemostasis and in the chemical chain of clotting reactions factor VIII appears to act as a co-factor during the activation of factor X by factor IX, in the presence of calcium ions and phospholipid. The catastrophic bleeding that can occur in pathological deficiency states clearly illustrates how vital is factor VIII to haemostasis.

Factor-VIII-related antigen is present in normal human blood plasma and wholly or partially absent in patients with von Willebrand's disease (Zimmerman *et al*, 1971). However, unlike factor VIII activity, it is present in plasma from haemophiliacs. As with normal subjects, the actual concentration varies between individuals but on average the amount in the haemophiliac population is probably little different from that in the normal population. Some estimates suggest it may even be a little higher. Presence of this antigen is demonstrated, as its name suggests, by raising heterologous antibodies in animals to factor VIII concentrates and using these in immunoelectrophoresis. Antigen-antibody precipitin lines reveal the presence of antigen.

A third function called ristocetin co-factor is also absent in von Willebrand's disease but present in haemophilia and in the normal state. This co-factor is required for the aggregation of normal human platelets by ristocetin (an antibiotic which is no longer used because it precipitates protein *in vitro*; Howard & Firkin, 1971; Bouma *et al*, 1972; Weiss *et al*, 1973a, 1973b; Meyer *et al*, 1974; Gralnick *et al*, 1975). Factor VIII, factor-VIII-related antigen and ristocetin co-factor are normally found together and only by special chromatographic procedures can the factor VIII activity be separated from the other two. Antigen and ristocetin co-factor are almost always associated together and cannot be separated in the laboratory. This may suggest that they are two functions of the same molecule but no such proof exists at present. The biological significance of the absence of factor-VIII-related antigen and ristocetin co-factor in von Willebrand's disease is as yet unknown and efforts are being made to find relationships between the levels of these two functions and such measurements as glass adhesion of platelets (Bouma et al, 1972; Weiss et al, 1973c), bleeding time and clinical condition (Weiss et al, 1975).

Table 2.1. The occurrence of factor VIII functions.

Material	Material contains		
	Factor VIII activity	Factor-VIII-related antigen	Ristocetin co-factor
Normal plasma	Yes	Yes	Yes
Plasma from severe haemophiliac	No	Yes	Yes
Plasma from severe von Willebrand's disease patient	No	No	No
Normal human serum	No	Yes	Yes
Plasma adsorbed with alumina	Yes	Yes	Yes
Plasma reacted with homologous haemophilic antibody	No	Yes	Yes
Platelet granules	No	Yes	Yes
Endothelial cells	None detected	Yes	Yes

It can be seen that, in considering the properties of factor VIII, it is necessary to refer to three functions or activities which may or may not be normally separate entities. These are factor VIII activity (i.e. clotting activity), factor-VIII-related antigen and ristocetin co-factor and these terms will be used throughout this chapter. Table 2.1 shows a brief summary of materials in which the three functions are normally found. Since they are particularly difficult to separate it is likely that early work on factor VIII purification and identification concerned materials which contained all three functions.

Measurement of factor VIII

The absolute amount of factor VIII in blood plasma is unknown although estimates have been made. Factor levels in the past have been measured as a percentage of the average normal human level or else in units/ml where 1 unit/ml was defined as the amount in 1 ml of fresh citrated normal human plasma. These are still the best units for expressing concentrations of factor-VIII-related antigen or ristocetin co-factor but in the case of factor VIII activity an international standard is now available. Results expressed in terms of international units ml are numerically fairly similar to those expressed in the old units/ml although different laboratories disagree about the exact inter-relation. In the absence of an international standard, the provision of a standard of measurement for any of the three factor VIII functions can be something of a problem. Levels in individual plasma samples vary from 45% to 180% of the average normal level making it necessary to prepare pools of very large numbers of samples before a satisfactory standard is obtained.

At present it is not possible to use any of the known chemical structure of active factor VIII to devise a quantitative biochemical assay and those assays which are used are all based upon the clotting reaction. They are extremely sensitive and adequately precise but they can only express the factor VIII level as a percentage of a standard sample (Biggs et al, 1955; Austen & Rhymes, 1975). These clotting tests are discussed in Chapter 3. Factor-VIII-related antigen is mostly measured by the Laurell technique (Zimmerman et al, 1971; Laurell, 1972). Other methods are available, all based upon an antibody-antigen reaction. There are radioactive techniques (Hoyer, 1972; Paullsen et al, 1975; Ruggeri et al, 1976), using either a single or a double antibody technique and there is a method in which a sensitive colour reaction detects antibody-antigen complex (Bartlett et al, 1976). The new methods are probably more sensitive but for everyday analysis it is difficult to compete with the simple elegance of the Laurell technique. Detection by haemoglutination is also possible but this is not sensitive (Stites et al, 1971). Ristocetin co-factor is assayed by mixing the sample with washed human platelets and observing the degree of platelet aggregation (Weiss et al, 1973b).

Factor VIII in the body

As mentioned above, factor VIII activity, factor-VIII-related antigen and ristocetin co-factor can all vary in the individual normal human from about 45% of the average level to about 180%. The variation is further heightened because fear, stress and vigorous exercise increase the levels of all three functions (approximately in proportion) and, in subjects exercised to the point of mild exhaustion, levels can easily increase to more than double their starting values (Rizza, 1961; Rizza & Eipe, 1971; Bennett & Ratnoff, 1972; Prentice et al, 1972). Haemophiliacs are of course deficient in factor VIII activity but their levels of factor-VIII-related antigen and ristocetin co-factor are similar to those of normal people regardless of the severity of the disease. This also applies to haemophiliacs with factor VIII antibodies and patients who have developed spontaneous antibodies to factor VIII. The amount of factor-VIII-related antigen and ristocetin co-factor in plasma from patients with von Willebrand's disease is roughly proportional to the amount of factor VIII activity. The same appears to hold for normal subjects and so, when this relationship is expressed graphically, von Willebrand's disease appears as an extension of the normal

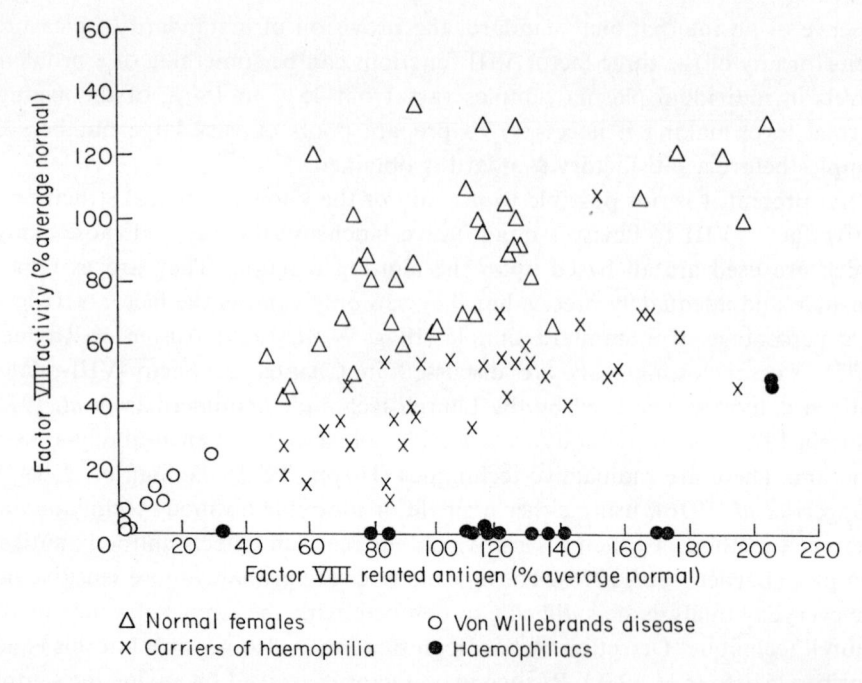

Figure 2.1. Factor VIII activity and factor-VIII-related antigen in pathological deficiency states.

condition and haemophilia appears as an anomaly. This is illustrated in Figure 2.1 together with results for carriers of haemophilia.

The female carrier of haemophilia on average will have 50% of the factor VIII clotting activity of the average normal female and this can be used as a basis for diagnosis. However, such levels are subject to a similar spread between individuals as observed with normal subjects and so it is only for a limited number of carriers that a diagnosis on this basis can be made with any confidence at all. However, increased confidence can be obtained if diagnosis is made on the basis of a ratio of clotting activity to factor-VIII-related antigen (Zimmerman et al, 1971; Ekert et al, 1973; Rizza et al, 1975). A carrier will have normal antigen levels and so an average ratio of 0·5 is to be expected compared to an average ratio of 1 for a normal female. Probably the reason for improvement is that antigen and clotting activity are similarly affected by fear, stress and exercise and use of a ratio provides a method by which such extraneous effects are cancelled out.

When factor VIII concentrates are infused into haemophiliacs during replacement therapy, the subsequent half life of the factor VIII activity is approximately 12 hours. If factor VIII is infused into a normal subject, the clotting activity in excess of the subject's normal amount has a half life which is considerably shorter than this. However, it cannot be concluded that this represents the normal turnover of factor VIII since levels in excess of normal may be subject to additional regulatory mechanisms. A similar problem arises when studying the factor-VIII-related antigen levels in haemophiliacs after infusion.

The levels of factor VIII clotting activity in von Willebrand's disease patients after infusion is even more complicated since the factor VIII level obtained after infusion is often maintained for many hours before a significant fall-off is observed and, in extreme cases, the factor VIII clotting activity can even rise as though the patient were beginning to synthesise activity. Some workers have reported that factor-VIII-related antigen and ristocetin co-factor after infusion into von Willebrand's patients do not persist as long as the clotting activity so that, for a period following infusion, the patient's plasma contains proportionately less antigen and co-factor than it does clotting activity (Bennett et al, 1972; Bloom et al, 1973; Sultan et al, 1976). Other workers have not observed this effect with their patients (Kernoff et al, 1974). After infusion in patients with von Willebrand's disease Sultan et al (1976) also find that the electrophoretic mobility of the antigen increases as its level falls.

Factor VIII synthesis *in vivo*

Recently, interest has centred around the possible presence of factor VIII in platelets and in endothelial cells but so far all positive findings have been confined to factor-VIII-related antigen and ristocetin co-factor and not to clotting activity. Immunofluorescence studies have shown that, *in vivo*, endothelial cells, megakaryocytes and platelets contain factor-VIII-related antigen. Both the antigen and ristocetin co-factor have been detected on the platelet membrane (Nachman & Jaffe, 1975) as well as in the granules (Howard et al, 1974). That which is in the platelet interior cannot be exchanged with that in the blood plasma since the two functions are present within the platelets of patients with von Willebrand's disease (Howard et al, 1974; Sonia et al, 1974). The amount present in platelets is very significant and has been estimated as equal to 15% of the amount in platelet-poor plasma (Nachman & Jaffe, 1976).

Endothelial cells have been successfully cultured and it has been shown that they synthesise and release the antigen as well as ristocetin co-factor (Jaffe et al, 1973). In patients with von Willebrand's disease the factor-VIII-related antigen in their endothelial cells is reduced or absent (Holmberg et al, 1974), unlike that in their platelets. These observations strongly suggest that endothelial cells are a major site for the synthesis of factor-VIII-related antigen and ristocetin cofactor. Antigen from endothelial cells appears to have identical properties to that circulating in plasma and it has a similar sub-unit structure (Jaffe & Nachman, 1975). It seems significant that no factor VIII clotting activity has been observed to be released during any of the endothelial cell experiments. Thus while the endothelial cells can be implicated in antigen and ristocetin co-factor production there is no proof of their involvement in production of factor VIII clotting activity. If the cells are involved in synthesis of clotting activity then it suggests that some extra step is required before activity is finally achieved.

A similar hypothesis is suggested by the inheritance of factor VIII deficiency. Haemophilia is determined by an X-linked recessive mechanism whereas von Willebrand's disease is inherited as an autosomal dominant condition. As far as is known, there is no inherited deficiency of antigen alone and the concentration of antigen in normal people and most patients with von Willebrand's disease is roughly proportional to their factor VIII activity. These various relationships could suggest that the production of factor-VIII-related antigen and factor VIII activity proceed, *in vivo*, by a common route at some stage.

A further and important clue is that the infusion of haemophilic plasma into a patient with von Willebrand's disease produces factor VIII activity in that patient. Thus the power to synthesise factor VIII activity must be at least partially present in von Willebrand's disease even though the ability to synthesise factor-VIII-related antigen and ristocetin co-factor is absent. Furthermore the substance needed to initiate this apparent synthesis of factor VIII activity is present in haemophilic plasma but absent in the von Willebrand's disease plasma. Factor-VIII-related antigen and ristocetin co-factor are in that category.

The purification of factor VIII

The purification of factor VIII has fascinated scientists for many years. Its concentration in plasma is low and its instability during purification has been a major stumbling block. In particular it is unstable during ion exchange chromatography and to be unable to use such a powerful separation technique represents a severe limitation. Factor VIII adsorbs well enough onto ion exchange columns; the problem arises in trying to elute the factor in reasonable yield while retaining its activity. Moreover, factor VIII which has been prepared by this method has been reported to be of reduced stability as though some damage to the molecule had been incurred. Luckily, factor VIII concentrates after purification can be maintained in a stable condition when they are freeze dried. In this form the activity is much more stable than for example in deep frozen solution. Freeze dried preparations are best stored at 10°C and there is no advantage in the use of very low temperatures; some reports suggest that lower temperatures even decrease stability.

The simplest method of factor VIII concentration is that of cryoprecipitation and a large proportion of concentrates used in the United Kingdom are prepared this way. The basis of the method is to thaw frozen plasma at 2 to 6°C (Pool & Robinson, 1959; Pool et al, 1964; Pool & Shannon, 1965) and the yield in large scale practice is 35 to 45%.

Precipitation by organic solvents is another powerful tool in factor VIII purification. Usually this involves ethanol (Cohn et al, 1946) or ether at low temperatures and valuable separation techniques have been devised which incorporate these stages (Blombäck, 1958; Kekwick & Mackay, 1954; Maycock et al, 1963; Newman et al, 1971). Precipitation by amino acids is another method which is often employed (Wagner et al, 1964; Roberts et al, 1964). Glycine is the most popular of the amino acids but β-alanine and γ-amino butyric acid can also be used. Using a selection of these precipitation techniques, useful therapeutic concentrates of intermediate potency can be prepared (Hershgold et al, 1966; Brinkhous et al, 1968), and if an additional stage of polyethylene glycol precipitation is introduced (Johnson et al, 1966; Brinkhous et al, 1968; Newman et al, 1971) further improvement can be made. Purifications of up to 380-fold are reported.

The successful use of tannic acid (Simonette et al, 1961), aluminium hydroxide (Wagner et al, 1957) and bentonite in factor VIII separation have been reported, the last two being used particularly to separate factor VIII and fibrinogen. However, the results with all three seem to vary widely, depending on the source of the material, and so they have not found wide application for large scale production. Other substances which have been applied successfully are calcium phosphate (Niemetz et al, 1961) and calcium citrate (Simonetti et al, 1972; Blombäck et al, 1962; Legaz et al, 1973) but again they are not extensively used at present. A modern precipitant for factor VIII is concanavalin A which precipitates glycoproteins; several workers are currently using this (Kass et al, 1969).

One of the most difficult parts of factor VIII purification is the separation of fibrinogen which has similar precipitation properties. Originally this led to the hypothesis that the two were bound together in some way and that fibrinogen was essential for factor VIII stability. More recently factor VIII preparations have been reported which are claimed to be free of fibrinogen and to be completely stable (Schmer et al, 1972; Legaz et al, 1973). However, there has been a counter-claim that all factor VIII samples contain trace fibrinogen and so the problem is not entirely resolved. Certainly, factor VIII activity is found in the plasma of patients with afibrinogenaemia and in addition, the venom of certain snakes (Ankistrodon rhodostoma and Crotalus terrificus) will coagulate fibrinogen leaving factor VIII unaffected. Some of the small scale preparative techniques for the highest purity factor VIII use the step of bentonite adsorption mentioned above to reduce fibrinogen levels and Arvin or Chymotrypsin digestion has also been used (Green, 1971; Marchesi et al, 1972).

Very significant improvement in purity can be obtained in small scale preparations by the use of gel filtration chromatography. Under normal conditions factor VIII appears to be a very large molecule and it separates in the first fraction, the so-called exclusion volume. Fibrinogen leaves the column a little later and some of the factor VIII can be collected which is apparently free of fibrinogen except possibly for traces. Most of the other proteins leave the column later still and gel filtration alone can result in high purifications of the factor (Ratnoff et al, 1969).

Combinations of techniques mentioned above can yield highly purified products (Ratnoff et al, 1969; Shanbrom, 1970; Casillas et al, 1970; Hershgold et al, 1971; Marchesi et al, 1972; Legaz et al, 1973; Schwitzer & McKee, 1976) and purification of up to 20,000 to 40,000-fold has been obtained for human factor VIII and up to 10,000-fold for animal factor VIII (Michael & Tunnah, 1966; Schmer et al, 1972).

The stability of factor VIII

Instability has been such a major problem with factor VIII that many workers have turned their attention to the possibility of a stabilising additive. Many stabilisers have been suggested which no doubt were effective under the particular conditions of investigation but no additive has yet received universal acclaim. Ratnoff et al (1969) suggested ε-aminocaproic acid, glycerol, glycine or gelatin while Kass et al (1969) found some advantage for magnesium chloride, manganese chloride, calcium chloride, cysteine or fructose. Casillas et al (1969) were in favour of ε-aminocaproic acid, glucose or glycine. Citrate or EDTA have been reported to give some stabilisation over a narrow concentration range (Hynes et al, 1969). However, there is no doubt that higher concentrations of citrate (Simonette et al, 1972) or oxalate or EDTA (Mustard, 1958) cause a loss of activity and that a certain minimum amount of calcium is vital to factor VIII stability (Stibbe et al, 1972). It might be expected that factor VIII would be susceptible to oxidation since it contains thiol groups associated with, or close to the sites of clotting activity (Austen, 1970). Certainly some of the successful reagents mentioned above are reducing agents such as cysteine and fructose. In addition Pennell et al (1962) found that ascorbic acid can stabilise factor VIII. However, there is insufficient data to allow any firm conclusion. As discussed earlier it is now believed that highly purified factor VIII can be stable in the absence of fibrinogen. Previously fibrinogen had been thought to be an essential stabiliser (Schmer et al, 1972; Legaz et al, 1973). This rather unexpected stability of the pure factor suggests that some of the instability experienced during purification procedures may be due to the presence of an impurity, for example a proteolytic enzyme.

When factor VIII decomposes, the activity first decreases rapidly and then subsequently at a much reduced rate (Stibbe et al, 1972). It is not known whether this indicates some heterogeneity in factor VIII or whether some stabilising entity can accumulate during inactivation. The first phase of inactivation appears to accelerate if the calcium ion level is low but the second phase is largely unaffected.

Buffers for factor VIII

Buffers which have been most used in the experimental study of factor VIII are those made with Tris (i.e. Tris-(hydroxymethyl)-methylamine), barbitone or imidazole (syn:-glyoxaline). Phosphate buffers have been employed but their presence complicates any subsequent assays by reducing calcium ion concentration. Tris is popular in purification procedures and for elution of chromatographic columns although it is possible that the stability of factor VIII can be impaired by using high concentrations of Tris for chromatographic elution. Most workers appear to use a level of about 0·02 Molar for this work.

Recently, wide acceptance has been gained for buffers which incorporate HEPES (N-2-hydroxyethylpiperazine-N'-2-ethanesulphonic acid; Good et al, 1966; Zucker et al, 1970). These have good buffering action around neutral pH levels and have satisfactory low levels of enzymic inhibition. Their use appears to improve the stability of factor VIII on storage (Denson, 1970) and collecting blood directly into a mixture of HEPES and trisodium citrate is reported to give significant stabilisation (Godfrey et al, 1975). The expense of HEPES relative to other buffers has probably limited some of its application but increased demand seems to be improving the price position.

It has recently been suggested (Roberts et al, 1976) that HEPES buffer can shorten the clotting times in some factor assays including the one-stage assay of factor VIII. No evidence is available to suggest it is reacting with the factor and the inference is that acceleration of clotting occurs at a later point in the reaction chain where factor VIII is not directly involved. However, it does illustrate the need for correct control samples when using this buffer.

Animal factor VIII

Since the blood of cows or pigs can fairly easily be obtained from slaughter houses, this represents a convenient source of factor VIII. An additional advantage in animal products is that factor VIII activity in the blood plasma is 5 to 6 times that in human plasma. It is not known whether the extra activity is due to an increased concentration or whether the molecules of animal factor VIII have greater activity than those of the human species. Much higher levels of factor VIII are sometimes recorded in the literature for cow plasma which may indicate there are variations between cows of different age or breed. Alternatively it may represent variations in fear and stress at slaughter.

Fractional precipitation by phosphate and then citrate ions leads to high potency therapeutic concentrates (Bidwell, 1955a and 1955b) and polyethylene glycol precipitation gives additional improvement. In this way it is simple to obtain products of good solubility which have an activity of 30 units/ml or more (human units of activity). Animal plasma and factor concentrates apparently contain factor-VIII-related antigen and ristocetin co-factor in the same way as the human materials but unlike factor VIII activity it is not possible to relate them numerically with the human antigen. Measurements of their levels are made by comparison with the amount present in the average normal pig or in the average normal cow (in practice by having pools of such plasmas). In immunoelectrophoretic methods of measurement, cross reaction between the antigen and antibody of different species is not observed. If von Willebrand's disease is unknown for a particular animal species then the existence of factor-VIII-related antigen and ristocetin co-factor can only be postulated by analogy with other species and this is the case for the cow. Von Willebrand's disease is described in the pig and the dog and, as with the human disease it is characterised by reduced levels of antigen and ristocetin co-factor as well as factor VIII activity. In the absence of plasma from an animal with von Willebrand's disease the characteristic of antigen and co-factor which aids identification is that they are concentrated together with the factor VIII activity during purification, for example during gel filtration.

In the use as a therapeutic material, animal factor VIII concentrates have three particular disadvantages. They cause thrombocytopenia (Macfarlane *et al*, 1954; Forbes *et al*, 1972) in the patient; they may cease to be effective after several days of treatment due to a 'resistance' developing and in addition, they may cause a series of undesirable symptoms such as rigors and sweating during infusion. However, they are used in treatment, either in cases where human material is not available or else where the patient has developed an antibody to the human product which does not cross react with animal material.

An animal product which did not have these problems would find wider application and some laboratories are investigating the possibility of reducing side effects. The problem of rigors may present a difficult, if not impossible, problem but at least it would be directionally correct to eliminate all traces of pyrogens. A slaughter house, particularly in the summer months, is not the best place for collecting aseptic samples and even though filtering removes bacteria, cell debris can pass into the product. It should be possible to improve this situation.

Development of resistance to treatment is apparently complex. No effect of factor VIII infusion is detected in the patient and yet blood plasma from the patient will not destroy factor VIII *in vitro*. A reasonable explanation is that an antibody develops which can attach itself to active factor VIII and yet not neutralise its clotting activity. Such antibody-antigen complexes would be removed by the body, negating treatment, and yet the antibody would fail to neutralise activity *in vitro*. In support of this, antibodies to animal proteins have been detected in the plasma of such patients although exact identification of the antibody has not yet been made.

The third problem of animal products, that of causing platelet aggregation and thrombocytopenia, is definitely associated with a material related to factor VIII but is not due to the active clotting factor itself. The substance in question has been termed platelet aggregating factor (PAF) and is very similar to animal factor-VIII-related antigen (Forbes & Prentice, 1973; Griggs *et al*, 1973; Brown *et al*, 1974; De Gaetano, 1974; Griggs *et al*, 1974). Whether it is identical is unproven. However, it has been shown to be concentrated with the antigen during purification procedures, to be similar immunologically and to remain with the antigen when active factor VIII is split into sub-units and removed (Evans & Austen, 1977). It is reduced or absent in porcine von Willebrand's disease. Since active factor VIII can be separated from the antigen and like molecules (discussed later) then the problem of causing thrombocytopenia is one which at least in principle could be eliminated from animal factor concentrates.

The chemical structure of factor VIII

Factor VIII appears to be a glycoprotein. This might be inferred from free film electrophoresis experiments (Bidwell *et al*, 1966) in which the mobility of factor VIII increased with the presence of borate in the buffer and it might also be inferred from the evidence that concanavalin A precipitates factor VIII (Kass *et al*, 1969). Factor-VIII-related antigen and ristocetin co-factor are precipitated in the same way. Highly purified factor VIII has been subjected to chemical analysis and carbohydrate contents of between 5 and 10% have been reported for the human material (Hershgold *et al*, 1971; Marchesi *et al*, 1972; Legaz *et al*, 1973) and 20% for the bovine factor (Schmer *et al*, 1972). Of course, these analyses were carried out on a material which contained factor VIII activity, factor-VIII-related antigen and ristocetin co-factor and so the exact interpretation depends upon which hypothesis is adopted for the inter-relation of those three functions. In addition, although samples analysed by the different laboratories were highly purified they appear to have been of different purity levels so that not all of the results can be given equal weight. It is, however, reasonable to conclude that a carbohydrate moiety appears to be associated with one of the functions of factor VIII and this has been confirmed by work using glycolytic enzymes where it was shown that a carbohydrate moiety is associated with factor VIII clotting activity. In this work a wide-range glycolytic enzyme from Trichomonas Foetus was found to inactivate factor VIII clotting activity in a reaction which was inhibited by glycoproteins and by some simple sugars (Austen & Bidwell, 1972).

Because of the differences in the degrees of purification of the investigated samples it is best at this stage not to recount the specific classes of sugar which have been analysed in factor VIII samples. Similarly it is better not to list the amino-acid analyses (Hershgold *et al*, 1971; Marchesi *et al*, 1972; Legaz *et al*, 1973; Shapiro *et al*, 1973). Attempts have been made to detect a lipid component in the factor VIII molecule but no evidence has been found for the presence of significant amounts (Schmer *et al*, 1972; Marchesi *et al*, 1972; Legaz *et al*, 1973).

Thiol groups have been shown to be present in factor VIII at or near to the active site of clotting (Austen, 1970). The sodium salt of p-chloromercuribenzoic acid inactivates clotting ability but application of a reducing agent such as cysteine restores activity. It follows that some sensitivity to oxidation might be expected and an example of particular interest is the reaction with haematoporphyrin. This substance in very low concentration (10^{-5} molar) destroys factor VIII clotting activity (Davis *et al*, 1967) providing the reaction is carried out in the light (usually with a tungsten lamp). In the dark the factor is not inactivated. Almost certainly this is an example of photo-oxidation but it is very interesting that it should occur at such low concentration and suggests that the reaction may have some measure of specificity. Factor VIII clotting activity is destroyed by thrombin, plasmin and many other proteolytic enzymes and activity is not present in human blood serum (factor-VIII-related antigen and ristocetin cofactor are present). Variations of pH, both acid and alkaline, destroy clotting activity and maximum stability is achieved in the range of pH 6·2 to 7·4.

Thrombin, at levels below that required for the destruction of activity, will give an apparent activation of factor VIII providing the measurements are made by a one-stage method of assay. Levels recorded by the two-stage methods give no indication of activation (Ozge Anivar *et al*, 1965; Ozge Anivar, 1970; Osterud *et al*, 1971; Anderson & McKee, 1972; Legaz *et al*, 1973). Trypsin shows a similar effect. Plasmin and chymotrypsin do not cause apparent activation although both will destroy factor VIII activity at higher concentrations. Ancrod and Reptilase are reported neither to activate nor destroy the activity. When apparent activation by thrombin or trypsin is obtained there is no change in molecular weight of factor VIII or its sub-unit as measured by SDS gel electrophoreses. Neither are there any new peptides detected. However, in a later section dealing with molecular weight in polyacrylamide gels it is suggested that there are distinct limitations to these analytical techniques when applied to factor VIII activity.

The electrophoretic mobility of factor VIII is that of a globulin but it has been shown by different workers to migrate with the α, β or γ globulins depending on the condition of the experiment. This may be consistent with the view that factor VIII is a large and complex molecule. Under free film conditions factor VIII moves as an α-globulin (Bidwell et al, 1966) although the mobility is increased by the presence of borate.

Factor VIII is adsorbed slightly by barium sulphate, aluminium hydroxide and bentonite when these adsorbents are employed in excess. It is strongly adsorbed to ion exchange materials including the popular chemically-treated celluloses and is difficult to remove without gross inactivation. This property also makes factor VIII difficult to use in experiments involving affinity chromatography where the column materials are made from cyanogen-bromide-treated sepharose. Factor VIII adheres non-specifically to these columns by means of hydrophobic interaction with the spacers and probably also due to attachment to charged groups on the gel. It can be removed in poor yield from some of these columns by high ionic strength such as 1 molar sodium chloride and it is vitally important in work with affinity chromatography to distinguish this effect from the intended specific absorption.

Molecular weights, sub-units and the segregation of factor VIII activity

If the molecular weights of active factor VIII, factor-VIII-related antigen or ristocetin co-factor, are measured under normal isotonic conditions, either by sedimentation techniques or by gel filtration, then values in excess of a million are obtained (Hershgold & Sprawls, 1966; Ratnoff et al, 1969; Hershgold et al, 1971; Schmer et al, 1972; Legaz et al, 1973). This is supported by the fact that in polyacrylamide gel electrophoresis factor VIII will not enter a 3% gel. However, there is now a great deal of evidence that factor VIII can exist in more than one molecular weight form. Using ultracentrifuge techniques, it can be shown that the diffusion coefficient decreases when ionic strength is increased by using for example 0·4 M or 1·0 M saline (Thelin & Wagner, 1961; Johnson et al, 1966; Weiss & Kochwa, 1970) and this is confirmed using gel filtration chromatography. Under conditions of normal isotonic elution factor VIII appears in the first fractions to leave the column, in the so called 'exclusion volume', indicating a molecular weight in excess of a million (Hershgold et al, 1967; Kass et al,

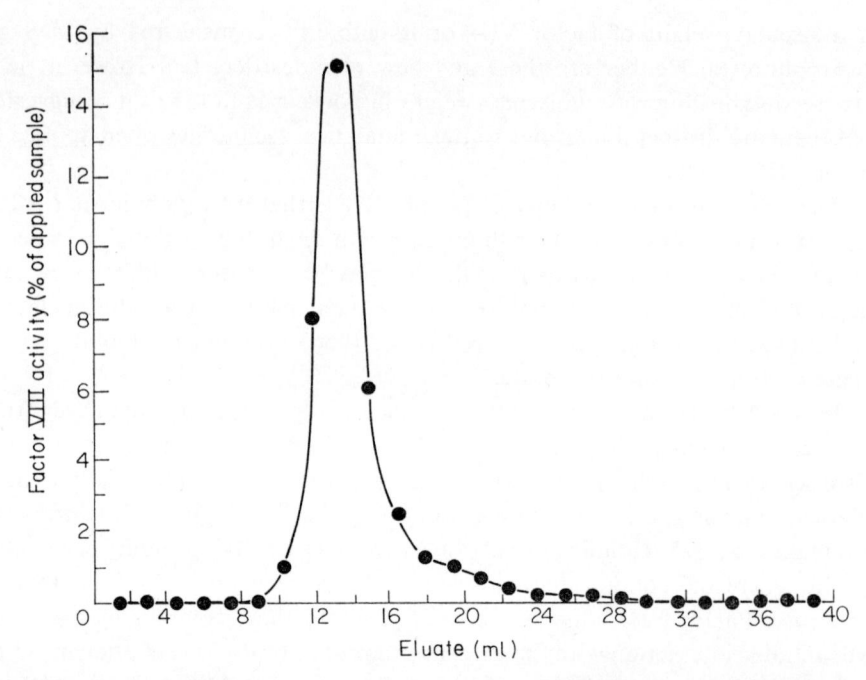

Figure 2.2. Factor VIII activity after gel filtration chromatography of normal factor VIII.

1969; Ratnoff *et al,* 1969). Clotting activity, the antigen and the ristocetin cofactor are all present in these fractions and this is illustrated in Figures 2.2 and 2.3. However, a different result is obtained if the factor VIII preparation remains for a period in a solution of 0·8 to 1·3 molar sodium chloride (Weiss *et al,* 1972; Weiss & Hoyer, 1973) or 0·25 molar calcium chloride (Owen & Wagner, 1972; Griggs *et al,* 1973; Rick & Hoyer, 1973) and is then subjected to gel filtration chromatography using the same hypertonic solution to elute the chromatography columns. Then factor VIII activity emerges from the column at a much later point corresponding to a considerable reduction in molecular weight, while factor-VIII-related antigen and ristocetin co-factor still appear in the exclusion volume. Similar results have been obtained using succinic anhydride (Barrow & Graham, 1972), low ionic strengths (van Mourik *et al,* 1974), proteolytic enzymes (Anderson & McKee, 1972; Weiss & Kochwa, 1970; McKee *et al,* 1975), sodium periodate (Kaelin, 1975) and levels of the reducing agent dithiothreitol up to 3×10^{-4} molar (Austen, 1974). Figure 2.4 illustrates the disaggregation by high ionic strengths and the change in molecular size can be seen by comparing this with Figure 2.2. Values of molecular weight for the active factor VIII sub-unit have been variously reported as shown in Table 2.2. A wide divergence of results is evident but there does seem to be considerable support for a value between 150,000 and 250,000. Recent work by Schwitzer &

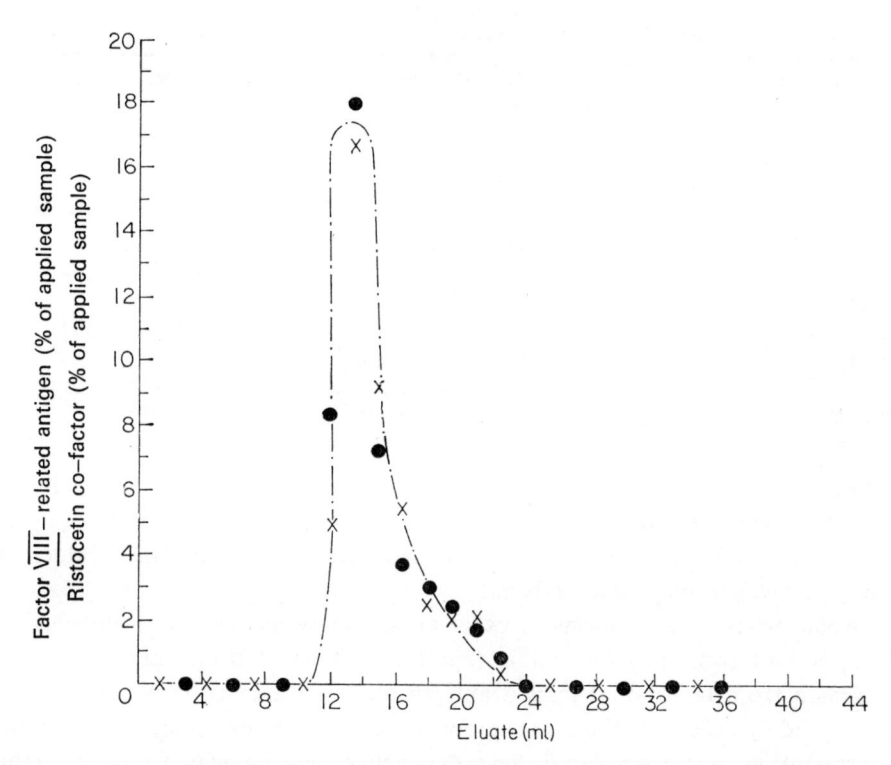

Figure 2.3. Factor-VIII-related antigen (●) and ristocetin co-factor (×) after gel filtration chromatography of normal factor VIII.

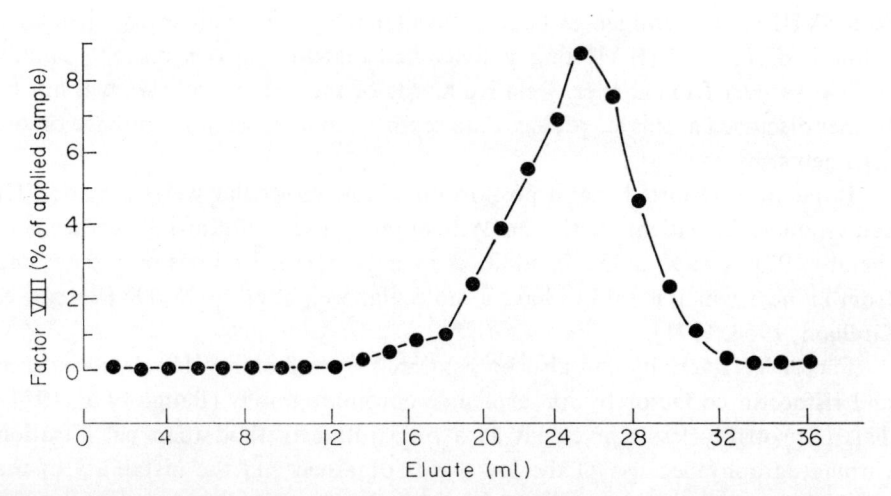

Figure 2.4. Factor VIII activity after reaction with 1·3 molar sodium chloride and followed by gel filtration chromatography.

Table 2.2. Sub-unit size of active factor VIII.

Sub-unit size	Reagent used	Reference
'Comparable to albumin'	0·4 to 1·65 M NaCl	Thelin & Wagner 1961
'Comparable to fibrinogen'	1·0 M NaCl	Weiss & Kochwa 1971
100,000 to 150,000	Succinic anydride/Mn^{++}/ thrombin	Barrow & Graham 1972
25,000 to 100,000	0·25 M CaCl$_2$	Owen & Wagner 1972
169,000 to 194,000	1·0 M NaCl	Weiss et al 1972
100,000	0·25 M CaCl$_2$	Griggs et al 1973
'Between fibrinogen and albumin'	1·0 M NaCl	Rick & Hoyer 1973
230,000	1·3 M NaCl or 1 to 3 × 10^{-4} M dithiothreitol	Austen 1974
690,000	Sodium periodate	Kaelin 1975

McKee (1976) has illustrated that caution is necessary. They show that the position at which factor VIII is eluted from a column can vary with the amount of protein applied and this could mean that some of the published values of molecular weight may need revision.

Apart from considerations of exact molecular weight, the vital conclusion from gel filtration experiments is that factor VIII clotting activity can be separated from factor-VIII-related antigen and ristocetin co-factor. Although this is widely accepted, there are important differences of opinion concerning interpretation. Some workers believe that active high molecular weight factor VIII is made up of several low molecular weight sub-units which are disaggregated by the various reagents discussed, leaving factor-VIII-related antigen and ristocetin co-factor circulating separately and unchanged. Others believe that factor-VIII-related antigen of large molecular weight is a carrier for the active sub-unit of factor VIII clotting activity and that the various reagents simply sever passenger from carrier. Relative merits of the two hypotheses will not be further discussed at this stage since data reported in later sections impinge on the arguments.

It has been reported that a proportion of low molecular weight factor VIII can circulate in patients with von Willebrand's disease following replacement therapy (Bloom et al, 1973). In addition an active factor VIII has been separated from kidneys which is said to have a molecular weight of 25–28,000 (Barrow & Graham, 1968, 1971).

Factor VIII activity can also be separated from factor-VIII-related antigen and ristocetin co-factor by ion exchange chromatography (Baugh et al, 1974). This is probably less convenient as a preparative method than gel filtration chromatography because of the low yields obtained and the instability of the product, so often associated with ion exchange chromatography of factor VIII. It is interesting because it raises the possibility of separating factor VIII activity

Factor VIII

without disaggregation, but since elution in these experiments was by saline gradient it cannot be assumed that no disaggregation took place.

Sub-units of factor-VIII-related antigen and ristocetin co-factor

As reported above, factor-VIII-related antigen and ristocetin co-factor remain as large molecules when active factor VIII is separated into its sub-units by changes in ionic strength or by mild reducing conditions. Increase in ionic strength will not reduce the molecular size associated with the other two functions although such experiments are complicated by protein precipitation at high solute levels. Increasing the severity of reduction conditions does, however, have a profound effect and factor-VIII-related antigen and ristocetin co-factor now split into sub-units which appear to be the same size as the active factor VIII sub-units (Austen

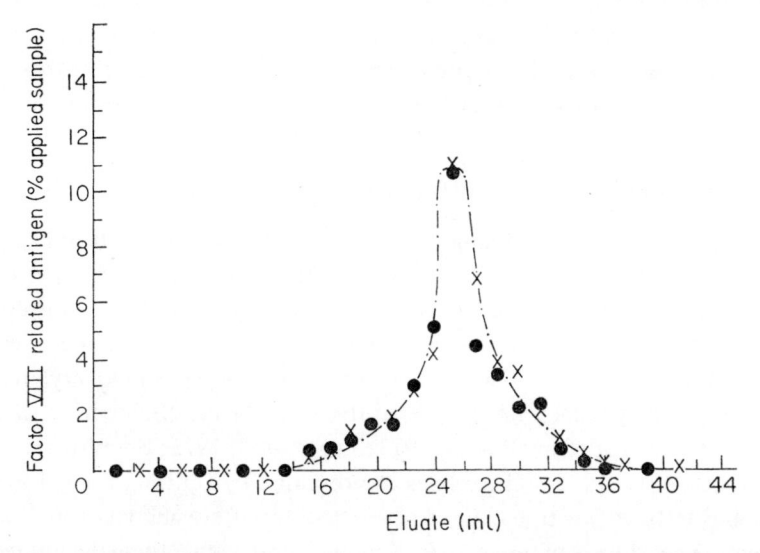

Figure 2.5. Factor-VIII-related antigen (●) and ristocetin co-factor (×) after reaction with 10^{-3} molar dithrothreitol and followed by gel filtration chromatography.

et al, 1975). This is illustrated in Figure 2.5 and the change in molecular size can be seen by comparing this with Figure 2.3. The level of reducing agent employed in this work was 10^{-3} to 3×10^{-3} molar dithiothreitol although the purity of the factor VIII can affect the actual level of reducing agent which is needed. Other workers confirm this reductive cleavage of factor-VIII-related antigen into sub-units and they additionally found a change in electrophoretic mobility (Peeke & Bloom, 1976). A similar size of sub-unit is also recorded by polyacrylamide gel electrophoresis as shown in Table 2.3. Disaggregation into

Table 2.3. Sub-unit size of factor-VIII-related antigen or factor VIII with clotting activity destroyed

Sub-unit size	Reagent used	Reference
85,000	β-Mercaptoethanol-SDS	Schmer *et al* 1972
240,000	Dithioerythritol-SDS	Marchesi *et al* 1972
240,000	β-Mercaptoethanol-SDS	Legaz *et al* 1973
105,000	β-Mercaptoethanol	Legaz *et al* 1973
195,000	β-Mercaptoethanol-SDS	Shapiro *et al* 1973
202,000	β-Mercaptoethanol	Shapiro *et al* 1973
200,000	β-Mercaptoethanol	Bennett *et al* 1973
230,000	Dithiothreitol	Austen *et al* 1975
235,000	α-Chymotrypsin	Gralnick *et al* 1975

sub-units demonstrates such a marked similarity between factor-VIII-related antigen and ristocetin co-factor that one suspects they may represent two functions of the same molecule. Active factor VIII also seems to have the same sub-unit size as these two and although there is considerable error in this type of measurement it suggests a similar identity.

The molecular weight of factor VIII in polyacrylamide gels

Several reports are now available showing that factor VIII will not enter the normal gels used for polyacrylamide gel electrophoresis (3 to 5% gel concentration) confirming that the factor is of high molecular weight. If, however, the factor is first reduced with β-mercaptoethanol or dithiothreitol it does then enter and it appears as a single line on polyacrylamide or SDS/polyacrylamide gel providing highly purified factor preparations are used (Schmer *et al*, 1972; Marchesi *et al*, 1972; Bennett *et al*, 1973; Legaz *et al*, 1973; Shapiro *et al*, 1973: Gralnick & Coller, 1975). These lines are revealed by staining the gel to detect protein and tests of function cannot be carried out after such vigorous chemical treatment. The values of molecular weight found using these techniques are included in Table 2.3; they mostly fall in the range of 200,000 to 250,000.

Similar results are obtained by isoelectric focusing which again uses polyacrylamide gel but now detects minute differences in isoelectric point and usually reveals small differences in molecular structure. Again a single line is obtained by protein staining, providing the highest purity preparations of factor VIII are used. This might suggest that the sub-units of factor VIII, factor-VIII-related antigen and ristocetin co-factor are intimately similar or even identical, at least after vigorous reduction. Alternatively it could be that one (or more) of these substances and in particular the active factor VIII, is not being detected at all because it is present in a concentration far below that of the others. Such an alternative should not be ruled out at this stage because some workers have reported difficulties in staining the protein associated with factor VIII activity (Veder, 1966; Baugh et al, 1974). In addition it has been shown that concentrates of factor-VIII-related antigen and ristocetin co-factor, which are prepared from haemophilic plasma and so contain no factor VIII activity, give identical results to those which do contain factor VIII activity, when examined by SDS gel chromatography or by isoelectric focusing (Shapiro et al, 1973). Thus whatever entity is needed to produce factor VIII clotting activity, be it the introduction of a specific grouping or a separate molecule, these methods of analysis do not register the presence of that entity.

The reaggregation of factor VIII

Experiments have been reported on the reaggregation of factor VIII sub-units and results vary. Some workers have claimed that reaggregation of active factor VIII can be achieved only in the presence of factor-VIII-related antigen (Cooper et al, 1973) and, of course, this has implications for those who believe the antigen to be a carrier of factor VIII activity. Reversal of any sort has only been achieved where the original disaggregation was caused by an ionic strength effect. No effects of chemical reduction have been reversed.

One paper claims the reaggregation of active factor VIII in the absence of factor-VIII-related antigen (Austen, 1974) and here the agent which facilitated reaggregation was ε-aminocaproic acid, although no specificity was claimed for that material. Here the reversal was observed when no antigen was measurable but this lacks meaning until the amounts of factor VIII and antigen in plasma are known in absolute terms. Relative methods by which the two are measured need not have the same sensitivity, and when antigen is measured as zero, the amount which is still present may be quite large when compared to normal levels of active factor VIII.

Antibodies to factor VIII

In haemophiliacs, antibodies to factor VIII activity can arise in response to therapeutic treatment with the factor. Approximately 6% of haemophilic patients are affected in this way. Similar antibodies can occur, although rarely, in people who are not haemophiliacs but are suffering from such diseases as rheumatoid arthritis, penicillin allergy or certain collagen disorders. Occasionally they develop immediately after childbirth. All of these antibodies, both haemophilic and non-haemophilic, are of a non-precipitating variety and appear to be entirely specific for factor VIII activity. They have no demonstrable action upon factor-VIII-related antigen or ristocetin co-factor. Another somewhat unusual feature is that their reaction with factor VIII activity can easily be followed with time, providing the antibody is not excessively concentrated. Antibodies are more usually instantaneous in their action. When the courses of reaction of these factor-VIII antibodies are investigated they are seen not to be identical in their kinetics. At one extreme, reactions follow a simple second order equation which, when studied in antibody excess, resolves into a pseudo-first order equation and a useful assay can be evolved based on such an equation (Biggs & Bidwell, 1959; Biggs *et al*, 1972a). However, at the other extreme reactions are far more complex in that they exhibit an extremely fast first stage followed by a much slower second stage. This can be for the most part explained by the hypothesis that antibody–antigen complexes resulting from the reaction retain some measure of clotting activity (Biggs *et al*, 1972b). Basic equations can be evolved and a suitable assay devised (Rizza & Biggs, 1973) but complete kinetics can, of course, never be worked out until the reactant concentrations are known in terms of molarity. Information like this is not yet available.

Across the haemophiliac population, antibodies which develop can vary between the extremes mentioned but there is a marked tendency for each patient to produce a consistent variety of antibody and not to alternate from one type to another. An antibody developed to human factor VIII may or may not cross react with factor VIII from animal sources and again there is a tendency for a given patient to consistently produce antibodies broadly of the same degree of cross reaction.

Patients with severe von Willebrand's disease have been reported to produce antibodies (Stratton *et al*, 1975; Manucci *et al*, 1976) and these are of the precipitating variety directed against factor-VIII-related antigen with only a low level of reaction towards factor VIII activity.

Antibodies to factor VIII preparations can be raised in experimental animals and those in rabbits have been the subject of many papers. They can vary in quality and quantity depending on the individual animal, and can be produced against factor VIII activity, factor-VIII-related antigen and ristocetin co-factor. They do not normally cross react with the substances from another animal species. In rabbits, the antibody directed against factor-VIII-related antigen develops independently of the antibody directed against factor VIII activity (Kernoff & Rizza, 1973). That directed against clotting activity does not precipitate the antigen in immunoelectrophoresis nor affect ristocetin aggregation. Moreover factor-VIII-related antigen does not normally block the action of an antibody to factor VIII activity. Thus the site of activity in factor VIII must be discretely separate from those of the other two functions.

There is less agreement about the extent to which antibodies to factor-VIII-related antigen will cross react with factor VIII activity. Some workers report evidence of cross reaction while others have prepared antibodies which do not cross react (Gralnick et al, 1973; Sonia et al, 1974) and in one paper (Ratnoff et al, 1976) there is evidence presented of cross reaction with the large molecular weight factor VIII but not with the smaller sub-unit.

A particular complication of precipitating antibodies is illustrated in a paper by Kernoff (1973) which shows that the precipitate made by factor-VIII-related antigen and its antibody incorporate active factor VIII and the precipitated complex retains factor VIII activity. As a result, apparent inactivation was obtained if the supernatant liquid was assayed after centrifugation, but no inactivation was recorded if the precipitate was re-suspended prior to assay. An analogous result was seen in immunoelectrophoresis experiments (Bird & Rizza, 1975) in which the actual precipitin lines (Laurell 'rockets') formed by factor-VIII-related antigen and its antibody were shown to possess factor VIII activity (the sample being tested contained both antigen and activity). These two sets of experiments demonstrate that factor-VIII-related antigen and active factor VIII have antigenic determinants in common or alternatively the two are in some way combined together.

Hougie et al (1974) used antibodies to illustrate separate identity of factor VIII activity and antigen. Their experiments indicate that the complex made by inactivating factor VIII with haemophilic antibody (non-precipitating, specific for activity) could be precipitated by an antibody to human γ globulins leaving antigen and ristocetin co-factor in the supernatant liquid (without clotting activity). By making the antibody radio-active they showed that the precipitation had in fact been virtually complete.

Chemical conclusions about factor VIII

In conclusion, the data reported under different headings will be selected to build up a chemical picture of factor VIII. In previous sections an attempt has been made to report several points of view although, in the light of so much conflicting data, total impartiality has not been entirely possible. Now the strain of impartiality will be abandoned in favour of the luxury of personal bias.

The first point which needs to be considered is the triple identity of factor VIII. Three functions of the factor are described: factor VIII clotting activity, factor-VIII-related antigen and ristocetin co-factor. Out of all of the information presented, there is little to suggest that the last two, antigen and ristocetin co-factor, are separate molecules. Ristocetin co-factor may have limited stability so that a molecule could be devoid of this activity and yet still register as an antigen. However, this apart, the two may be considered identical at this stage in our knowledge, and no distinction will be made between them in the remainder of this section.

On the other hand, factor VIII activity does have a claim to separate identity. It can be separated from the antigen by gel filtration or by ion exchange chromatography. Antibodies raised in rabbits can be directed against clotting activity or factor-VIII-related antigen or against both indicating that these two have some antigenic sites which are in common and that, in addition, each has individual antigenic sites which are peculiar to themselves.

Thus there does seem to be considerable evidence against factor-VIII-related antigen and active factor VIII being two functions of the same identical molecule. This being so, it becomes important to know how different they are and whether they could be bonded as a molecular complex. They are exceedingly difficult to separate and so they must either be similar in molecular structure or be joined together. Certainly the theory of attachment, in which active factor VIII is carried by factor-VIII-related antigen has a wide measure of support. However, based on that theory it seems a coincidence that active factor should be of similar size to an antigen sub-unit. Furthermore, it has been shown that antibody precipitation can separate clotting activity from factor-VIII-related antigen, which illustrates that any attachment could only be of a very low order, and separation of activity from antigen by ion exchange chromatography also suggests a similar conclusion.

If then active factor VIII is not bonded to factor-VIII-related antigen it must resemble it in basic chemical structure to account for the difficulties encountered in separation. Active factor VIII would then have some additional grouping which is responsible for clotting activity. Using this hypothesis, the main problem is to account for the fact that active factor VIII alone does not form a precipitate with its antibody in immunoelectrophoresis. It could be that it is present in too minute a quantity or that for some reason it is only univalent with respect to the particular antibody.

Active factor VIII of small molecular weight can be obtained by the action of various reagents and following the above hypothesis this means that active factor VIII of molecular weight greater than 1 million is split into sub-units of about 230,000 leaving factor-VIII-related antigen still circulating as a large molecule (the alternate theory requires the small active passenger to be split off from the large carrier antigen).

By chemical reduction factor-VIII-related antigen can also be split into subunits suggesting that disulphide bonds are involved in the structure. Such bonds could link the sub-units together and reduction would simply sever these bonds of attachment. However, an alternative possibility is that the disulphide bonds are intra-molecular, connecting different parts of the same sub-unit. Reduction would then alter the geometry of the sub-units possibly to a point where electrostatic forces could no longer hold the sub-units together. Either hypothesis could apply to the sub-units of active factor VIII or of factor-VIII-related antigen but with active factor VIII the dissociation can be effected by change in ionic strength alone (as well as by reduction) and this would favour the hypothesis involving intra-molecular bonds.

Thiol groups are present in active factor VIII close to, or associated with, the site of clotting activity. Quite possibly, other thiol groups are also present, not associated with any particular activity and the same would apply to factor-VIII-related antigen. Both molecules possess carbohydrate moieties and probably have little, if any, lipid structure.

In von Willebrand's disease, a quantitatively similar deficiency of both active factor and antigen is inherited but in haemophilia a deficiency of the active factor alone is inherited, this time by a completely different inheritance mechanism. It seems, therefore, that the routes by which active factor VIII and factor-VIII-related antigen are produced in the body must have some reaction steps which are in common. Again a similarity between the two substances is suggested.

Finally it has been demonstrated that infusion of haemophilic plasma into a patient with von Willebrand's disease produces factor VIII activity in that patient. The trigger must be contained in those substances which the two plasmas do not have in common and with present knowledge that is factor-VIII-related antigen (plus ristocetin co-factor and other associated activities). If it were not a trigger, it would have to be a precursor and that would be even more exciting since it would point to new treatment in haemophilia.

References

Austen D.E.G. (1970) Thiol groups in the blood clotting action of factor VIII. *British Journal of Haematology*, **19**, 477.

Austen D.E.G. & Bidwell E. (1972) Carbohydrate structure in factor VIII. *Thrombosis et Diathesis Haemorrhagica*, **28**, 464.

Austen D.E.G. (1974) Factor VIII of small molecular weight and its aggregation. *British Journal of Haematology*, **27**, 89.

Austen D.E.G., Carey M. & Howard M.A. (1975) Dissociation of factor VIII-related antigen into sub-units. *Nature (London)*, **253**, 55.

Austen D.E.G. & Rhymes I.L. (1975) *A Laboratory Manual of Blood Coagulation*, p. 53. Blackwell Scientific Publications, Oxford.

Anderson J.C. & McKee P.A. (1972) The effects of proteolytic enzymes on the coagulant properties and molecular structure of human factor VIII. *Circulation* (Suppl. 2), **46**, 52.

Barrow E.M. & Graham J.B. (1968) Kidney antihemophilic factor. Partial purification and some properties. *Biochemistry*, **7**, 3917.

Barrow E.M. & Graham J.B. (1971) Antihemophilic factor activity isolated from kidneys of normal and haemophilic dogs. *American Journal of Physiology*, **220**, 1020.

Barrow E.M. & Graham J.B. (1972) Factor VIII (AHF) activity of small size produced by succinylating plasma. *American Journal of Physiology*, **222**, 134.

Bartlett A., Dormandy K.M., Hawkey C.M., Stableforth P. & Voller A. (1976) Factor-VIII-related antigen: measurement by enzyme immunoassay. *British Medical Journal*, **1**, 994.

BAUGH R., BROWN J., SARGEANT R. & HOUGIE C. (1974) Separation of human factor VIII activity from the von Willebrand's antigen and ristocetin platelet aggregating activity. *Biochimica et Biophysica Acta*, 371, 360.

BENNETT B. & RATNOFF O. (1972) Studies on the response of patients with classic haemophilia to transfusions with concentrates of antihemophilic factor. *Journal of Clinical Investigation*, 51, 2593.

BENNETT B., RATNOFF O. & LEVIN J. (1972) Immunologic studies in von Willebrand's disease. *Journal of Clinical Investigation*, 51, 2597.

BENNETT B., FORMAN W.B. & RATNOFF O.D. (1973) Studies on the nature of antihemophilic factor (factor VIII). Further evidence relating the AHF-like antigens in normal and hemophilic plasma. *Journal of Clinical Investigation*, 52, 2191.

BIDWELL E. (1955a) The purification of bovine antihaemophilic globulin. *British Journal of Haematology*, 1, 35.

BIDWELL E. (1955b) The purification of antihaemophilic globulin from animal plasma. *British Journal of Haematology*, 1, 386.

BIDWELL E., DIKE G.W.R. & DENSON K.W.E. (1966) Experiments with factor VIII separated from fibrinogen by electrophoresis in free buffer film. *British Journal of Haematology*, 12, 583.

BIGGS R. & BIDWELL E. (1959) A method for the study of antihaemophilic globulin inhibitors with reference to six cases. *British Journal of Haematology*, 5, 379.

BIGGS R.P., EVELING J. & RICHARDS G. (1955) The assay of antihaemophilic globulin activity. *British Journal of Haematology*, 1, 20.

BIGGS R., AUSTEN D.E.G., DENSON K.W.E., RIZZA C.R. & BORRETT R. (1972a) The mode of action of antibodies which destroy factor VIII. 1. Antibodies which have second order concentration graphs. *British Journal of Haematology*, 23, 125.

BIGGS R., AUSTEN D.E.G., DENSON K.W.E., BORRETT R. & RIZZA C.R. (1972b) The mode of action of antibodies which destroy factor VIII. 2. Antibodies which give complex concentration graphs. *British Journal of Haematology*, 23, 137.

BIRD P. & RIZZA C.R. (1975) A method for detecting factor-VIII clotting activity associated with factor-VIII-related antigen in agarose gels. *British Journal of Haematology*, 31, 5.

BLOMBÄCK M. (1958) Purification of antihemophilic globulin. *Arkiv für Kemi*, 12, 387.

BLOMBÄCK B., BLOMBÄCK M. & STRUWE I. (1962) Studies on factor VIII. *Thrombosis et Diathesis Haemorrhagica*, 7 (Suppl. 1), 172.

BLOOM A.L., PEAKE I.R. & GIDDINGS J.C. (1973) The presence and reaction of high and lower molecular weight procoagulant factor VIII in the plasma of patients with von Willebrand's disease after treatment: significance for a structural hypothesis for factor VIII. *Thrombosis Research*, 3, 389.

BOUMA B.N., WIEGERINCK Y., SIXMA J.J., VAN MOURIK J.A. & MOCHTAR I.A. (1972) Immunological characterisation of purified anti-haemophilic factor (factor VIII) which corrects abnormal platelet retention in von Willebrand's disease. *Nature New Biology*, 236, 104.

BRINKHOUS K.M., SHANBROM E., ROBERTS H.R., WEBSTER W.P., FEKETE L. & WAGNER R.H. (1968) A new high-potency glycine-precipitated antihemophilic factor (AHF) concentrate. *Journal of the American Association*, 205, 613.

BROWN J.E., BAUGH R.F., SARGEANT R.B. & HOUGIE C. (1974) Separation of bovine factor-VIII-related antigen (platelet aggregating factor) from bovine antihaemophilic factor. *Proceedings of the Society for Experimental Biology and Medicine*, 147, 608.

CASILLAS G., SIMONETTI C. & PAVLOVSKY A. (1969) Chromatographic behaviour of clotting factors. *British Journal of Haematology*, 16, 363.

CASILLAS G., SIMONETTI C. & PAVLOVSKY A. (1970) Molecular sieving experiments on human factor VIII. *Coagulation*, 3, 123.

COHN E.J., STRONG L.E., HUGHES W.L., MULFORD D.J., ASHWORTH J.N., MELIN M. & TAYLOR H.L. (1946) A system for the separation into fractions of the protein and

lipoprotein components of biological tissue and fluids. *Journal I the American Chemical Society,* **68,** 459.
COOPER H.A., GRIGGS T.R. & WAGNER R.H. (1973) Factor VIII recombination after dissociation by CaCl$_2$. *Proceedings of the National Academy of Sciences, U.S.A.,* **70,** 2326.
DENSON K.W.E. (1970) *Standardisation of methods for the determination of antihaemophilic factors.* Abstracts of the VIth Congress of the World Federation of Haemophilia, Baden, 25th July, 1970, p. 82.
DEGAETANO G., DONATI M.B. & VERMYLEN J. (1974) Evidence that human platelet-aggregating activity in porcine plasma is a property of von Willebrand factor. *Thrombosis et Diathesis Haemorrhagica,* **32,** 549.
EKERT H., HELLIGER H. & MUNTZ R.H. (1973) Detection of carriers of haemophilia. *Thrombosis et Diathesis Haemorrhagica,* **30,** 255.
EVANS R.J. & AUSTEN D.E.G. (1977) Assay and characterisation of the factor in porcine and bovine plasma which aggregates human platelets. *British Journal of Haematology,* **36,** 117.
FORBES C.D., BARR R.D., MCNICOL G.P. & DOUGLAS A.S. (1972) Aggregation of human platelets by commercial preparations of bovine and porcine antihaemophilic globulin. *Journal of Clinical Pathology,* **25,** 210.
FORBES C.D. & PRENTICE C.R.M. (1973) Aggregation of human platelets by purified porcine and bovine antihaemophilic factor. *Nature New Biology,* **241,** 149.
GODFREY R., RHYMES I. L., BIDWELL E. & BARROWCLIFFE T.W. (1975) The buffering of anticoagulant for blood collection. *Thrombosis et Diathesis Haemorrhagica,* **34,** 879.
GOOD N.E., WINGET G.D., WINTER W., CONNOLLY T.H., IZAWA S. & SINGH R.M.M. (1966) Hydrogen ion buffers for biological research. *Biochemistry,* **5,** 467.
GRALNICK H.R., COLLER B.S. & MARCHESI S.L. (1973) Immunological studies of factor VIII in hemophilia and von Willebrand's disease. *Nature New Biology,* **244,** 281.
GRALNICK H.R., COLLER B.S. & MARCHESI S.L. (1975) Studies of the human factor VIII/von Willebrand's factor protein. I. Comparison of the protein found in normal, von Willebrand's disease and haemophilia A. *Thrombosis Research,* **6,** 93.
GRALNICK H.R. & COLLER B.S. (1975) Studies of the human factor VIII/von Willebrand's factor protein. II. Identification and characterisation of the von Willebrand protein. *Blood,* **46,** 417.
GREEN D. (1971) A simple method for the purification of factor VIII (antihemophilic factor) employing snake venom. *Journal of Laboratory and Clinical Medicine,* **77,** 153.
GRIGGS T.R., COOPER H.A., WEBSTER W.P., WAGNER R.H. & BRINKHOUS K.M. (1973) Plasma aggregating factor (bovine) for human platelets: a marker study of antihaemophilic and von Willebrand factors. *Proceedings of the National Academy of Sciences, U.S.A.* **70,** 2814.
GRIGGS T.R., WEBSTER W.P., COOPER H.A., WAGNER R.H. & BRINKHOUS K.M. (1974) Von Willebrand factor: gene dosage relationship and transfusion response in bleeder swine: a new bioassay. *Proceedings of the National Academy of Sciences, U.S.A.,* **71,** 2087.
HERSHGOLD E.J. & SPRAWLS S. (1966) Molecular properties of purified human, bovine and porcine antihemophilic globulin (AHG). *Federation Proceedings,* **25,** 317.
HERSHGOLD E.J., POOL J.G. & PAPPENHAGEN A.R. (1966) The potent antihemophilic globulin concentrate derived from a cold insoluble fraction of human plasma. *Journal of Laboratory and Clinical Medicine,* **67,** 23.
HERSHGOLD E.J., SILVERMAN K., DAVISON A. & JANSZEN M. (1967) Native and purified factor VIII. Molecular and electron microscopical properties and a comparison with hemophilic plasma. *Federation Proceedings,* **26,** 488.
HERSHGOLD E.J., DAVISON A.M. & JANSZEN M.E. (1971) Isolationand some chemical properties of factor VIII (anti-hemophilic factor). *Journal of Laboratory and Clinical Medicine,* **77,** 185.
HOLMBERG L., MANUCCI P.M., TURESSON I., REIGGERI Z.M. & NILSSON I.M. (1974) Factor VIII antigen in the vessel walls in von Willebrand's disease and Haemophilia A. *Scandinavian Journal of Haematology,* **13,** 33.

HOUGIE C., SARGEANT R.B., BROWN J.E. & BAUGH R.F. (1974) Evidence that factor VIII and the ristocetin aggregating factor (VIII rist) are separate molecular entities. *Proceedings of the Society for Experimental Biology and Medicine*, **147**, 58.

HOWARD M.A. & FIRKIN B.G. (1971) Ristocetin—a new tool in the investigation of platelet aggregation. *Thrombosis et Diathesis Haemorrhagica*, **26**, 362.

HOWARD M.A., MONTGOMERY D.C. & HARDISTY R.M. (1974) Factor VIII related antigen in platelets. *Thrombosis Research*, **4**, 617.

HOYER L.W. (1972) Immunologic studies of antihemophilic factor (AHF, factor VIII) III. Comparative binding properties of human and rabbit anti-AHF. *Blood*, **39**, 481.

HYNES H.E., OWEN C.A., BOWIE E.J.W. & THOMPSON J.H. (1969) Citrate stabilisation of chromatographically purified factor VIII. *Blood*, **34**, 601.

JAFFE E.A., HOYER L.W. & NACHMAN R.L. (1973) Synthesis of antihemophilic factor antigen by cultured human endothelial cells. *Journal of Clinical Investigations*, **52**, 2757.

JAFFE E.A. & NACHMAN R.L. (1975) Sub-unit structure of factor VIII antigen synthesised by cultured endothelial cells. *Journal of Clinical Investigation*, **56**, 698.

JOHNSON A.J., NEWMAN J., HOWELL M.B. & PUSZKIN S. (1966) *The preparation and some properties of a clinically useful high purity antihemophilic factor (AHF)*. XIth Congress of the International Society of Blood Transfusion. Abstracts of papers, Sydney, Australia, p. 1109.

KAELIN A.C. (1975) Sodium periodate modification of factor VIII procoagulant activity. *British Journal of Haematology*, **31**, 349.

KASS L., RATNOFF O.D. & LEON M.A. (1969) Studies on the purification of antihemophilic factor (factor VIII). I. Precipitation of antihemophilic factor by concanavalin A. *Journal of Clinical Investigation*, **48**, 351.

KEKWICK R.A. & MACKAY M.E. (1954) *The separation of protein fractions from human plasma with ether*. Special Report Series Medical Research Council, London, p. 286.

KERNOFF P.B.A. (1973) Affinity of factor VIII clotting activity for antigen detectable immunologically. *Nature New Biology*, **244**, 148.

KERNOFF P.B.A. & RIZZA C.R. (1973) The specificity of antibodies to factor VIII produced in the rabbit after immunisation with human cryoprecipitate. *Thrombosis et Diathesis Haemorrhagica*, **29**, 652.

KERNOFF P.B.A., RIZZA C.R. & KAELIN A.C. (1974) Transfusion and gel filtration in von Willebrand's disease. *British Journal of Haematology*, **28**, 357.

LAURELL C.-B. (1972) Electroimmunoassay. *Scandinavian Journal of Clinical and Laboratory Investigation*, **29** (Suppl. 124), 21.

LEGAZ M.E., SCHMER G., COURTS R.B. & DAVIE E.W. (1973) Isolation and characterisation of human factor VIII (antihemophilic factor). *Journal of Biological Chemistry*, **248**, 3946.

MACFARLANE R.G., BIGGS R.P. & BIDWELL E. (1954) Bovine antihaemophilic globulin in the treatment of haemophilia. *Lancet*, **i**, 1316.

MANUCCI P.M., MEYER D., RUGGERI Z.M., KOUTTS J., CIAVARELLA N. & LAVERGNE J.-M. (1976) Precipitating antibodies in von Willebrand's disease. *Nature*, **262**, 141.

MARCHESI S.L., SHULMAN N.R. & GRALNICK H.R. (1972) Studies on the purification and characterisation of human factor VIII. *The Journal of Clinical Investigation*, **51**, 2151.

MAYCOCK W.d'A., EVANS S., VALLET L., COMBRIDGE B., WOLF P., MACGIBBON B., FRENCH E.E., WALLETT L.H., DACIE J.V., BIGGS R., HANDLEY D. & MACFARLANE R.G. (1963) Further experience with a concentrate containing human antihaemophilic factor. *British Journal of Haematology*, **9**, 215.

MCKEE P.A., ANDERSEN J.C. & SWITZER M.E. (1975) Molecular structural studies of human factor VIII. *Annals of the New York Academy of Sciences*, **240**, 8.

MEYER D., JENKINS C.S.P., DREYFUS M.D., FRESSINAND E. & LARRIEU M.J. (1974) Willebrand factor and ristocetin II. Relationship between Willebrand factor, Willebrand antigen and factor VIII activity. *British Journal of Haematology*, **28**, 579.

MICHAEL S.E. & TUNNAH G.W. (1966) The purification of factor VIII (anti-haemophilic globulin) II. Further purification and some properties of factor VIII. *British Journal of Haematology*, **12**, 115.

MUSTARD J.F. (1958) Some *in vitro* effects of various concentrations of disodium ethylenediamine tetra acetate, potassium oxalate and sodium citrate in coagulation of blood, *American Journal of Clinical Pathology*, **30**, 498.

NACHMAN R.L. & JAFFE E.A. (1975) Subcellular platelet factor VIII antigen and von Willebrand factor. *Journal of Experimental Medicine*, **141**, 1101.

NACHMAN R.L. & JAFFE E.A. (1976) The platelet-endothelial cell-VIII axis. *Thrombosis and Haemostasis*, **35**, 120.

NEWMAN J., JOHNSON A.J., KARPATKIN M.H. & PUSZKIN S. (1971) Methods for the production of clinically effective intermediate and high purity factor VIII concentrates. *British Journal of Haematology*, **21**, 1.

NIEMITZ J., WEILLAND C. & SOULIER J.P. (1961) Preparation of a human plasma factor rich in factor VIII. *Nouvelle Revue Française d'hématologie*, **1**, 880.

OSTERUD B., RAPAPORT S.I., SCHIFFMAN S. & CHONG M.M.Y. (1971) Formation of intrinsic factor-x-activator activity, with special reference to the role of thrombin. *British Journal of Haematology*, **21**, 643.

OZGE-ANWAR A.H., CONNELL G.E. & MUSTARD J.F. (1965) The activation of factor VIII by thrombin. *Blood*, **26**, 500.

OZGE-ANWAR A.H. (1970) Slow activation of factor VIII by thrombin and other enzymes at low temperature. *Scandinavian Journal of Haematology*, **7**, 5.

OWEN W.G. & WAGNER R.H. (1972) Antihemophilic factor: separation of inactive fragments following dissociation by salts or detergents. *Thrombosis et Diathesis Haemmorrhagica*, **27**, 502.

PAULLSEN M.M.P., VAN DE GRAAF-WILDSCHUT M., KOLHORN A. & PLANJE M.C. (1975) Radioimmunoassay of antihaemophilic factor (factor VIII) antigen. *Clinica Chimica Acta*, **63**, 349.

PEAKE I.R. & BLOOM A.L. (1976) The dissociation of factor VIII by reducing agents, high salt concentration and affinity chromatography. *Thrombosis and Haemostasis*, **35**, 191.

PENNELL B., MELIN M., ROTHSTEIN F. & SARAVIO C.A. (1962) *The influence of low levels of ascorbic acid on the isolation of biologically active plasma proteins by precipitation techniques*. Proceedings of the 8th Congress of the International Society of Blood Transfusion, Tokyo, 1960, p. 140.

POOL J.G. & ROBINSON J. (1959) Observations on plasma banking and transfusion procedures for haemophilic patients using a quantitative assay for anti-haemophilic globulin (AHG). *British Journal of Haematology*, **5**, 24.

POOL J.G., HERSHGOLD E.J. & PAPPENHAGEN A.R. (1964) High potency antihaemophilic factor concentrate prepared from cryoglobulin precipitate. *Nature*, **203**, 312.

POOL J.G. & SHANNON A.E. (1965) Production of high-potency concentrates of anti-hemophilic globulin in a closed-bag system. *New England Journal of Medicine*, **273**, 1443.

PRENTICE C.R.M., FORBES C.D. & SMITH S.M. (1972) Rise in factor VIII after exercise and adrenaline infusion measured by immunological and biological techniques. *Thrombosis Research*, **1**, 493.

RATNOFF O.D., KASS L. & LANG P.D. (1969) Studies on the purification of antihemophilic factor (factor VIII) II. Separation of partially purified antihemophilic factor by gel filtration of plasma. *Journal of Clinical Investigation*, **48**, 957.

RATNOFF O.D., SLOVER C.C. & POON M.-C. (1976) Immunologic evidence that the properties of human antihemophilic factor (factor VIII) are attributes of a single molecular species. *Blood*, **47**, 657.

RICK M.E. & HOYER L.W. (1973) Immunologic studies of antihemophilic factor (AHF, factor VIII) V. Immunologic properties of AHF sub-units produced by salt dissociation. *Blood*, **42**, 737.

RIZZA C.R. (1961) Effect of exercise on the level of anti-haemophilic globulin in human blood. *Journal of Physiology*, **156**, 128.

RIZZA C.R. & BIGGS R. (1973) The treatment of patients who have factor-VIII antibodies. *British Journal of Haematology*, **24**, 65.

RIZZA C.R. & EIPE J. (1971) Exercise, factor VIII and the spleen. *British Journal of Haematology*, **20**, 629.

RIZZA C.R., RHYMES I.L., AUSTEN D.E.G., KERNOFF P.B.A. & ARONI S.A. (1975) Detection of carriers of haemophilia: a blind study. *British Journal of Haematology*, **30**, 447.

ROBERTS H.R., GRAHAM J.B., WEBSTER W.P. & PENICK G.D. (1964) In: *The Hemophilias* (Ed. Brinkhous, K.M.), p. 323. University of North Carolina Press, Chapel Hill.

ROBERTS P.S., HUGHES H.N. & FLEMING P.B. (1976) The effect of hepes buffer on clotting tests, assay of factor V and VIII and on the hydrolysis of esters by thrombin and thrombokinase. *Thrombosis and Haemostasis*, **35**, 202.

RUGGERI Z.M., MANNUCCI P.M., JEFFCOATE S.L. & INGRAM G.I.C. (1976) Immunoradiometric assay of factor-VIII-related antigen with observations in 32 patients with von Willebrand's disease. *British Journal of Haematology*, **33**, 221.

SCHMER G., KIRBY E.P., TELLER D.C. & DAVIE E.W. (1972) The isolation and characterisation of bovine factor VIII (antihemophilic factor). *Journal of Biological Chemistry*, **247**, 2512.

SHANBROM E. (1970) Rapid correction of AHF deficiency by antihemophilic factor—method four with special reference to inhibitors. In: *The hemophiliac and his world.* Proceedings of the 5th Congress of the World Federation of Hemophilia, Montreal, p. 52.

SHAPIRO G.A., ANDERSEN J.C., PIZZO S.V. & MCKEE P.A. (1973) The sub-unit structure of normal and hemophilic factor VIII. *Journal of Clinical Investigation*, **52**, 2198.

SHEARN S.A.M., GIDDINGS J.C., PEAKE I.R. & BLOOM A.L. (1974) A comparison of five different rabbit antisera to factor VIII and the demonstration of factor-VIII-related antigen in normal and von Willebrand disease platelets. *Thrombosis Research*, **5**, 585.

SIMONETTI C., CASILLAS G. & PAVLOVSKY A. (1961) Purification du factor VIII anti-hémophilique (AHF). *Hémostase*, **1**, 57.

SIMONETTI C., CASILLAS G. & PAVLOVSKY A. (1972) Studies on the adsorption of factor VIII: application to the purification of bovine factor VIII. *British Journal of Haematology*, **23**, 29.

STIBBE J., HEMKER H.C. & v. CREVELD S. (1972) The inactivation of factor VIII *in vitro*. *Thrombosis et Diathesis Haemorrhagica*, **27**, 43.

STITES D.P., HERSHGOLD J.D., PERLMAN J.D. & FUNDENBERG H.H. (1971) Factor VIII detection by hemagglutination inhibition: hemophilia A and von Willebrand's disease. *Science*, **171**, 196.

STRATTON R.D., WAGNER R.H., WEBSTER W.P. & BRINKHOUS K.M. (1975) Antibody nature of circulating inhibitor of plasma von Willebrand factor. *Proceedings of the National Academy of Sciences, U.S.A.*, **72**, 4167.

SULTAN Y., SIMEON J., MAISONNEUVE P. & CAEN J.P. (1976) Immunologic studies in von Willebrand's disease. *Thrombosis and Haemostasis*, **35**, 110.

SWITZER M.E. & MCKEE P.A. (1976) Studies on human anti-hemophilic factor. Evidence for a covalently linked subunit structure. *The Journal of Clinical Investigation*, **57**, 925.

THELIN G.M. & WAGNER R.H. (1961) Sedimentation of plasma antihemophilic factor. *Archives of Biochemistry and Biophysics*, **95**, 70.

VAN MOURIK J.A., BOUMA B.N., LABRUYÈRE W.T., DE GRAFF S. & MOCHTAR I.A. (1974) Factor VIII. A series of homologous oligomers and a complex of two proteins. *Thrombosis Research*, **4**, 155.

VEDER H.A. (1966) Further purification of the antihemophilic factor (AHF). *Thrombosis et Diathesis Haemorrhagica*, **16**, 738.

WAGNER R.H., RICHARDSON B.A. & BRINKHOUS K.M. (1957) A study of the separation of fibrinogen and anti-hemophilic factor (AHF) in canine, porcine and human plasmas. *Thrombosis et Diathesis Haemorrhagica*, **1**, 1.

WAGNER R.H., MCLESTER W.D., SMITH M. & BRINKHOUS K.M. (1964) Purification of antihemophilic factor (factor VIII) by amino acid precipitation. *Thrombosis et Diathesis Haemorrhagica*, **11**, 64.
WEISS H.J. & KOCHWA S. (1970) Molecular forms of anti-hemophilic globulin in plasma, cryoprecipitate and after thrombin activation. *British Journal of Haematology*, **18**, 89.
WEISS H.J., PHILLIPS L.L. & ROSNER W. (1972) Separation of sub-units of antihemophilic factor (AHF) by agarose gel chromatography. *Thrombosis et Diathesis Haemorrhagica*, **27**, 212.
WEISS H.J. & HOYER L.W. (1973) Von Willebrand factor: dissociation from antihemophilic factor procoagulant activity. *Science*, **182**, 1149.
WEISS H.J., ROGERS J. & BRAND H. (1973a) Defective ristocetin-induced platelet aggregation in von Willebrands disease and its correction by factor VIII. *Journal of Clinical Investigation*, **52**, 2697.
WEISS H.J., HOYER L.W., RICKLES F.R., VARMA A. & ROGERS J. (1973b) Quantitative assay of a plasma factor deficient in von Willebrands disease that is necessary for platelet aggregation. *Journal of Clinical Investigation*. **52**, 2708.
WEISS H.J., ROGERS J. & BRAND H. (1973c) Properties of the platelet retention (von Willebrand) factor and its similarity to antihemophilic factor (AHF). *Blood*, **41**, 809.
WEISS H.J. (1975) Abnormalities of factor VIII and platelet aggregation—use of ristocetin in diagnosing the von Willebrand syndrome. *Blood*, **45**, 403.
ZIMMERMAN T.S., RATNOFF O.D. & LITTELL A.S. (1971) Detection of carriers of classical haemophilia using an immunologic assay for antihaemophilic factor (factor VIII). *Journal of Clinical Investigation*, **50**, 255.
ZUCKER S., CATHEY M.H. & WEST B. (1970) Preparation of quality control specimens for coagulation. *American Journal of Clinical Pathology*, **53**, 924.

Chapter 3. The Laboratory and Clinical Diagnosis of Patients with Coagulation Defects

ROSEMARY BIGGS

The diagnosis of coagulation defects involves a general clinical and laboratory assessment of each individual patient. Exact diagnosis has become important since the use of concentrated materials for specific treatment became practicable. For satisfactory management it is necessary to know as exactly as possible the nature of the defect and the extent of the deficiency. The main conditions considered in this book are haemophilia A and von Willebrand's disease (factor VIII deficiency) and Christmas disease (factor IX deficiency). Of over 1,000 patients having coagulation defects known at the Oxford Haemophilia Centre 96% have abnormality of factors VIII or IX. In practice the accurate measurement of factors VIII or IX and the measurement of anti-factor VIII antibodies are by far the most important laboratory skills to acquire. These three measurements are thus considered in more detail than other laboratory test systems. In addition deficiencies of factors I, II, V, VII, X, XI, XII and XIII do occur. Patients may also have excess or deficiency of natural blood clotting inhibitors or may have abnormal inhibitory substances. Brief reference will be made to these less common coagulation defects.

The diagnosis of a severe hereditary haemorrhagic state in a patient means that the patient will be in need of specialised medical care for the rest of his or her life. In the United Kingdom such care is provided by special Centres, called Haemophilia Centres for the diagnosis and treatment of patients having haemorrhagic states. When the diagnosis has been made the patient should be registered at one of the centres and be given a special identification card for persons having serious haemostatic defects. The card states the exact diagnosis, the name and address of the Director of the centre to which the patient is attached, the blood group and other information which may be important for that particular patient. The patient should be instructed to carry the card at all times and to show it to medical and dental personnel whenever any question of illness, accident or treatment arises. The patient should also carry a pocket booklet about emergency treatment which is called 'Notes on the Care of Patients with Haemophilia & Christmas disease' and is issued by the Department of Health and Social Security. As more complete and up-to-date handbooks for patients become available the doctors should bring these books to the patient's notice.

Clinical history and diagnosis

Laboratory tests judged entirely by themselves may sometimes give misleading information about the nature and severity of a patient's haemostatic defect. Many laboratory tests give information which must be taken in context with the clinical history. Some techniques, particularly those which give general evidence of abnormality, must be considered in conjunction with the results of other more specific tests. For example a patient who has haemophilia and a prolonged whole blood clotting time is severely affected. On the other hand the long whole blood clotting time of Hageman (factor XII) deficiency presages no haemostatic abnormality. At the other extreme completely normal laboratory findings do not assure haemostatic normality. The patient may have an abnormality which cannot be detected by present test systems though this kind of patient is not often seen today if all of the known laboratory tests are carried out.

Since total reliance cannot be put on the results of laboratory tests it is particularly important to take a complete and careful clinical history. There are two main groups of symptoms which afflict patients having haemostatic efects. One group occurs typically in patients having coagulation defects and the other occurs in patients suffering from von Willebrand type of abnormality. The symptoms are listed separately in Table 3.1. This table is a good guide to the questions which should be asked when taking a clinical history.

Patients having von Willebrand's disease in its most severe form are quite easy to identify, they have dominant inheritance, a long bleeding time, failure of platelet adhesion to glass, failure of aggregation of platelets in the presence of ristocetin, absent factor-VIII-related antigen and a low plasma concentration of factor VIII activity (see also Chapter 8). But von Willebrand's disease as usually conceived contains a broad range of clinical entities many of which were classified by us in the past as 'capillary defects'. In the mildly affected patient in this general group only some of the laboratory tests give abnormal results. The milder forms of this syndrome, where factor VIII is normal in amount, have bleeding which is well controlled by pressure on the site of bleeding. These mildly affected patients are quite often seen.

The items noted in Table 3.1 are mostly self-explanatory but one or two notes about eliciting the clinical history may be helpful. These will follow the headings listed in Table 3.1.

Patients, particularly women and children, are often said to bruise easily and an answer of 'yes' to the question 'do you bruise easily?' has little significance. The questioner should make a specific enquiry as to the size of the largest

Table 3.1. The clinical assessment of patients having haemostatic defects.

Nature of enquiry	Coagulation defect	von Willebrand defect
Bruising	Large bruises occur	Small bruises common
Haemarthroses	Common in severely affected patients and often the main feature	Very uncommon
Epistaxis	Seldom a predominant symptom	Often a major source of bleeding
Gastrointestinal bleeding	Seldom a predominant symptom unless peptic ulceration is also present	Often a major source of bleeding
Haematuria	Common	Uncommon
Menorrhagia	Uncommon because most patients are males	Common
Dental extraction bleeding	Starts 1–4 hours post-operative; lasts 3–40 days and is not controlled by pressure	Starts immediately. Lasts 24–48 hours and is often controlled by pressure
Post-operative bleeding	Late bleeding with wound haematoma formation is characteristic	Bleeding mainly occurs at the time of operation and is less severe than in patients with coagulation defects
Onset of bleeding after trauma	Usually late (1–4 hours after the event)	Usually immediate
Symptoms of the mildly affected patient	Large haematomata following injury. Persistent and often dangerous bleeding after trauma	Epistaxis and menorrhagia
Inheritance	Most are sex-linked and recessive	Mainly dominant

recollected bruises. Bruises larger than 3 inches in diameter are uncommon in normal people and it is very unusual for a bruise in a normal person to cover a hard subcutaneous lump.

Haemarthroses and muscle haematomata leave no blue discoloration of the skin. Enquiry should be about painful swelling in joints and muscles and not about 'bleeding' into joints or muscles.

The blood lost in menorrhagia is not easily assessed and women often associate normality with what is usual to themselves. It may be helpful to ask if the patient has ever had to take iron pills or been treated for anaemia as a consequence of menorrhagia.

The extent of bleeding after dental extraction depends on the number and location of teeth removed. The removal of lower wisdom teeth usually causes more trauma than the removal of other teeth. The questions should ask exactly which teeth were removed and for how long the bleeding lasted and what measures were taken to stop it.

The patient should also be asked about tonsillectomy. If he or she has undergone this operation without undue bleeding then the patient was unlikely to have been suffering from a significant haemostatic defect at the time of the operation.

The nature of inheritance can only be determined by an exact record of all members of the family in the form of a family tree. It is not enough to ask 'does anyone else in your family bleed abnormally?'

A few examples of clinical histories are given below.

Case 181. At the age of 10 months the patient was brought to hospital with bruises on his legs and a stiff swollen elbow following a fall. He was, at the time of the visit, bleeding from eruption of teeth. No other members of the family were known to bleed abnormally. He is a haemophiliac with 0% of factor VIII.

Case 66. This 9-year-old boy was well until the age of 5, when 5 teeth were removed. He bled sufficiently to require hospital admission and remained in hospital for 10 days from which it can be deduced that local pressure on the sockets failed to control the bleeding. At another time 1 tooth was removed and the socket was plugged, two days later bleeding started despite the plug and he was again admitted to hospital, on this occasion for a week. Tonsillectomy was performed at the age of 8. He bled excessively and was kept in hospital for 5 days. Two days after discharge bleeding recurred and he was re-admitted and transfused with 2 pints of blood. There was no record of large bruises, epistaxis, haematuria or joint swellings. No other members of the family were known to bleed excessively.

This is the record of a mildly affected bleeder of the clotting defect variety. This patient has 15% of factor VIII.

Case 67. The patient, a man aged 41, was referred to us as a known case of haemophilia. His history revealed very numerous episodes of epistaxis as a child, frequently necessitating transfusion. There was also a 12-year-old history of severe and dangerous gastrointestinal bleeding. He had previously had an operation for the gastrointestinal bleeding, at which no lesion was found. The surgical wound burst and 2 transfusions were given. There was no history of massive bruising, joint swelling or haematuria. One brother was said to be affected similarly.

This history was very suggestive of a severe von Willebrand type abnormality. Investigation showed a grossly prolonged bleeding time and a plasma factor VIII concentration of less than 4%. He has von Willebrand's disease.

Case 68. This 10-year-old girl had a history of rather profuse bleeding for 5 hours following the extraction of 2 molar teeth. Her mother had a history of bleeding for 24 hours after dental extraction but the bleeding was well-controlled by plugging the tooth sockets. The mother also suffered from menorrhagia. The grandmother also bled after dental extraction but had an uneventful appendicectomy. Laboratory results showed a bleeding time of 5–8 minutes for the child. Her mother also had a bleeding time of 5–8 minutes and a weakly positive tourniquet test. In our laboratory most normal bleeding times are less than 5 minutes. Coagulation tests were normal. Tonsillectomy was performed on the child with special care about immediate haemostasis which involved packing the tonsillar fossae for 5 minutes at the end of the operation.

This case was probably one of mild von Willebrand's disease since the inheritance was likely to have been dominant and the bleeding time was slightly prolonged. On the other hand the symptoms were so mild that many might consider the family to be within normal limits from the haemostatic point of view. Tests such as those for factor-VIII-related antigen, ristocetin aggregation of platelets and adhesion of platelets to glass beads were not done. Even if these tests had shown abnormal results the assessment of the clinical symptoms would have been the same. In this sort of case operation is safe provided that immediate attention is paid to haemostasis. If immediate attention is not paid to haemostasis a proportion of patients will bleed. The majority of doubtful cases referred to the coagulation laboratory for an opinion about the danger of bleeding after operation are of this sort.

Case 135. A female patient aged 48. The patient had always bruised easily and in the last two years had had two very large bruises the size of which were quite disproportionate to the trauma. At the age of 20 excessive bleeding followed dental extraction and the extraction of 3 teeth was followed by such severe bleeding that 4 pints of blood were given, from which it can be concluded that simple pressure on the tooth sockets was ineffective. Laboratory tests of haemostatic function at the time were normal apart from a platelet count consistently higher than 600,000 mm^3.

This patient was seen by us many years ago now and at the time, the normality of laboratory tests blinded the physicians to the undoubted history of severe post traumatic bleeding. She was submitted to vaginal hysterectomy which was followed by severe and dangerous postoperative bleeding. Subsequent tests showed abnormal platelet function of the kind seen in thrombasthenia.

The next case had a rather complicated clinical story and the mother was sure that his troubles were all due to roughness and fighting.

Case 69. This 5-year-old Italian boy had a history of sub-arachnoid haemorrhage following a severe fall on the head at the age of 13 months. At 4 he was admitted to hospital with 14 days record of pyrexia and some pain over, but not involving the right shoulder. He also had a cystic swelling on the forehead. He was found to have an erythrocyte sedimentation rate of 65 mm/hour and a positive tuberculin test. The swelling on the head subsided gradually with some skin discoloration, suggesting that it had been a large bruise. Later he had a swollen knee joint, thought to have been caused playing football. His mother said that he was quite excessively rough, fighting on slight provocation and playing football most of the time and she did not think that he bruised excessively. No other members of the family were known to bleed excessively. The history was confused by the positive tuberculin test and probability of exposure to unusual trauma.

He is a haemophilic patient with 4% of factor VIII.

Laboratory diagnosis

Having obtained the history, the next problem is to establish as exact a diagnosis as possible, with the aid of laboratory tests. Unfortunately, there are no simple 'screening' tests which will include or exclude all significant bleeders. It is necessary to use intelligent judgement for each individual patient. It is our general practice to carry out the following tests in all patients:

Whole blood clotting time
Prothrombin consumption index (PCI)
Kaolin-cephalin clotting time (KCCT)
One-stage prothrombin time
Factor XIII test
Bleeding time
Tourniquet test
Platelet count
Haemoglobulin and white cell count
Examination of blood film
Blood Group

These tests constitute a minimum procedure and the extent of further tests will depend entirely on the clinical history. A rough guide to appropriate testing is given below.

**Patients with a clear history of previous severe
bleeding of the coagulation defect variety**

In these cases there is no doubt about the existence of a congenital haemorrhagic state, the problem is simply to define it and over 96% of these patients will be found to have haemophilia, Christmas disease or von Willebrand's disease. Diagnosis may be reached according to the scheme outlined below.

A. CLOTTING TIME OR KCCT PROLONGED

(a) One-stage prothrombin time normal;
   Assay of factor VIII or IX
      Abnormal—haemophilia or Christmas disease
      Normal—contact defects defined by specific tests
(b) One-stage prothrombin time grossly prolonged:
   Factor V, II, X or fibrinogen deficiency: confirmed by specific assays.

B. CLOTTING TIME NORMAL

(a) One-stage prothrombin time normal:
   Assay of factors VIII or IX abnormal: haemophilia or Christmas disease
(b) One-stage prothrombin time prolonged:
   Probably factor VII deficiency: confirmed by specific assay.

Specific assays are required at this stage because they provide the most certain evidence about the defect and because it is necessary to know in each case the extent of the deficiency.

**Patients with a history of bleeding of the coagulation defect
variety but of a moderate or mild degree**

It is in this group of patients that most difficulty in diagnosis arises. Many laboratory tests such as the whole blood clotting time Kaolin Cephalin Clotting Time (KCCT), prothrombin consumption test and the thromboplastin generation test may give normal results. In factor VIII deficiency for example, the whole blood clotting time may be normal with plasma factor VIII concentrations as low as 1%. The prothrombin consumption test may be normal with factor VIII concentrations above 5% and then thromboplastin generation test and KCCT give normal results with factor VIII concentrations above 10%. Excessive post-traumatic bleeding may occur with factor VIII concentrations up to 30% of normal. Thus a proportion of patients with factor VIII levels between 10 and

30% will be recorded as normal by all these tests. On occasion the kaolin-cephalin clotting time is more reliable but this is not the case with all plasma samples.

Thus for the mildly affected patients it is particularly important to carry out assay procedures particularly assays for factors VIII and IX since, in the United Kingdom, most of the patients will be found to have one or other of these defects.

Assay of factor VIII

There are two methods of carrying out the assay of factor VIII; the one-stage and the two-stage methods. It is not proposed to describe these methods in detail here but merely to outline the principles of the two methods. Detailed description is given by Austen & Rhymes (1975).

In principle *the one-stage method* is based on the Kaolin Cephalin Clotting Time (KCCT). All reagents are placed in one tube and the clotting time of the contents by this method becomes proportional to factor VIII. Dilutions of normal plasma, in the range 1 in 10 to 1 in 1,000, are added to haemophilic plasma. To the mixture is added kaolin and phospholipid after a standard period of incubation (2 to 5 min) at 37°C, the mixture is recalcified and the clotting times of the mixtures are recorded. This forms the normal dilution curve used to assess the abnormal. The procedure is repeated with a sample from the patient. The clotting times are plotted on double logarithmic paper when parallel straight lines should be obtained. The results of one such test are shown in Table 3.2

Table 3.2. One-stage factor VIII assay.

Sample tested	Plasma dilution tested			Control haemophilic plasma alone	u/ml
	1 in 10	1 in 30	1 in 100		
Standard normal dried plasma 0·91 u/ml	82·7	98·4	112·3		0·91
Frozen normal plasma	74·3	93·6	108·8	155·2	1·45
Patient before treatment	132·6	143·5	146·9		<0·03
Patient during treatment: (a) before dose (b) after dose	89·5 80·6	107·6 99·7	121·1 114·3		0·45 0·91

Test system: 0·1 ml haemophilic plasma 0·1 ml dilution in glyoxalline buffer of test sample 0·1 ml chloroform extract of brain 0·1 ml kaolin. The mixture was incubated 3 min and then 0·1–0·025 M $CaCl_2$ was added and the clotting time in seconds was recorded.

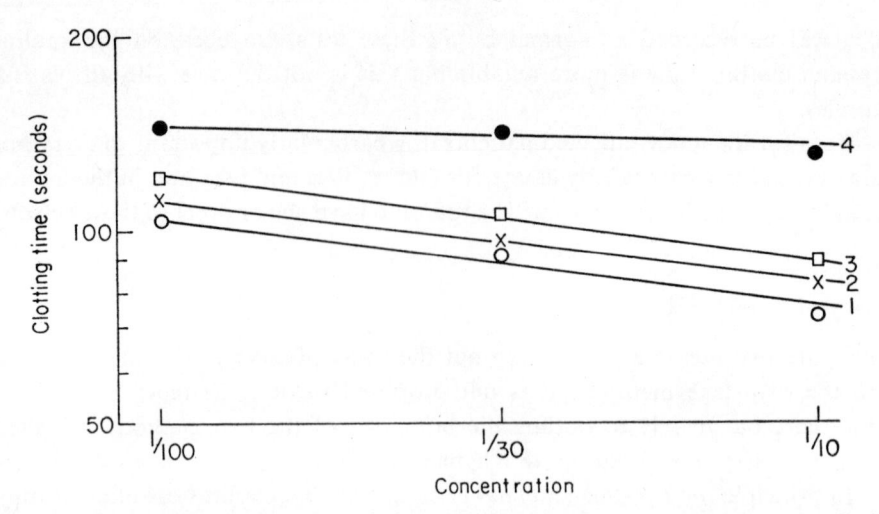

[Figure: plot of clotting time (seconds) versus concentration, with lines labeled 1, 2, 3, 4]

Figure 3.1. One-stage assay of factor VIII from Table 3.2. Line 2 is derived from the clotting times of a standard plasma containing 0·91 u/ml. Line 1 represents the results for a sample having 1·45 u/ml. Line 4 represents the results for an untreated haemophilic patient. Line 3 represents the results for a haemophilic patient during a course of treatment but before a dose was given (see Table 3.2).

and Figure 3.1. The clotting times are the means for duplicate observations. The results are expressed as percentages of normal or units per ml.

Several comments may be made about these results. In the first place the clotting time of the haemophilic plasma without the addition of any factor VIII was 155 secs. This 'blank' time limits the reliability of the method. The definite blank clotting time derives from one of two possibilities. The plasma sample may contain some factor VIII. Extrapolation of the result from the normal standard (0·91 u/ml) suggests that if the haemophilic plasma contains some factor VIII this is likely to be about 1% of normal. Alternatively the clotting in the absence of factor VIII may be brought about by the extrinsic clotting system. Whichever of these alternatives is correct the observation means that it will not be possible to assess factor VIII levels below 5% with any reliability. This is shown in Table 3.2 and Figure 3.1 by the results for the untreated patient. When the clotting times for a sample with low factor VIII are plotted the line is not parallel to the standard plasma line. The clotting times are too near the 'blank' time for reasonable assessment. This is a minor disadvantage since it is not very important to measure low factor VIII levels at all accurately.

The second comment concerns the difference between the clotting time for the 1 in 10 dilution of standard and that for the 1 in 100 dilution. This difference amounts to 30 seconds. Since values above 120 seconds are likely to approach too nearly to the blank time this means that there is rather a narrow range of clotting times (about 70–120 seconds), from which to judge the abnormality.

The effect of this narrow range on the results is illustrated in Figure 3.1 by the closeness between the lines representing 0·45 u/ml, 0·91 u/ml and 1·45 u/ml. It is the conclusion of long experience that the error, expressed as coefficient of variation, of determining the clotting time is of the order of 5% of the clotting time for duplicate readings. This means that results for repeated duplicate clotting times on a single sample may vary by about 7% of the observed clotting time. Even if the only error conceived in this method is that due to the actual recording of the clotting time then the effect such an error is likely to have on the results interpreted as percentage of normal factor VIII must nevertheless be large. A clotting time of 100 secs. in the system used for Figure 3.1 corresponds to 26% of factor VIII, 107 seconds corresponds to about 15% and 93 seconds to about 45%. Thus at a true clotting time of 100 seconds chance variations in observed clotting time could give results interpreted within the range of 15 to 45% of factor VIII.

The error in observing the clotting time is, of course, not the only error. Quite large errors can be introduced by very minor deviations in technique such as allowing test dilutions to stand longer or shorter periods of time before testing. Different haemophilic plasma samples used as substrate may also affect the results. In fact duplicate assays carried out in one laboratory on a single day may well differ from each other by as much as 50% of the true value (Bangham et al, 1971).

It may seem that such errors are so large as to render the method useless. In fact, if one considers values of factor VIII in the range 0–20% of factor VIII the clotting times of the 3 dilutions will differ very substantially from the normal. Thus for recognition of haemophiliacs the method is quite reliable. Moreover the carrying out of assays on 3 dilutions and assessing the results from parallel lines on double logarithmic paper also reduces the error to some extent. Allowing for the unavoidable errors it is unwise to test less than 3 dilutions of the standard plasma and 3 of the test plasma. In basing clinical decision on the result the magnitude of the error must be taken into account. It is our opinion that when patients are submitted to surgery the two-stage method of measuring factor VIII should be used in preference to the one-stage method.

The *two-stage method* for measuring factor VIII requires more reagents than the one-stage method and is procedurally more complex to carry out. Very reasonably there is a tendency to prefer the one-stage method particularly in those laboratories where tests are not carried out every day and indeed where sometimes several weeks may pass in which no tests are required. In addition, as previously noted, the one-stage test is quite adequate for the diagnosis of haemophilia.

The two-stage test is based on the thromboplastin generation test. In this test system factor Xa is formed in the first stage mixture and the amount formed is tested in the second or substrate stage. The amount of factor Xa formed is found, under the controlled conditions of the test, to be proportional to the amount of factor VIII in the initial mixture. A mixture is made of reagents required to generate factor Xa. These reagents are:

1 citrated plasma absorbed with $Al(OH)_3$ which is regarded as the source of factor VIII;
2 normal serum, a source of factors XII, XI, IX and X;
3 factor V;
4 phospholipid; and
5 $CaCl_2$.

At least 3 dilutions of the absorbed plasma (source of factor VIII) are mixed with constant and optimal amounts of the other reagents and the mixtures are incubated for a predetermined time and the amount of factor Xa is measured by adding a sample to normal whole plasma with enough additional calcium for optimal clotting. Two incubation times, for example 20 and 25 mins, are selected and the substrate clotting times should agree with one another within 1 or 2

Table 3.3. Two-stage factor VIII assay.

Sample tested	Dilution tested	Incubation time in minutes 20	25
Normal plasma	1 in 8	11	12
	1 in 16	15	15
	1 in 32	16	18
	1 in 64	20	22
	1 in 128	25	25
	1 in 256	29	30
Haemophilic plasma	1 in 2	25	25
	1 in 4	29	30
	1 in 8	35	35
Buffer		50	51

0·1 ml absorbed plasma dilution was mixed with 0·1 ml diluted normal serum, 0·1 ml of factor V, and 0·1 ml of phospholipid. 0·1 ml 0·05M $CaCl_2$ was added and after 20 and 25 minutes 0·1 ml samples were removed and added to 0·1 ml volumes 0·025 M $CaCl_2$, to which 0·1 ml amounts of normal plasma were added and the clotting times of the normal plasma were recorded.

Calculation (see Figure 3.2):
1 normal sample = 0·91 u/ml;
2 haemophilic plasma = 1·5% normal
    = 0·014 u/ml.

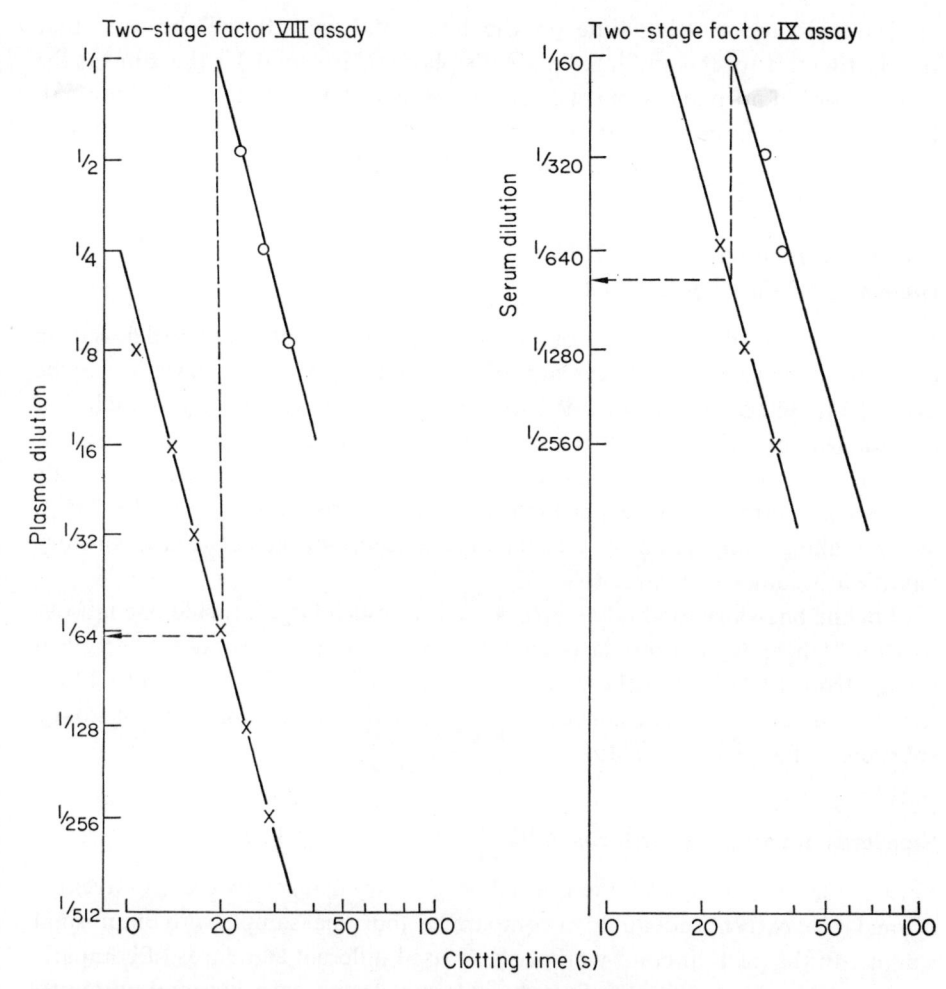

Figure 3.2. Two-stage assays of factor VIII and factor IX data derived from Tables 3.3 and 3.4. For both factor VIII and factor IX assays x———x indicates the results for normal plasma and ○———○ indicates the results for the patient's plasma.

seconds since the objective is to record the minimum clotting time. The incubation times selected will depend on the reagents and must be determined for each test system. Various sorts of reagents may be used for phospholipid or factor V. The details of some versions of this method are described by Biggs & Macfarlane, 1962; Denson, 1976 and Austen & Rhymes, 1975.

The results of the two-stage method are assessed by plotting the clotting times against plasma concentration on double logarithmic paper. It is found that the graphs resulting are linear and parallel. The clotting times of the example of Table 3.3 are plotted in Figure 3.2. In this diagram concentration is on the vertical axis and clotting time on the horizontal axis. It will be seen that the clotting time of the undiluted patient's plasma (21 seconds) is the same as the clotting time of normal plasma at a concentration of 1·5% of the original normal. If the normal plasma has 0·91 u ml factor VIII then the patient's plasma contains (0·015 × 91)/100 = 0·014 u/ml of factor VIII activity.

Errors in measuring factor VIII by the two-stage and one-stage methods

In routine use inside one laboratory it is our experience that a standard deviation of ±10% (expressed as percentage of the mean) covers the variation to be expected in all comparisons made using the two-stage method. This conclusion accords with experience at other Centres (Bangham et al, 1971). Comparison of like substances (plasma with plasma or concentrate with concentrate) the results between laboratories are less reliable but within reasonable range (13–26%). When making comparisons of plasma with concentrate the between laboratory variation becomes very large (68–76%).

For the one-stage method all errors are very much larger. Inside one laboratory on a single day the standard deviation expressed as percentage of the mean ranged from 17–26% and the variation between laboratories from 26 to 138% for comparison of like substances and 138 to 376% for comparisons of unlike substances (Bangham et al, 1971).

Standards of normality for factor VIII

Since the levels of factor VIII in normal people vary from 50 to 200% of average normal it is clearly not adequate to compare an abnormal sample with one normal sample. In the past different workers have used different standards of comparison. Some have used pools of normal plasma deep frozen in small amounts. Some have used freeze dried semi-purified preparations of human or animal factor VIII which have been standardised over a period of time against many normal samples.

The unit of factor VIII was originally defined as the amount of activity contained in 1 ml of average normal plasma as collected for testing in the laboratory by mixing 1 ml of 3·8% sodium citrate solution with 9 parts of blood and subsequent centrifugation. The whole definition is important since one would not expect to find 1 unit of factor VIII in 1 ml of plasma if twice the amount of citrate solution were used for the collection of blood. The unit is now established in a dried International Standard preparation of known activity (Bangham et al, 1971). The value attached to this standard was based on a study at many centres involving the comparison of the dried preparations with a total of 167 samples of normal plasma. The various laboratories did not agree exactly on the value to be attributed to the activity of the standard in relation to average normal plasma and a mean value was accepted. In some laboratories (e.g. that at Oxford) the International Standard Unit does not have exactly the same factor VIII activity as average normal plasma. Normal plasma samples tested against the International Standard give an average 0·8 u/ml and not 1 u/ml. A difference of this sort is of little clinical significance but affects the number of 'units' of factor VIII that can be made from a given amount of plasma by plasma fractionation laboratories (see also Chapter 4), and effects the estimation of factor VIII activity in commercial factor VIII preparations. In the United Kingdom a calibrated freeze dried plasma sample is available for use in assessing the activity of laboratory standards. For daily use in the laboratory several commercial preparations (e.g. Hyland plasma) have been found to be reliable.

The assay of factor IX

Factor IX may be assayed by one-stage or two-stage methods. As with the assay of factor VIII, the one-stage method for factor IX requires the use of factor IX deficient plasma containing no factor IX. Since factor IX deficiency is very rare and patients with no factor IX tend to have frequent treatment it is not easy to obtain suitable substrate plasma for the test. In our experience the one-stage assay for factor IX is less reliable than the one-stage factor VIII assay. We have little experience of the one-stage method in recent years and cannot give any actual data about the use of this method.

The two-stage method is more complex than the two-stage factor VIII assay since factor IX is assayed in serum which must be prepared from a normal standard plasma and from the patient's plasma and from a patient with severe factor IX deficiency. The factor IX deficient serum supplies the factor X required by the assay and must be free of factor IX. The system also requires factors VIII and V which are usually provided by absorbed normal plasma. This reagent introduces variation in the results since low factor VIII levels give too long clotting times and high factor VIII too short blank clotting times. The activation of factor IX is brought about by contact product and is an essential stage in the measurement of factor IX. This stage also needs to be controlled in some way. In principle the test (like the factor VIII assay) is based on the thromboplastin generation test. The first step in the reaction consists in the preparation of sera by clotting of plasma carried out under standard conditions. The test system proper consists of a mixture of the test serum (normal or that of the patient, supplying factor IX) of Christmas disease serum (supplying factor X) $Al(OH)_3$ absorbed normal plasma (supplying factors V, VIII), phospholipid and $CaCl_2$.

Some test systems also make an addition of contact product (factor IXa) or kaolin to ensure rapid and complete activation of factor IX to factor IXa. The details of the method now used at the Oxford Haemophilia Centre are given by Austen & Rhymes (1975). The results of an assay given by Sen *et al* (1967) for their method are given in Table 3.4 and Figure 3.2. If the normal plasma is assumed to have 1 u/ml factor IX then the test plasma has 0·2 u/ml.

Table 3.4. Two-stage factor IX assay (adapted from Sen *et al*. 1967)

	Factor IX = 1 u/ml		Factor IX = 0·2 u/ml
Dilution of serum	Mean clotting time	Dilution of serum	Mean clotting time
1 in 640	22·7	1 in 160	24·8
1 in 1280	27·1	1 in 320	31·7
1 in 2560	34·4	1 in 640	35·7
Control no serum	48 secs.		

0·1 ml normal serum dilution was mixed with 0·1 ml diluted absorbed normal plasma, 0·1 ml diluted factor IX deficient serum, 0·1 ml factor V, and 0·1 ml phospholipid. 0·1 ml 0·05 M $CaCl_2$ is added. After 2 incubation times 0·1 ml of each mixture is added to 0·1 ml 0·025 M $CaCl_2$, and 0·1 ml normal plasma is added. The clotting times are recorded and are the average of the 2 incubation times.

The intrinsic complexity of the technique and the relative infrequency of its use (since factor IX deficient patients are so rarely seen) necessarily give rise to large differences of results from time to time inside one laboratory and are likely to give very large differences between laboratories. An example of the effects of different methods of controlling the contact phase of clotting are given by Sen *et al* (1967). These authors compared test systems in which contact activation was provided during the clotting of the plasma to make serum and the other in which the serum was prepared without contact but contact factor was added in the incubation stage. The experiment which involved the testing of samples from a patient following surgery are produced in Table 3.5. It will be seen that the two modifications of the method did not give exactly the same results. The rise in factor IX and the dose (expressed as u/kg) were both apparently higher when the contact factor was included in the test incubation mixture than when contact was supplied during the preparation of the serum. An interesting point is that the recovery of the factor IX in the patient's plasma after infusion expressed as percentage factor IX/u/kg was the same in both methods.

Clearly these two methods used in different laboratories on the same factor IX preparation would be likely to give statistically highly significant differences

Table 3.5. Comparison of two modifications of the two-stage factor IX assay (adapted from Sen *et al*, 1967).

	Contact factor in incubation mixture			Contact activation of serum		
Day	Dose u/kg	Rise % factor IX	Rise % /u/kg	Dose u/kg	Rise % factor IX	Rise % /u/kg
1	69	57	0·83	64	49	0·76
2	53	37	0·70	40	32	0·80
3	66	51	0·77	53	34	0·64
4	52	42	0·81	28	20	0·71
5	60	46	0·77	57	35	0·61
6	43	60	1·39	28	30	1·07
7	47	53	1·12	32	33	1·03
8	38	59	1·55	29	33	1·14
9	37	32	0·86	36	37	1·03
10	32	48	1·50	37	38	1·03
11	44	35	0·79	33	46	1·39
12	37	43	1·16	18	10	0·55
Mean	48·2	46·9	1·02	37·9	33·1	0·90

and to provide large components of 'between laboratory' variation. Nevertheless each of these methods could be used in one laboratory and each might give very reasonable results each of which could be correlated with the clinical condition of the patient. It is because the sort of difference demonstrated in Table 3.5 is probably quite common that the value of a method for clinical use is best judged on its reproducibility inside one laboratory rather than its general reproducibility between different laboratories.

There is at present little good evidence about the reliability and reproducibility of the factor IX assay. It is our impression that replicate observations in our laboratory have a standard deviation of about 20% of mean values when the test is operating well. The test is much more liable to days of total breakdown for ill defined reasons than is the factor VIII assay. Factor IX is rather a stable substance stored in plasma and thus pools of large numbers of normal samples may be made and aliquots may be stored frozen for considerable periods of time (6 months to a year). Such plasma pools have proved very satisfactory standard preparations for clinical use. An International Standard preparation is under study.

The diagnosis of patients having anti-factor VIII antibodies

About 6% of all haemophilia A patients develop antibodies directed against factor VIII. A similar sort of anti-factor VIII antibody may also occasionally develop in previously normal people. These antibodies are very important since the presence of antibody greatly complicates the treatment of haemophilic patients and causes a serious haemorrhagic state when it appears in normal people (see Chapter 9). The measurement of antibody is not easy but it is essential to be able to identify patients who have antibody in their blood and if possible to measure the antibody quantitatively. Before describing the technique some discussion will be given of the general principles underlying this assay.

THE KINETICS OF FACTOR VIII AND ANTIBODY INTERACTION

When factor VIII is mixed with antibody and the amount of residual factor VIII is measured after different periods of incubation the factor VIII disappears progressively. From experiments in which bovine factor VIII (VIII) and antibody (Ab) were incubated together Biggs & Bidwell (1959) thought that the pattern of disappearance suggested a simple bimolecular reaction of the type:

$$VIII + Ab \longrightarrow VIII.Ab$$

From these observations Biggs & Bidwell thought that if antibody were present in excess the reaction could be expressed by the equation:

$$K = \frac{1}{t\text{Ab}} \log \frac{100}{\text{VIII}_R}$$

where t = incubation time
Ab = antibody concentration
VIII_R = residual factor VIII after incubation time t
K = constant

If, in the reaction between antibody and factor VIII, antibody were in excess, and if a constant incubation time were taken, a graph relating log residual factor VIII and antibody concentration should be linear. Biggs & Bidwell (1959) defined the unit of antibody as the amount which would destroy 75% of the added factor VIII in 1 hour. They used a graph relating antibody concentration to the logarithm of the amount of residual factor VIII after 1 hour incubation with antibody as a standard by which to measure unknown antibodies (Figure 3.3). The method worked quite well so long as bovine factor VIII was used as the source of factor VIII to be destroyed. When human factor VIII is used the method of Biggs & Bidwell is often not satisfactory. Table 3.6 shows the results of incubating human factor VIII with antibodies from 5 different patients and of calculating the antibody concentration using the graph of Biggs & Bidwell. It will be seen that antibody units calculated for different dilutions of antibody often gave different results. The method thus cannot be relied upon to measure anti-factor VIII antibody in all samples.

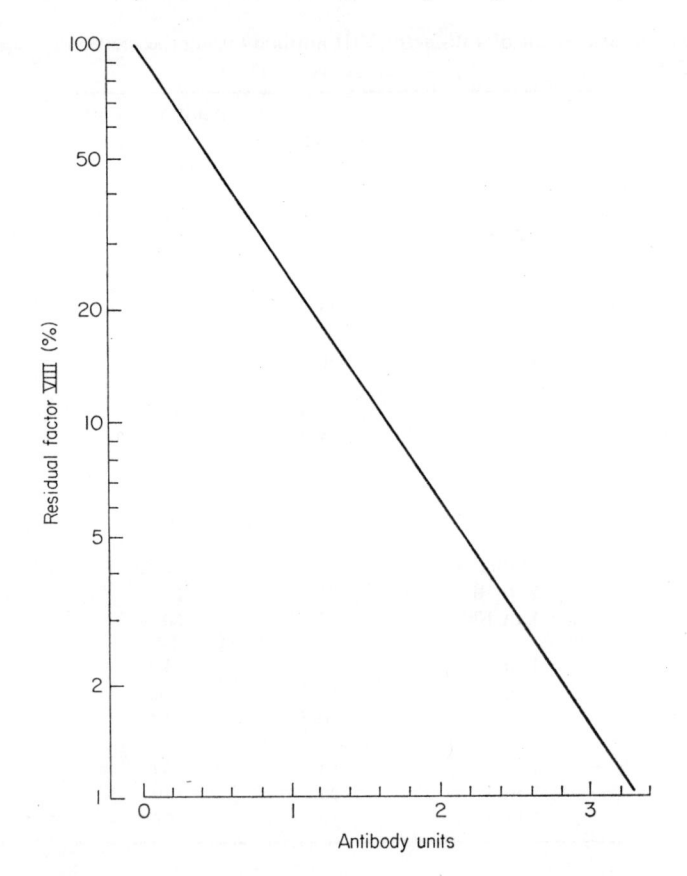

Figure 3.3. Calibration graph for the measurement of antifactor VIII antibody used by Biggs & Bidwell (1959).

A study was made of the disappearance of human factor VIII after various periods of incubation. Sometimes the initial disappearance of factor VIII was very rapid but after a certain period of time a much slower disappearance of activity was observed (Figure 3.4). Sometimes this flattening of the time course graph could be attributed to the using up of antibody during the reaction. This was not the only explanation. In the experiment illustrated in Figure 3.4, for example, more factor VIII was added after the flattening out of the graph. This newly added factor VIII was rapidly destroyed. A more probable explanation in this case was that when factor VIII and antibody had reacted together the complex (VIII.Ab) retained some factor VIII activity which was much more slowly destroyed by antibody possibly by forming further complexes such as VIII.2 Ab and VIII.3 Ab and so on.

The affinity of antibody for factor VIII is high; this is indicated by the fact that we have not been able to demonstrate reversibility between factor VIII and

Table 3.6. The measurement of anti-factor VIII antibody using the method of Biggs & Bidwell (1959).

Sample	Dilution of antibody tested	Residual factor VIII % after 1 hour	Antibody u/ml according to Biggs & Bidwell (1959)
1a	1 in 512	6·6	1024
	1 in 1024	28	973
1b	undiluted	11	1·6
	1 in 2	21	2·3
	1 in 3	40	1·98
2	1 in 20	7·5	38
	1 in 40	8·4	72
	1 in 80	21	92
	1 in 160	50	83
	1 in 320	70	80
3	undiluted	7·2	1·95
	1 in 10	21	11·5
	1 in 100	52	50
4	1 in 2	9·7	3·5
	1 in 4	16·5	5·2
	1 in 8	26·5	7·6
5	1 in 2	15	2·8
	1 in 4	26	3·8
	1 in 8	32	6·8

antibody for any of the antibodies whose reactions with factor VIII we have studied (Biggs *et al*, 1972a and b). Affinity between antibody and antigen is said generally to increase with repeated immunisation. It may be that patients who have demonstrable antibodies to factor VIII have all had repeated immunisation and it may be that a reversible antibody to factor VIII would not be easy to detect and thus not recorded. A patient who had a reversible antibody to factor VIII might simply be said to 'respond poorly' to factor VIII in that his plasma level of factor VIII might fail to show the expected rise following an infusion or the factor VIII activity might disappear unusually fast after infusion.

The importance of trying to understand the mechanism of interaction of factor VIII and antibody lies in the need to have a reasonably reliable method for measuring antibody potency. The main reasons for measuring antibody are to have an idea of the rate of formation and subsequent disappearance of antibody following treatment and to have an idea of the amount of factor VIII which might have to be given to a patient having an antibody to achieve a measurable level of factor VIII in his plasma despite the presence of antibody.

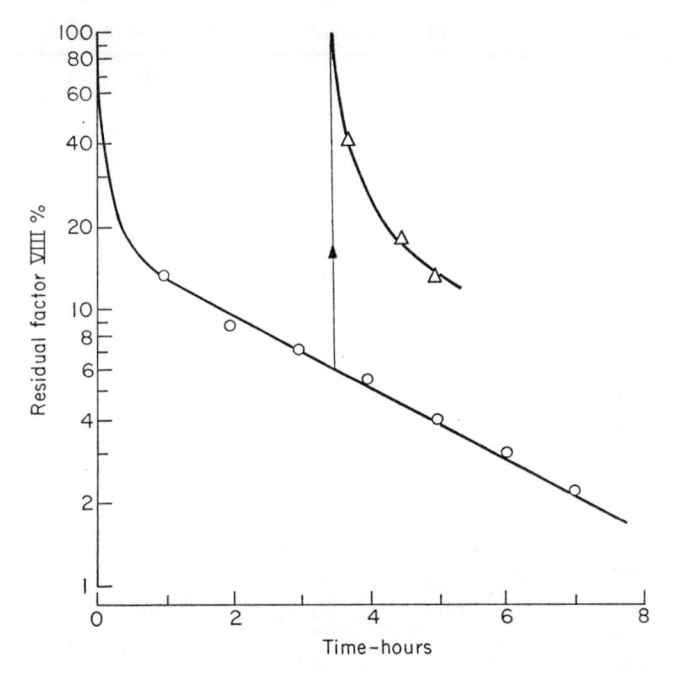

Figure 3.4. The levels of factor VIII in a mixture of factor VIII and factor VIII antibody after various periods of incubation. After four hours of incubation some more factor VIII was added (after Kernoff, 1972).

THE MEASUREMENT OF ANTI-FACTOR VIII ANTIBODIES

Rizza & Biggs (1973) concluded that the most generally comparable method was likely to be one in which the reaction between antibody and factor VIII was studied in factor VIII excess. They defined a new unit of antibody as the amount which leaves 50% of the initial factor VIII after 4 hours of incubation between antibody and 1 unit of factor VIII. The whole of this definition is important. The method, like all others, involves assumptions and may be far from ideal. Examples of the use of this method, taken from Rizza & Biggs, is given in Table 3.7 and Figure 3.5. Using the unit as defined by Rizza & Biggs at least 2 units of antibody should be absorbed by 1 unit of factor VIII. Under experimental conditions of antibody excess about 4 units of antibody can be absorbed by 1 unit of factor VIII. When factor VIII is administered to a patient who has a factor VIII antibody it is found that a dose of 20 u/kg of factor VIII is usually enough to neutralise 1 u/ml antibody.

In detail the method consists in mixing various dilutions of antibody contained in absorbed plasma with a known concentration of factor VIII for 4 hours at 37°C. At the end of this time the mixtures are put in an ice bath and the amount of residual factor VIII is measured. The concentration of antibody

Table 3.7. The assay of anti-factor VIII antibodies using the method of Rizza & Biggs (1973)

Plasma sample	Concentration* of antibody plasma tested	Control factor VIII concentration (u/ml)	Residual factor VIII (%)	Antibody plasma concentration giving 50% residual factor VIII	Antibody u/ml in undiluted plasma
a	0·01	2·5	1·3	0·0032	$\dfrac{1 \times 2\cdot 5}{0\cdot 0032} = 781$
	0·005		21		
	0·0025		63		
b	0·04	0·46	3·1	0·005	$\dfrac{1 \times 0\cdot 46}{0\cdot 005} = 92$
	0·02		9·1		
	0·01		23·8		
	0·005		51·5		
c	0·066	1·0	3·4	0·009	$\dfrac{1}{0\cdot 009} = 111$
	0·033		7·1		
	0·016		27		
	0·008		56		
	0·004		80		
d	0·1	1·0	6	0·0058	$\dfrac{1}{0\cdot 0058} = 172$
	0·05		5·7		
	0·025		5·1		
	0·0125		13·5		
	0·0062		46		
	0·0031		76		

* The concentration of whole plasma is taken as 1·0.

plasma is then plotted against the logarithm of the residual factor VIII taking the initial factor VIII to be 100% (Figure 3.5). The concentration of antibody which leaves half of the initial factor VIII is then determined from the graph. The antibody concentration is calculated by dividing the initial factor VIII concentration by the antibody plasma concentration in which 50% of the initial factor VIII remained after 4 hours (see Table 3.7).

This method is time consuming and it is not always necessary to make a quantitative measurement. The quantitative assay procedure is in any case a laborious waste of time when no antibody is present. A simple screening procedure may be used to detect the presence of antibody. The undiluted patients plasma may be incubated at 37°C with a known concentration of factor VIII. At various time intervals samples are removed from the mixture and the amount of residual factor VIII is measured. A rapid disappearance of factor VIII indicates the presence of anti-factor VIII antibody.

Having considered the three most important coagulation techniques in some detail, problems which arise in the diagnosis of specific types of coagulation defect will be considered.

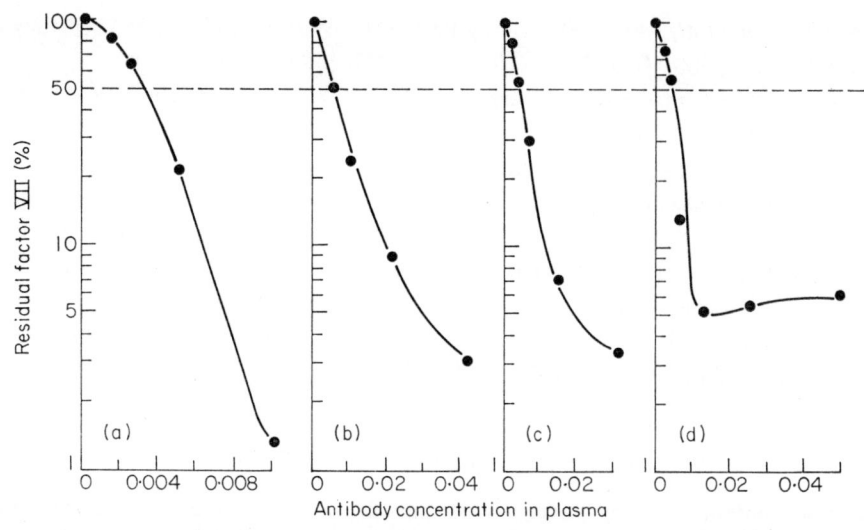

Laboratory and Clinical Diagnosis of Coagulation Defects 79

Figure 3.5. The determination of antibody units in 4 samples a, b, c and d. This figure was used to obtain the data for Table 3.6. Several concentrations of antibody in an absorbed haemophilic plasma sample are incubated with a known concentration of factor VIII. After 4 hours the amounts of residual factor VIII are determined (see Table 3.6). The concentrations of residual factor VIII are plotted against plasma concentration on semilogarithmic paper. From the graph the plasma concentration giving 50% of the original factor VIII concentration is determined. These values for the 4 samples are given in Table 3.6. The antibody concentration is calculated by dividing the initial factor VIII concentration in units by the plasma concentration which produces 50% of the initial factor VIII (see Table 3.6).

The diagnosis of carriers of haemophilia using the level of factor VIII activity as criterion

Were it possible to make a certain diagnosis of the carrier state it might be possible ultimately to reduce the population of haemophiliacs by genetic counselling (see Chapters 10 and 11). It has been known for some time that the factor VIII level in female carriers of haemophilia taken as a group is about 50% of that of a comparable group of normal women. In a recent study by Rizza *et al* (1975) a group of 34 normal women was compared to a group of 34 known carriers of haemophilia. The mean level of factor VIII in the normal women was 95% and that of the carriers was 54%. This statistical information is of little help in diagnosis since in each group the range was very large. In the normal women the levels were from 44 to 163% and in the carriers from 22 to 116%. Of the carriers 12 had factor VIII levels of 40% or less and no such levels could be found in the normals. Thus one could say that, taking the evidence of factor VIII levels, it should be possible to diagnose 12 of 34 (35%) of carriers. Estimates based on factor VIII levels alone by other workers were 90% (Bentley & Krivit,

1960; Nilsson *et al*, 1962), 50% (Alagille & Prou Wartelle, 1960), 55% (Pitney & Arnold, 1959), 30% (Ikkala, 1960) and 0% (Gardikas *et al*, 1957).

In recent years increasing evidence has supported the idea that the defect in haemophilia is not a simple absence of factor VIII but that many if not most of these patients have a protein variant equivalent to normal factor VIII but lacking factor VIII clotting activity (see Chapter 2). The fact that the level of factor VIII in the carriers of haemophilia is about 50% of normal gives rise to the idea that half of the factor VIII in the plasma of carriers may be in the inactive form which is thought to occur in the haemophiliac. It has been thought that this inactive factor VIII could be identified and measured by a technique of antibody adsorption such as that used in the study of viruses.

THE ABSORPTION OF ANTIBODY BY FACTOR VIII

Antibody absorption by factor VIII has aroused considerable interest but attempts to use this method to detect and measure a protein similar to factor VIII but lacking coagulant activity have given astonishingly variable results. The reliability of measuring antibody absorbed must depend on the amount of antibody that can be absorbed by each factor VIII molecule. When considering virus antibody Dulbecco *et al* (1956) showed that the attachment of one molecule of antibody to each virus particle was enough to destroy the virus but as many as 20 antibody molecules could be attached to each virus particle after its activity had been destroyed. Thus there must have been 20 or more sites to which antibody could be attached on each virus particle for the virus types studied. The very considerable ability of virus particles to absorb virus antibody means that the presence of virus can quite readily be detected by antibody neutralisation tests. The difficulty that has arisen in measuring absorption of antibody by factor VIII lies in the fact that factor VIII absorbs little or no more antibody than is required to destroy the factor VIII.

In principle the method of measuring antibody absorption consists in mixing antibody with factor VIII (or factor VIII related antigen) and incubating the mixture for 4 hours at 37°C and storing the mixture overnight at 4°C. This initial mixture must contain antibody excess so that all of the availabile sites on the factor VIII can be occupied by antibody and as much antibody as possible is absorbed. The mixture is then heated to 56°C and centrifuged to remove any remaining trace of factor VIII activity and to remove antibody attached to inactivated factor VIII. The amount of antibody in the supernatant is then measured and the amount of absorbed antibody is obtained comparison with antibody which has not been incubated with factor VIII. It seems (Pool, Biggs & Miller, 1976 and Biggs, 1973) that each factor VIII molecule has attachment sites for 1–3 antibody molecules only. Thus in conditions of antibody excess the

Table 3.8. An experiment to illustrate antibody absorption by factor VIII from Pool, Biggs & Miller (1976).

Test sample	Concentrations of antibody tested	Residual factor VIII	Antibody concentration u/ml
Control No factor VIII incubated with antibody	0·016 0·04 0·08	84 64 32	19·6
1·08 units factor VIII incubated with antibody	0·04 0·08 0·16	77 42 12	15·4
2·17 units factor VIII incubated with antibody	0·04 0·08 0·16	82 55 17	11·9

Antibody absorbed per unit of factor VIII was:

$$1 \quad \frac{19·6 - 15·4}{1·08} = 3·9;$$

$$2 \quad \frac{19·6 - 11·9}{2·17} = 3·54.$$

In this experiment the concentration of factor VIII used to test for antibody concentration was 1·08 u/ml.

differences in antibody level before and after absorption are small. For example, if about 20 units of antibody (Pool & Biggs, 1976) are mixed with about 1 unit of factor VIII and the amount of residual antibody measured, it may be found that about 15 units of antibody remain. The difference in actual clotting time measurement between about 20 and 15 units of antibody is shown in Table 3.8. It is clear that such small differences cannot be measured reliably without unacceptable replication. The observer is thus forced to consider conditions where antibody is not present in large excess. For example, the use of about 2 u/ml factor VIII in the experiment of Table 3.8 resulted in 12 u/ml residual antibody and a more measurable difference in antibody concentration as a result of absorption. The technique of antibody absorption thus has a very narrow range for reliable measurement. The relative concentrations of antibody and antigen must be arranged so that nearly but not more than half of the initial antibody will be absorbed. If more than half is absorbed then there is no antibody excess.

The difficulty in arranging conditions for the reliable measurement of antibody absorption by normal factor VIII explains the contradictory results which have been obtained when trying to distinguish between the absorption ability of different types of antigen such as the antigen resembling factor VIII that might be present in plasma samples from haemophilic patients. Consensus in this branch of study would now suggest that most haemophilic antibodies are not absorbed by protein in most haemophilic patients' plasma. A minority of patients, whose plasma shows some factor VIII activity, do retain some ability to absorb haemophilic antibody. These patients have been said to be haemophilia A+ in distinction from the majority who are haemophilia A−. There is no recorded difference in the incidence of anti-factor VIII antibodies in patients who are A+ when compared to those who are A−.

The method of antibody absorption has not proved useful in the diagnosis of carriers of haemophilia since the test is clearly not sufficiently reliable.

Factor-VIII-related antigen and the detection of carriers of haemophilia

In 1971 Zimmerman *et al* produced a rabbit antibody to purified human factor VIII which formed a precipitate with normal factor VIII. The amount of precipitate could conveniently be measured by the immuno electrophoretic technique described by Laurell (1966). The antibody demonstrated a normal amount of precipitate in all tested samples of haemophilic plasma, in heated normal plasma, in serum and in outdated stored plasma. If this protein is connected in some way with the defect in haemophilia then its properties are very different from those of factor VIII. It might have been thought that the precipitated protein respresented an irrelevant contaminant of the purified factor VIII used to immunise the rabbit. However, Zimmerman *et al* demonstrated complete absence of this protein in patients severely affected with von Willebrands disease and these latter patients also lack factor VIII. Since 1971 evidence has been accumulating which suggests that the precipitable protein, called factor-VIII-related antigen, has some definite though not precisely defined connection with factor-VIII activity (see Chapter 2).

The levels of factor-VIII-related antigen have been measured by Rizza *et al* (1975) in the 34 carriers and 34 normal women referred to above. Taken as groups the factor-VIII-related antigen was the same in both groups (97% in the normals and 105% in the carriers). The range of observations was also about the same in the 2 groups (46% to 219% in normals and 49 to 215% in the carriers). There was a definite correlation between factor VIII and factor-VIII-related antigen in both groups. This correlation means that on the whole a high level of factor VIII is associated with a high level of factor-VIII-related antigen. This correlation is illustrated from the data of Rizza *et al* (1975) in Figure 3.6. The correlation means that even if the factor VIII level is within the normal range the ratio of factor VIII to factor-VIII-related antigen may be less than that observed in normal women because the factor-VIII-related antigen may be well above normal. Taking the ratio of factor VIII to factor-VIII-related antigen as a criterion it was found that 24 of the 34 (71%) carriers studied by Rizza *et al*

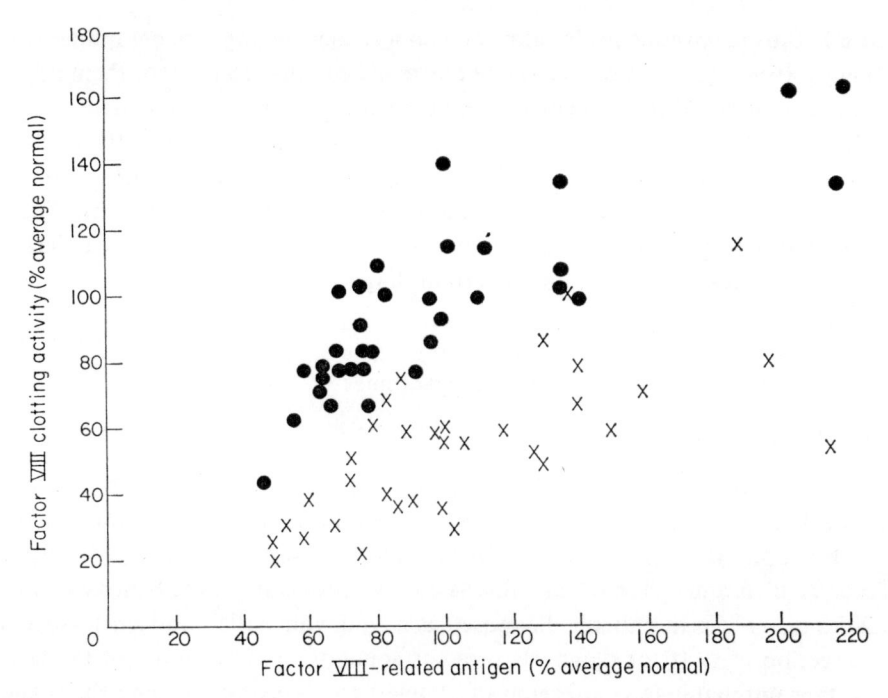

Figure 3.6. Correlation between factor VIII clotting activity and factor-VIII-related antigen both expressed as percentage of average normal in 34 normal women (●) and 34 carriers of haemophilia (x).

(1975) had ratios of less than 0·6 whereas no normals had values below this figure. One carrier whose ratio was more than 0·61 had 39% of factor VIII. Thus in our experience 25 of the 34 (73%) of carriers were distinguished from normal women by carrying out both factor VIII and factor-VIII-related antigen tests. Thus in our hands the use of the two measurements does substantially increase the proportion of carriers who can be diagnosed with reasonable certainty. Other workers have also recorded improved diagnosis of carriers using tests for factor VIII and factor-VIII-related antigen. Zimmerman *et al* (1971) were able to distinguish 24 of 25 known carriers and by Meyer *et al* (1972) 9 out of 9 carriers were distinguished from normal.

This improvement of diagnosis is clearly helpful to the Clinician who is charged with advising female members of haemophilic families about the probability of having haemophilic sons. In fact unless the diagnosis is certain then the advice inevitably descends into a morass of increasingly complex probabilities. To take the least complex situation, we may suppose that one knows for certain that a woman is a carrier of haemophilia (for example her father may have haemophilia) then she has a 1 in 2 chance of having a son as the next born child and if she has a son a probability of 1 in 2 that he will have haemophilia.

There is thus an overall probability of 1 in 4 of her having a haemophilic son. Taking 100 children of such marriages one could say that 16 to 39 of them might have haemophilia. But when considering the next child in a single marriage even when the mother is known to be a carrier, the odds are 3 to 1 against the birth of a haemophilic child. Were it possible to diagnose with certainty those women who are *not* carriers then for them the case would be very different. These women will not have haemophilic sons. Thus although diagnosis of carriers is improving no tests are providing a certain diagnosis of normality.

Clinical syndromes

Von Willebrand's disease

Patients with von Willebrand's disease are considered in Chapter 8 since so much new evidence is coming to light about the aetiology of this condition. In the present chapter the practical tests which should be made to arrive at a diagnosis of von Willebrand's disease are discussed. As previously noted many abnormalities may occur in patients diagnosed as having von Willebrand's disease and the selection of tests for diagnosis presents some difficulties. Many of the tests are rather unreliable (e.g. adhesion of platelets to glass and bleeding time) and some rather newly introduced (factor-VIII-related antigen and ristocetin platelet aggregation), and thus not too well tried. We feel at the moment that the practical reasons for making the diagnosis and the consequences which stem from the diagnosis are the prime considerations. The syndrome undoubtedly includes a large number of mildly affected patients for whom one or several of the criteria are present but for whom the condition has little practical importance. It is probable that the most generally useful criteria are the clinical and family history, the long bleeding time, the plasma factor VIII level and the factor-VIII-related antigen. Cards carrying the implication of a serious hereditary haemorrhagic state should only be given to those who have serious symptoms. Patients who are so mildly affected clinically that the condition has little practical significance should not hold haemophilia cards.

Factor IX deficiency

The diagnosis of female carriers of Christmas disease is of the same importance as is the diagnosis of haemophilic carriers. In Christmas disease there is as yet no quantitative technique for measuring an inactive analogue of factor IX. The diagnosis of the carrier state thus depends on measuring factor IX. Of 53 proved carriers of factor IX deficiency Simpson & Biggs found 25 (47%) who had less than 50% of factor IX. Of 48 normal females tested at the same time only 2 had factor IX levels of less than 50%. Thus a value below 50% on two occasions for a female in a family known to have Christmas disease is an indication that the woman is likely to be a carrier. As with haemophilia a normal value does not exclude the carrier state.

Factor I (fibrinogen) deficiency

Complete absence of fibrinogen (afibrinogenemia) is a very rare condition inherited through an autosomal recessive gene. It is diagnosed by the complete failure of blood or plasma to clot using any of the simple test systems such as the whole blood clotting time, thrombin clotting time or one-stage prothrombin time. The total absence of fibrinogen can be confirmed immunologically. There have now been described a number of patients who have abnormal fibrinogen. A high proportion of these patients have no adverse symptoms. These cases have been reviewed by Ménaché (1973) and Mammen (1975).

Factor II (prothrombin) deficiency

Prothrombin deficiency is very rare as a single inherited coagulation defect. It is now well known that this particular abnormality is not well measured by the unmodified one-stage prothrombin time. By this test system a few seconds alteration in clotting time may be associated with a very marked alteration in level of prothrombin. The method may be modified by replacing the tissue extract of the one-stage prothrombin time by Taipan venom (Oxyuranus acutellatus) or Tiger snake venom (Notechis scutatus scutatus). The Taipan venom requires only phospholipid to complete the conversion of prothrombin to thrombin and thus, provided the test is well standardised, will give a measure of prothrombin. The Tiger snake venom requires the presence of both phospholipid and factor V.

The other method for measuring prothrombin is the two-stage method for which many modifications have been proposed. This method has the disadvantage that its validity depends on some way of allowing for the presence of antithrombin in the samples. Some methods attempt to reduce the effect of antithrombin by dilution and others state that constant antithrombin is a condition for carrying out the test (Biggs & Douglas, 1953). In fact there are possibly circumstances in which a balance between prothrombin and antithrombin is important and the two-stage test gives a composite picture of this balance.

In practice by far the most usually encountered patients having prothrombin deficiency are patients with acquired defects such as Vitamin K deficiency and liver disease and patients treated with vitamin K antagonists such as dicoumarin in whose plasma factors II, VII, IX and X are all reduced. In most cases the defect is well measured by an unmodified one-stage prothrombin time test which will record abnormality in 3 of the 4 factors implicated. The only danger arises in some patients having liver disease and who have been treated with vitamin K. Sometimes all factors return towards normal except prothrombin. In this event the unmodified one-stage prothrombin time may fail to indicate the gravity of the defect. A specific assay of prothrombin should be used in these cases.

Deficiency of factors V, VII and X

All of these abnormalities are easily detected using the one-stage prothrombin time, and, with the use of plasma from patients lacking one or other factor, a quantitative assay for each of the factors can be devised.

Defects in the contact phase of clotting (factors XI and XII)

These abnormalities are detected using the KCCT test system and quantitative assays are based on the use of deficient samples. Since both factors XI and XII can be absorbed onto celite and readily eluted therefrom in the presence of powerful inhibitors of coagulation a test based on celite absorption has been devised (Nossel, 1964).

Factor XIII deficiency

Factor XIII deficiency is very rarely encountered but the defect is extremely easy to detect and this abnormality should always be sought if the diagnosis is not easily made in other test systems (see Austen & Rhymes, 1975).

Abnormalities of coagulation due to the presence of inhibitors

Inhibitors of blood coagulation are of two main varieties. The first sort is represented by all of the natural inhibitory mechanisms by which the enormous coagulant potential of normal blood is held in check. The second variety of inhibitor consists in abnormal acquired inhibitors of clotting. The first variety involves the inhibition of the natural activated clotting factors such as factors XIa, IXa, Xa and IIa. It seems that these inhibitors are closely related and may act through a single inhibitory activity. To the best of our knowledge this type of inhibitor has never caused a haemorrhagic state by virtue of any constituent being present in excess. Reduction in this type of inhibitor may on the other hand predispose to thrombosis. From the diagnostic point of view there are now several methods of measuring anti-IIa and anti-Xa activity (see Austen & Rhymes, 1975).

The acquired inhibitors are of two main varieties. One consists of specific inhibitors which destroy certain coagulation factors particularly factor VIII and the second type of inhibitor arises in patients with DLE or macroglobulinaemia. The coagulation factor inhibitors which are antibodies to coagulation factors are important though rarely encountered; the treatment of patients having anti-factor VIII antibodies is considered in Chapter 9.

Concluding remarks

The present Chapter is intended to assist in establishing priorities for laboratories attached to haemophilia centres which are set up to diagnose haemostatic defects. In coagulation laboratories many tests are carried out on haemostatically normal patients to reassure surgeons or dentists about the safety of proposed surgical intervention. By far the most important safeguard in this type of case is a careful clinical history. If there is no history of bleeding very modest laboratory testing is all that is required.

Much emphasis has been put on the assay of factors VIII and IX in the present Chapter because these two assays are the most important and the most difficult that have to be undertaken and it seems to us important that these tests should be understood and their results correctly interpreted.

References

ALAGILLE D. & PROU-WARTELLE O. (1960) Etude des conductives d'hémophilie. *Vox Sanguinis*, **31**, 797.

AUSTEN D.E.G. & RHYMES I.L. (1975) *A Laboratory Manual of Blood Coagulation*. Blackwell Scientific Publications, Oxford.

BANGHAM D.R., BIGGS R., BROZOVIC M., DENSON K.W.E. & SKEGG J.L. (1971) A biological standard for measurement of blood coagulation factor VIII activity. *Bulletin of the World Health Organisation*, **45**, 337.

BENTLEY H.P. JR & KRIVIT W. (1960) An assay of antihaemophilic globulin activity in the carrier female. *Journal of Laboratory and Clinical Medicine*, **56**, 613.

BIGGS R. (1973) The absorption of human factor VIII neutralizing antibody by factor VIII. *British Journal of Haematology*, **26**, 261.

BIGGS R. (Ed) (1976) *Human Blood Coagulation in Haemostasis and Thrombosis*. Blackwell Scientific Publications, Oxford.

BIGGS R., AUSTEN D.E.G., DENSON K.W.E., RIZZA C.R. & BORRETT R. (1972a) The mode of action of antibodies which destroy factor VIII: I, antibodies which have second-order concentration graphs. *British Journal of Haematology*, **23**, 125.

BIGGS R., AUSTEN D.E.G., DENSON K.W.E., BORRETT R. & RIZZA C.R. (1972b) The mode of action of antibodies which destroy factor VIII: II, antibodies which give complex concentration graphs. *British Journal of Haematology*, **23**, 127.

BIGGS R. & BIDWELL E. (1959) A method for the study of antihaemophilic globulin inhibitors with reference to six cases. *British Journal of Haematology*, **5**, 379.

BIGGS R. & DOUGLAS A.S. (1953) The measurement of prothrombin in plasma. *Journal of Clinical Pathology*, **6**, 15.

BIGGS R. & MACFARLANE R.G. (1962) *Human Blood Coagulation and Its Disorders*. 3rd Edition. Blackwell Scientific Publications, Oxford.

DENSON K.W.E. (1976) In: *Human Blood Coagulation, Haemostasis and Thrombosis*. Blackwell Scientific Publications, Oxford.

DULBECCO R., VOGT M. & STRICKLAND A.G.R. (1956) A study of the basic aspects of neutralization of two animal viruses, western equine encephalitis virus and poliomyelitis virus. *Virology*, **2**, 162.

GARDIKAS, C., KATSIROUMBAS, P. & KOTTAS, C. (1957) The antihaemophilic globulin concentration in the plasma of female carriers of haemophilia. *British Journal of Haematology*, **3**, 377.

IKKALA, E. (1960) Haemophilia. A study of its laboratory, genetic and social aspects based on known haemophiliacs in Finland. *Scandinavian Journal of Clinical and Laboratory Investigation*, **12**, Supplement 46.

KERNOFF P.B.A. (1972) The relevance of factor VIII inactivation characteristics in the treatment of patients with antibodies directed against factor VIII. *British Journal of Haematology*, **22**, 735.

LAURELL C.-B. (1966) Quantitative estimation of proteins by electrophoresis in agarose gel containing antibodies. *Analytical Biochemistry*, **15**, 45.

MAMMON E.F. (1975) Congenital abnormalities of the fibrinogen molecule. *Seminars in Thrombosis and Hemostasis*, **1**, 184.

MÉNACHÉ D. (1973) Abnormal fibrinogens: a review. *Thrombosis et Diathesis Haemorrhagica*, **29**, 525.

MEYER D., LAVERGNE J.M., LARRIEU M.-J. & JOSSO F. (1972) Cross-reacting material in congenital factor VIII deficiencies (haemophilia A and von Willebrand's disease). *Thrombosis Research*, **1**, 183.

NILSSON I.M., BLOMBACK M., RAMGREN O. & VON FRANCKEN I. (1962) Haemophilia in Sweden II. Carriers of haemophilia A and B. *Acta Medica Scandinavica*, **171**, 223.

NOSSEL H.L. (1964) *The Contact Phase of Blood Coagulation*. Blackwell Scientific Publications, Oxford.

PITNEY W.R. & ARNOLD B.J. (1959) Plasma antihaemophilic factor AHF concentrations in families of patients with haemorrhagic states. *British Journal of Haematology*, **5**, 184.

POOL J.G., BIGGS R. & MILLER R. (1976) The estimation of the number of binding sites for antibody on antigen molecules with reference to factor VIII and its antibody. *Thrombosis et Diathesis Haemorrhagica*. In press.

RIZZA C.R. & BIGGS R. (1973) The treatment of patients who have factor VIII antibodies. *British Journal of Haematology*, **24**, 65.

RIZZA C.R., RHYMES I.L., AUSTEN D.E.G., KERNOFF P.B.A. & ARONI S.A. (1975) Detection of carriers of haemophilia: a 'blind' study. *British Journal of Haematology*, **30**, 447.

SEN N.N., SEN R., DENSON K.W.E. & BIGGS R. (1967) A modified method for the assay of factor IX. *Thrombosis et Diathesis Haemorrhagica*, **18**, 241.

SIMPSON N.E. & BIGGS R. (1962) The inheritance of Christmas factor. *British Journal of Haematology*, **8**, 191.

ZIMMERMAN T.S., RATNOFF O.D. & LITTLE A.S. (1971) Detection of carriers of classic haemophilia using an immunologic assay for antihaemophilic factor (factor VIII). *Journal of Clinical Investigation*, **50**, 255.

Chapter 4. The Amount of Blood Required Annually to make Concentrates to Treat Patients with Haemophilia A and B

ROSEMARY BIGGS

During the first 25 years of this century the effectiveness of blood transfusions in the treatment of haemophilia was established. During the next 25 years whole blood, and towards the end of this time, plasma in small amounts became available to treat the patients. Large scale fractionation of human blood before 1950 was considered quite impracticable. Blood collection was concerned with the provision of whole blood for the saving of lives of war casualties, to treat severe anaemia of various sorts and to prevent exsanguination following or during major surgical operations.

Improvements in transfusion techniques, particularly the use of plastic bags for collecting blood, have made it possible to consider the more effective use of plasma and red cells. The plasma can be removed from fresh whole blood in plastic containers without exposing the contents of the containers to contamination. A simple method (cryoprecipitation) to separate factor VIII from plasma was discovered (Pool & Shannon, 1965) which could be carried out in any blood bank. The discovery of cryoprecipitate has provided a widely available effective haemophilia treatment based on close co-operation between local physicians and Blood Bank organisers. In addition laboratories for protein fractionation have developed methods for preparing freeze dried clotting factors from plasma on a large scale. Such freeze dried products are now also made commercially from plasma collected by plasmapheresis.

It is now clear (NILH Survey, 1972) that very substantial amounts of blood are already being fractionated in the USA and other countries to produce factor VIII concentrates. For example it seems that 1·5 million litres of plasma were fractionated annually in the United States by commercial firms alone during 1970 and 1971. Most of this plasma was derived from plasmapheresis but if it were derived from single whole blood donations it would require at least 7·5 million single donations. In the United Kingdom between 1·5 and 2 million donations is the total amount collected annually by the Blood Transfusion Service.

The time seems appropriate to try and assess the amounts of factor VIII required in the United Kingdom and to make some decision about the best type of material to make. Viewed on a National scale there are many things which need to be taken into account. There is no need to consider the problem of supply of blood to make factor IX separately since sufficient factor IX to meet the needs of Haemophilia B patients can be derived from the same plasma which is processed to give factor VIII and other valuable plasma derivatives.

The main considerations which affect an assessment of the amounts of factor VIII required are:

1 the total number of patients in the population;
2 the average amounts given to each patient annually;
3 what type of material is it best to use?
4 how can the material be provided?

The number of patients with haemophilia A in the population

The prevalence of haemophilia in the population depends on the number of patients born with the disease and the number who survive into adult life. The number born with the disease (the incidence) depends on the number of families in which the abnormal gene is inherited and on the number of cases contributed by mutations. In 1935, when Haldane considered the inheritance of haemophilia, it was rare for haemophilic patients to reach adult life and the prevalence of haemophilia was estimated by Haldane to be about 2 per 100,000 of the population of London.

Estimates of the prevalence of haemophilia in different countries are given in Table 4.1. In most of these estimates of frequency it seems a little unlikely that all of the patients were known to the doctors making reports. The NILH Study is exceptional in that great care was taken to detect all of the patients in the United States. First of all a postcard was sent to all haematologists, all members of the American Medical Association thought to treat haemophilia and to selected populations of internists, paediatricians, pathologists, etc. The postcard served simply to identify those doctors who treated haemophilic patients in the years 1970 and 1971. The identified 'treaters' were then asked to complete much more detailed questionnaires and the answers were clarified by telephone if necessary. This is the most ambitious and comprehensive attempt to identify all of the patients in a very large population. This survey gives the highest present estimate for the incidence of the disease but it is not much higher than two other recent estimates for localities inside the USA.

In the United Kingdom the Directors of the Haemophilia Centres in the country were asked to make returns of the numbers of patients treated during the years 1969, 1970 and 1971 and a report of this work was published in 1974

Table 4.1. Prevalence of haemophilia in various populations.

Author	Country or city	Year	Prevalence per 100,000 of population
Haldane	London	1935	2·0
Andreassen	Denmark	1943	2·2
Sjølin	Denmark	1960	3·6
Ramgren	Sweden	1962	3·35
Nilsson	Sweden	1972	5·5
Nilsson	Sweden	1976	6·9
Ikkala	Finland	1960	3·7
Martin-Villar et al	Spain	1971	2·3
Martin-Villar et al	Spain	1976	3·3
Larrain et al	Chile	1972	3·5
Rosenberg	Brazil	1972	7–10
NHLI Study	U.S.A.	1972	9·0
Sulz	New York	1972	7·3
Hemophilia Foundation	Michigan	1971	7·3
Biggs	Great Britain	1974	6·0
Cash	Edinburgh	1975	6·3
Mandalaki	Greece	1976	6·25
Mannucci & Ruggeri	Italy	1976	9·8
Brackmann et al	West Germany	1976	9·2
Allain	France	1976	5·3
Soulier	France	1976	6·6
Davey	Australia	1976	5·9
Masure	Belgium	1976	4·6

(Biggs, 1974). During this time about 1700 haemophilia A patients are known to have been treated at these Centres. During these years no attempt was made to sample hospitals outside the haemophilia centres and in fact about half of the cryoprecipitate made in the Transfusion Service for the treatment of haemophilic patients was apparently not used at the Haemophilia Centres. It seems therefore that only about half of the patients were treated at the Haemophilia Centres. The 1700 patients represents about 3 per 100,000 of the population. Since this report, the survey has continued and the number of haemophilia A patients known at the U.K. Centres had increased to 2,600 in 1975 and there may still be patients who are not known at the Centres. Thus 3,300 haemophilia A patients, about 6 per 100,000 of the population, is unlikely to be an over estimate of the number of patients in the United Kingdom.

From Table 4.1 it will be seen that the prevalence of haemophilic patients has increased since the middle of the present century. This increase may be due to two causes:

1 As treatment has improved more patients may have presented for treatment at specialist centres where statistics are kept. There may not actually be more patients but more of the existing patients may be known.

2 The patients born with the condition may live longer than they did before infusion therapy was available. This is certainly a factor since the average age of death of haemophilia A patients is now probably about 40 whereas it was 16–20 years earlier in the century (Ramgren, 1962; Andreassen, 1943).

The increase attributable to longer survival in the United Kingdom is almost certainly not complete since the average age of patients known at the Haemophilia Centres is below that of the whole population. In comparison with the general population there is an excess of haemophilia A patients in the age group 10 to 30 (Biggs, 1974).

We must, therefore, expect a further increase in the number of haemophilic patients who require treatment. In addition, seen in the long term, a further increase will result from mutation. Haldane (1935) pointed out that any gene resulting from mutation must die out if it caused malfunction sufficient to cause death before puberty. Such a gene could not be passed to future generations since the affected persons would have no children. If contrary to expectation such a harmful trait is found to survive then its incidence must be maintained by mutation. The incidence will represent a balance between loss of genes through early death of patients and the formation of new genes by mutation. For a sex-linked condition like haemophilia, Haldane (1947) represented this balance by the equation:

$$I = \frac{3m}{1-f}$$

where I is the incidence of the condition at birth before selection due to early death has occurred and m is the mutation rate per generation, a generation being taken to be about 30 years.

f = fitness of haemophiliacs. The fitness refers to the number of children born to haemophiliac fathers in comparison to those born to normal males at the same era of time. Thus if 1 child is on average born to a haemophiliac where 2 are born to normal males then the fitness of the haemophiliac would be ½ or 0·5.

Haldane (1947) applied this equation to figures then available from Denmark (Andreassen, 1943). From these figures $I = 13·3 \times 10^{-5}$ live male births. Haldane calculated $m = 3·2 \times 10^{-5}$ per generation and $f = 0·280$. Subsequent estimates (Table 4.2) have given similar results with the exception of those of Barrai et al (1968). The calculations of Barrai et al are based on very low figures for the incidence of Haemophilia A which were derived from questionnaires to selected doctors. There is every reason to believe that the incidence of Haemophilia A was much higher than they supposed at the time.

Haldane took the incidence of Haemophilia A to be $13·3 \times 10^{-5}$ males which is identical to the modern estimate of the prevalence of haemophilia which

Table 4.2. Genetic data about haemophilia.

Author	Incidence at birth $\times 10^{-5}$	Prevalence $\times 10^{-5}$	Mutation rate $\times 10^{-5}$ males per generation	Fitness
Andreassen** (1943)	13·3	4·5	1·9	0·570
Haldane** (1947)	(13·3)*	(4·5)*	3·16	0·280
Ikkala (1960)	15·4	5·9	3·2	0·236
Ramgren (1962)	12·9	6·6	—	—
Vogel (1955)			2·7	0·386
Bitter (1964)	16·0		4·1	0·240
Barrai et al (1968)	(5·5)		(1·31)	(0·280)
Means	14·1		3·01	0·342

( ) not included in means
* copied from Andreassen
** Haemophilia A and B included.

is 6–7 × 10⁻⁵ in relation to the whole population both male and female. The improved survival of haemophiliac patients as a result of infusion therapy must improve the fitness of haemophiliacs. Using the above formula improved fitness of haemophiliacs to 0·50 or 0·80 from Haldane's figure of 0·28 would lead to an increased incidence of haemophiliacs from Haldane's figure of 13·3 × 10⁻⁵ to 19·2 or 48 × 10⁻⁵. It is in fact difficult to predict the extent to which improved survival will affect the fitness of haemophiliacs. The improved survival will be accompanied by pressure towards family limitation from the general trend in the population during the next 200 years and through genetic counselling. It can, however, confidently be predicted that any increase in the number of haemophiliacs from increased fitness will be slow. For one generation all the abnormal sex-linked genes transmitted by surviving haemophiliacs will pass to their daughters. Thus the increased incidence will await the birth of grandsons. After two generations the incidence will show an irregular tendency to increase for several centuries till the new equilibrium is reached.

For the present an estimate of 6 haemophilia A patients per 100,000 of the population will be assumed to give a fair estimate of the number of haemophilia A patients requiring treatment.

The amount of factor VIII expressed as units of activity required on average by each haemophiliac

The amount of factor VIII used for each haemophiliac in the United Kingdom has increased steadily year by year as more material has become available. In 1974 the average usage in the United Kingdom was about 12,500 units per patient per year. This is rather less than the amount of that used in the U.S. as recorded by the NILH study for 1790–1971 which was about 14,000 units. In 1975 the amount of factor VIII used per patient in the United Kingdom was 14,800 units.

The haemophilic patient receives factor VIII treatment for the control of spontaneous bleeding into muscles and joints, for the control of bleeding after accidents, dental extraction and operations. Ten years ago the main use was to protect patients after dental extraction, surgery and accidents but now 80% of the material used is for the control of spontaneous bleeding into joints and muscles. Current practice after dental extraction and surgery can readily be defined and the amounts of material likely to be needed for the safety of the patient is easily predictable.

In the case of so-called spontaneous bleeding the amounts needed are not so easily to be foreseen. The patients are treated for spontaneous bleeding either at hospital as out-patients or at home. The patients who attend as out-patients may have to be driven by car or ambulance for long distances to reach the special centre. This makes them hesitate to come to hospital especially in the case of a small child for whom a visit to hospital may be frightening. Older patients are also often hesitant to bother the doctor. Thus there are reasons to suppose that patients who are treated as hospital out-patients receive less than optimum treatment because they hesitate for various reasons to avail themselves of treatment. There may also be some reluctance on the part of some doctors to treat patients on a purely 'on demand' basis. It may be thought that if there is no obvious physical indication of bleeding, treatment should be withheld. The treatment given in the past to patients for spontaneous bleeding may also have been limited by the amounts of cryoprecipitate and NHS concentrate available at the haemophilia centres and by the prohibitive cost of commercial factor VIII concentrates.

There is thus reason to suppose that the present usage of factor VIII averaging about 12,500 units of factor VIII activity per patient annually is not the optimum amount required to treat haemophilia A patients.

The number of doses given per year to haemophilia A patients in Oxford

A concept which should be mentioned at this stage is the record of the amount of material given to haemophilia A patients in terms of the number of doses of material received by each patient every year. The number of doses given per year gives an idea of the work done at a centre and the number of units of activity per dose will reflect to some extent the amount of activity dispensed in each bottle or ampoule. The amount per dose will also reflect experience in the management of patients and is likely to be influenced by the predictability of the activity of a particular preparation.

Amount of Blood Required

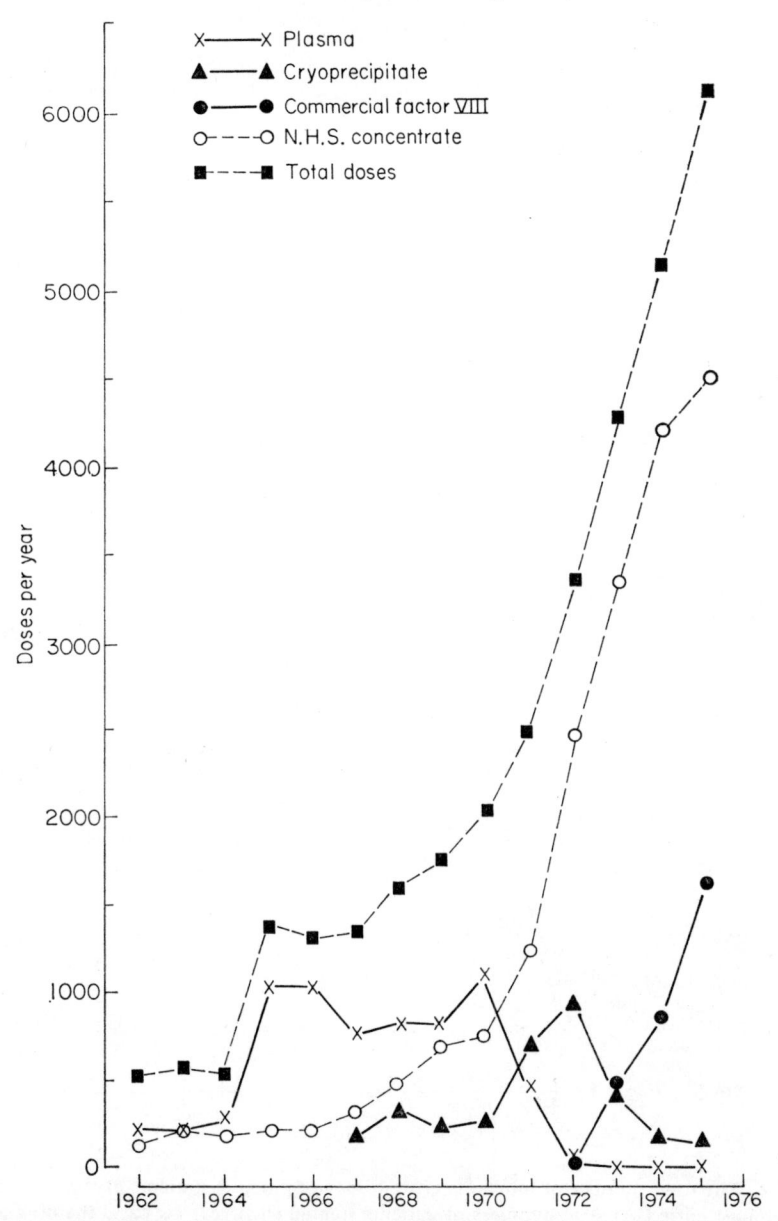

Figure 4.1. The numbers of doses of various sorts of factor VIII given to haemophilia A patients at the Oxford Haemophilia Centre from 1962 to 1975.

Since 1962 data have been collected about the number of doses of factor VIII given to haemophilic patients in Oxford. The information is summarised in Table 10.1, Figures 4.1 and 4.2. In Figure 4.1 the information is related to the different sorts of material used. It will be seen that from 1962 to 1964 small

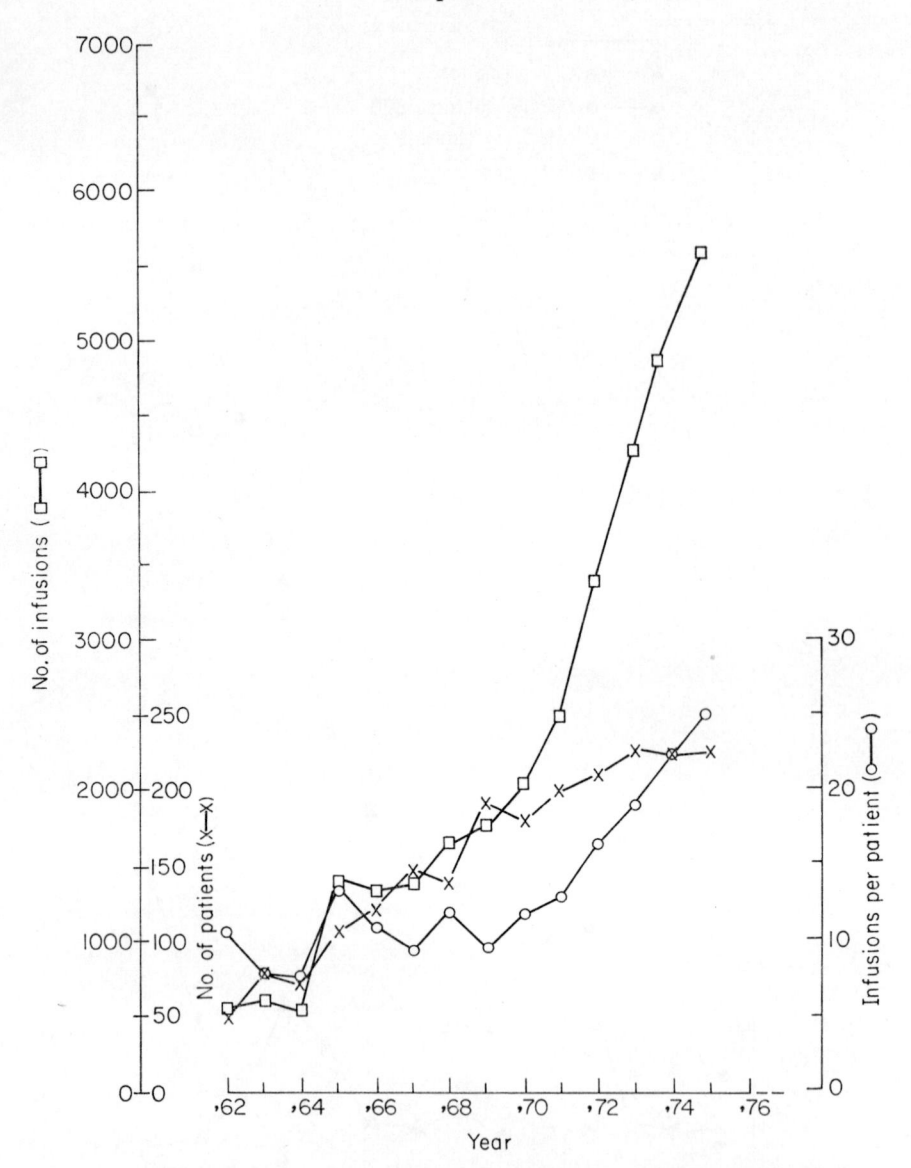

Figure 4.2. The total number of infusions given to haemophilia A patients at the Oxford Haemophilia Centre (□). The numbers of patients treated each year (×) and the number of infusions per patient (○) are also shown.

amounts of human factor VIII and concentrate were used. During this time and until cryoprecipitate was introduced in 1967, small amounts of animal factor VIII were also used for patients who did not have inhibitors. From 1964 to 1965 there was a large increase in the production of plasma by the Oxford Transfusion

Service. In 1967 there was an increase in the use of human concentrates associated with the start of production of freeze dried concentrate in Oxford and with the introduction of cryoprecipitate. The use of plasma was phased out in 1971 and in 1973 the freeze dried concentrate had largely taken over from cryoprecipitate.

In Figure 4.2 are shown the doses of factor VIII given in relation to the numbers of patients treated. There was an increase in the number of patients treated during the decade 1960 to 1970. Since 1969 there has also been an increase in the number of doses given per patient per year.

As would be expected this dual increase has been associated with a very marked increase in the total number of doses given annually. In 1975 the average number of doses per patient per year for haemophilia A patients was 24·4 (Table 10.1). Inspection of Figure 4.2 suggests that there is likely to be an increase in the future if enough therapeutic material is made available. Since 1972 there has been a rapid increase in home therapy for Oxford patients. By 1975 nearly all of the very severely affected patients who live in the Oxford Region were on home therapy and thus the number of doses given at the Centre have decreased slightly.

Information can also be derived from the treatment of 60 haemophilic boys at the Lord Mayor Treloar College in 1973 (Table 4.3 and Rainsford & Hall, 1973). Each boy had on average 26.4 observed bleeds per year and these required 32.5 doses of factor VIII. Once again it could be claimed that these boys also must have been very severely affected. In fact 7 were mildly affected and had measurable levels of factor VIII and only 17 were classed as severely affected. Information is also available from the NILH (1972) survey of haemophilic patients in the United States (Table 4.3). In this survey the average number of treatments per year per patient for severe and moderately affected patients works out at 34 per patient per year. This is not very different from the number of treatments given to the boys at the Treloar College.

Table 4.3. Amounts of factor VIII used to treat haemophilic patients.

	Average values		
	Treloar College 1973	Oxford 1973	NILH 1970–1971
u/kg/dose	9·21*	9·6	12
doses/year	32·5	19	34
wt of patient	—	55·7	34·6
units/patient/year u/dose	15,073	10,160	14,117

* assuming an average weight of 50 kg.

The average units of factor VIII given per infusion

The size of the dose in u/kg varies greatly with the reason for giving the infusion. Since more than 80% of infusions are given for the spontaneous type of bleeding the dosage schedule for this type of bleeding will predominate. The aim of therapy for spontaneous bleeding in Oxford is to raise the plasma concentration of factor VIII between 15 and 20% of normal. Study of modern therapeutic materials suggest that a dose of 1 unit/kg produces a rise of about 1·6 to 2% (Chapter 5) in the level of factor VIII. Thus a dose of 10 u/kg should on average have the desired effect. In 1971 in Oxford the average dose given was 9·6 u/kg. The NILH Survey did not collect exactly this data but the calculations assume a dose of about 12 u/kg. For the boys at Treloar College an approximate idea of the units/patient/year can be derived from the total amounts of material used. About 9·2 u/kg may have been used per dose. The relevant data is given in Table 4.3.

The data outlined above may be used to calculate the probable factor VIII needs of haemophilic patients. The average weight of haemophilic patients is taken to be 50 kg and the average dose 10 u/kg. The number of doses per patient per annum may be assumed to lie between 25 and 30. The number of patients is assumed to be 6 per 100,000 of the population giving a total of 3,300 for the United Kingdom. The total factor VIII required, based on these data, would lie between 41,250,000 and 49,500,000 units.

There is now some evidence that the size of the single dose needed by patients having spontaneous bleeding may depend on the promptness with which the dose can be given after the episode of bleeding is first detected. A dose as low as 5 u/kg may be sufficient as a single dose for the immediate treatment of a spontaneous bleed. Thus more frequent treatment of bleeding episodes will not necessarily increase the total amount of factor VIII used.

The types of therapeutic material available to treat haemophilia A patients

The types of therapeutic material at present available to treat haemophilia A patients are:

(a) fresh frozen plasma;
(b) cryoprecipitate;
(c) intermediate potency NHS factor VIII;
(d) commercial human factor VIII concentrate;
(e) commercial animal factor VIII concentrate.

Before considering the comparative values of the various preparations certain general principles may be considered. One is the yield of factor VIII from the starting blood, the second is the purification of the factor VIII activity and the third concerns clinical considerations of safety for the patient and the recovery of administered activity in the patient's circulation.

THE YIELD OF FACTOR VIII

The yield of factor VIII from the starting material concerns the amount of activity which is lost during handling. Factor VIII is a very labile substance and if much time elapses between collection of blood and separation and processing of the plasma, activity may be lost. Similarly during storage of frozen plasma prior to fractionation activity may be lost. During fractionation and freeze drying further activity may be lost. In the case of cryoprecipitate, activity may be left inside the plastic bags if these are not carefully washed out when making up the dose. The yield is expressed as a percentage and is:

$$\frac{\text{Volume of concentrate} \times \text{activity of concentrate} \times 100}{\text{Volume of starting plasma} \times 0.9}$$

0.9 is a factor which makes allowance for the fact that the starting plasma contains a larger volume of citrate than the standard of laboratory plasma used for assay. This factor is for blood collected into plastic bags. For bottles in which 120 ml acid citrate dextrose is mixed with 420 ml blood the factor would be 0.8.

The concept of yield is of the utmost importance since the yield will determine the amount of blood from which a given amount of activity can be obtained.

PURIFICATION

The purification of factor VIII concerns the extent to which the protein carrying the factor VIII activity is separated from other irrelevant proteins. Purification is expressed as a ratio:

$$\frac{\text{Activity units per mg of protein in the preparation}}{\text{Activity units per mg of protein in the starting plasma}}$$

It is clear that this concept has nothing to do with yield and in general so far as factor VIII is concerned the higher the purification the less the yield. Purification affects clinical practice in several ways. Impure preparations may produce dangerous immunisation of the patient to proteins other than factor VIII and cause severe and even dangerous reactions. The greater the purification the less the volume in which the material must be dissolved. Thus plasma and large doses of cryoprecipitate must be given by slow intravenous infusion whereas the more concentrated preparations can always be given by syringe. In general the higher the purification the greater the convenience of the material in use. However, high purification as at present carried out for factor VIII, greatly reduces the yield on preparation and the best high purity preparations would require at least twice as much blood for their manufacture as cryoprecipitate or the intermediate purity factor VIII.

RESPONSE TO TREATMENT

The patient's response to treatment is expressed as percentage rise in factor VIII in the plasma per u/kg dose. Biggs, 1966 calculated that the maximum rise that could occur was about 2·44%/u/kg assuming a relation between plasma volume and weight of 41 ml/kg (see also Chapter 5). The various modern concentrates differ from each other very little in respect of their recovery in the patient's plasma; 75–85% of the activity is recovered.

With these few preliminary concepts it is possible to consider the relative merits of the three most usual varieties of factor VIII used in the United Kingdom which are cryoprecipitate, intermediate potency NHS factor VIII and commercial human factor VIII. General properties of the preparations discussed are given in Table 4.4.

Table 4.4. Recovery of factor VIII activity.

Preparation	Factor VIII u/ml	Purification ratio	Yield on preparation %	Overall yield in patient %
Plasma	0·6	nil	80	64
Cryoprecipitate	3–10	6–16	20–45	16–36
Intermediate purity Oxford factor VIII	7–8	15–20	35–40	28–32
Hemofil	25	65	15–20	12–16
High purity Oxford	15	130	20	16
Factor IX Oxford	33–50	300	60	17

Fresh frozen plasma

An essential requirement for a factor VIII preparation is that it shall be able to be given to the patient in small volume and shall cause a large enough rise in plasma factor VIII concentration. Fresh frozen plasma is plasma collected following centrifugation of whole blood within 6 hours of collection and then immediately frozen at $-40°C$ and stored at $-30°C$. Such plasma has an average factor VIII content of 0·6 u/ml (Table 4.4). The low potency of this preparation means that it can never be used to raise the plasma factor VIII above 20% of average normal and must always be used at the maximum dose compatible with safety. Plasma is not now often used to treat haemophilia A patients in the United Kingdom. Eighty per cent of the original activity is retained in fresh frozen plasma.

Cryoprecipitate

When plasma is frozen at $-40°C$ and then thawed at a temperature below $8°C$ a residue of gelatinous material amounting to 3% of the plasma proteins remains undissolved and can be separated by centrifuging in the cold (Bidwell, Dike & Snape, 1976). Pool & Shannon, 1965 realised that this cryoprecipitate contained much factor VIII activity. They devised a method for its separation from whole blood collected into plastic bags which allows the red cells to be used for anaemic patients and those suffering from acute haemorrhage. The plasma separated from the cryoprecipitate may be returned to the red cells or may be used in a comprehensive fractionation procedure to give other valuable therapeutic materials such as factors II, VII, IX and X, albumin, and gamma globulin.

From the point of view of yield of activity from the starting material cryoprecipitate cannot easily be assessed since small changes in technique will alter the results. In fact in a study of 5 different centres the value in units of factor VIII per donation of blood varied from 12 to 130 (Biggs et al, 1974). Moreover, the average value varied very much from one centre to another. Under carefully controlled conditions 45–50% of the activity of the starting plasma may be recovered in cryoprecipitate. But even under ideal conditions the value of individual cryoprecipitates must vary greatly since the normal level of factor VIII varies from 50–200%. Some differences between centres may be due to the removal of different amounts of plasma from each unit of whole blood and some is due to relaxation of the attention to detail required to get the best yield. For example if plasma is thawed at too high a temperature some activity may go into solution or if the separation of plasma from whole blood is delayed a proportion of activity is lost. In general preparation the yield is seldom more than 35%. Also of course, the least deviation from the ideal in making up a dose of cryoprecipitate will lead to mechanical loss of activity which is left behind in the bags.

The degree of purification of cryoprecipitate is such that large enough doses can always be given. The circulation is never overloaded. Patients very seldom have reactions to cryoprecipitate. The preparation cannot easily be used for home therapy.

The recovery of factor VIII activity from cryoprecipitate in the patient is usually about 80% of that administered which gives an overall recovery in the patient from 16 to 36% (Table 4.4). The major difficulty in the use of cryoprecipitate is that the exact value of a particular dose cannot be known before it is given. Since there is very much variation it is wise always to assume that the dose is low and to give higher amounts than would be safe for a more predictable preparation. This fact means that even if calculations suggest that the average yield of factor VIII is 70 units of factor VIII activity per donation this average cannot be used to calculate the dose for any particular patient. The dose must be calculated from previous experience of the *least* amount of factor VIII that the cryoprecipitate is likely to contain. Although cryoprecipitate may seem to give a better yield of factor VIII than is customary in many fractionation procedures the material may be wasteful in clinical use.

In addition to these basic features of cryoprecipitate it must be noted that the material is very inconvenient to use. A single dose may require the doctor to pool the contents of 20–30 plastic bags each one of which must be washed out and the washings added to the dose. If trained staff carry out this work the yield of factor VIII will be best but in many hospitals the doses are made up by staff with little experience of this particular work. This is likely to be the case for example, in hospitals where relatively few patients attend.

When cryoprecipitate was introduced it made it possible for all blood banks to provide some of this factor VIII concentrate and thus the total amount of available concentrate was quite rapidly increased and this increase not only made possible safe operations and dental extractions but opened up the possibility of much wider use of concentrates. It was really never envisaged that very large numbers of blood donations (e.g. 500,000) should be fractionated annually in the United Kingdom by this method.

Cryoprecipitate must be stored at a temperature not higher than $-30°C$.

The intermediate purity NHS factor VIII

The method used in Oxford is described in detail by Bidwell, Dike & Snape (1976). The properties of the preparation are given in Table 4.4. The yield on preparation tested over the year 1971–72 in Oxford was almost the same as that of cryoprecipitate made during the same time (Biggs *et al*, 1974). The results of this experiment should be emphasised because it is often thought that the yield of factor VIII in cryoprecipitate is always higher than in freeze-dried concentrates. The belief rests on experiments at centres of exceptional excellence for the preparation of cryoprecipitate. Were such centres to supply plasma for the preparation of intermediate potency factor VIII the product would be found to be correspondingly better than average.

The obvious difference between the freeze-dried preparation and cryoprecipitate from the point of view of yield and purification is the much greater reliability of the freeze dried preparation from one batch to another and from one time to another. The material is a white dried powder easily soluble in sterile pyrogen free distilled water and each bottle contains 250 or 500 units of factor VIII. The material is stable and may be stored for over a year at 4°C without loss of activity.

The material is best made on a large scale and is not well adapted for preparation in any blood bank. Thus the making of this material envisages adequate centralised large scale fractionation plants and the transport of fresh frozen plasma in refrigerated containers from the blood banks to the fractionation laboratories. The setting up of fractionation laboratories and the degree of co-ordination required to transport plasma to the fractionation laboratories means considerable initial cost.

In clinical use the freeze-dried intermediate purity factor VIII is very satisfactory both at hospital and for home therapy. Intermediate potency factor VIII is not quite so convenient in use as the commercial factor VIII since it is at present made up for administration in a larger volume than is the commercial factor VIII.

Commercial human factor VIII

There are now several sources of commercial human factor VIII in addition to hemophil which is listed in Table 4.4. All of these preparations are more purified than the intermediate potency NHS factor VIII. They are very convenient to use since a dose can be dissolved in a small volume. Commercial human factor VIII is very expensive to buy.

Animal factor VIII

Animal factor VIII is available as freeze dried commercial preparation. In the past it was used to protect patients requiring major surgical operations. Now it is seldom used for this purpose but may be needed for patients having antibodies directed against factor VIII activity. A proportion of such antibodies have higher potency against human than animal factor VIII activity. Thus the animal preparations given to these patients may have more chance of giving a detectable factor VIII level in the plasma than human preparations.

The total amount of factor VIII required annually for all haemophilia A patients in the United Kingdom and the number of blood donations required to provide this amount

If it is assumed that there are 6 haemophilia A patients per 100,000 of the population. Then there will be 6 × 550 = 3300 patients in the United Kingdom. The 1974 usage of factor VIII in the United Kingdom was about 12,500 units per year. Thus the known need is for:

$$3300 \times 12{,}500 = 41{,}250{,}000 \text{ units of factor VIII}$$

The 1975 figures for use of factor VIII per patient give:

$$14{,}800 \times 3{,}300 = 48{,}840{,}000 \text{ units}$$

These calculations agree well with that given earlier which were based on the average number of doses per patient per annum and the average dose value in u/kg.

The number of factor VIII units derived from each blood donation will depend on the amount of plasma removed from each donation of whole blood and on the skill in preserving this activity during the preparation of the concentrate. In the United Kingdom it is commonly assumed that each donation used for the preparation of cryoprecipitate or NHS concentrate, yields 70 units of factor VIII. This assumption is based on the yield in Oxford between 1970 and 1972. In Oxford 220 ml of plasma was removed from each donation. In 1975 it is much more usual to remove 180 ml thus it is probable that the present average yield of factor VIII is about 54 units per donation. The approximate number of donations needed to supply factor VIII is thus:

$$\frac{41{,}250{,}000}{54} \quad \text{or} \quad \frac{481{,}840{,}000}{54}$$

$$= 764{,}000 \text{ donations} \qquad\qquad = 904{,}444 \text{ donations}$$

The above calculations make no allowance for batches withdrawn from use for various reasons such as testing for pyrogenicity and sterility and for estimates of potency which could require the withdrawal of 10% of each batch. The calculation also takes no account of the high dosage often used when the factor VIII is presented as cryoprecipitate.

What is the best form in which the factor VIII should be presented?

From Figure 4.1 it will be seen that the first big increase in treatment given to haemophilic patients in Oxford from 1964 to 1965 was associated with an increased supply of fresh frozen plasma, the second spurt in treatment was provided by cryoprecipitate but that the tendency from 1971 has been to rely increasingly on freeze dried concentrate and by 1975 it nearly replaced all other forms of therapy in Oxford. Choice between the various kinds of concentrate for use nationally lies between cryoprecipitate, intermediate potency NHS freeze dried factor VIII and various commercial preparations. In 1975, 80% of all NHS factor VIII in the United Kingdom was in the form of cryoprecipitate. All users of factor VIII in the United Kingdom agree that the NHS freeze-dried preparation is much preferable to cryoprecipitate and it is to be hoped that before long plasma now used to provide cryoprecipitate will be used to make intermediate potency freeze-dried concentrate. There is no doubt that the higher potency commercial factor VIII is very convenient to use and particularly convenient for home therapy. A certain amount of high potency material is essential for the treatment of patients having anti-factor VIII antibodies for whom large doses of factor VIII are often used. If all the NHS factor VIII were provided in a form similar in purification to the commercial factor VIII then nearly twice as much blood would need to be fractionated to provide this factor VIII. It seems unlikely that such amounts of plasma could be made available except by plasmapheresis. It would seem that the most economic and reasonable plan at present should concern the provision of adequate amounts of NHS freeze-dried concentrate of intermediate potency.

Is it possible to provide the factor VIII from a wholly voluntary blood transfusion service?

This question has been considered in an International Forum organised by *Vox Sanguinis* (1976). The conclusion of all of those experts consulted was that it should be possible to provide the material. This optimism is based on estimates of the number of donations required to supply the factor VIII. In the United Kingdom plasma derived from one-third to half of all donations would require to be fractionated. Experience suggests that one-third to half of red cell transfusion may be acceptable as packed cells. Jeffrey (1976) has made definite estimates of the amounts of blood needed to supply various products in a population of 1 million based on studies in Scotland. Jeffrey calculates the need for 21,000 units of red cells, either as whole blood or as concentrated red cells. He states that in Scotland 35% of all red cell transfusions are at present given as red cell concentrates and that 200 ml of plasma is removed from each donation used to make the red cell concentrates. If 40% of red cell transfusions were given as concentrated red cells, Jeffrey estimates that 672,000 units of factor VIII activity could be provided. This calculation is based on an assumed recovery of

40% of the factor VIII present in the initial plasma. In a population of 1 million we calculate that there might be 60 haemophilia A patients and 672,000 units of factor VIII would provide on average 11,200 units of factor VIII per patient which approaches the present calculated need. Even if the recovery of factor VIII were 30–35% and if 180 ml of plasma were removed from each donation instead of 200 ml, a very large amount of factor VIII would be provided. Jeffrey points out that the number of donations needed to make albuminoid fractions is at least twice the number needed to supply factor VIII. Thus if the objective of supplying albuminoid fractions within the NHS were met there would be no shortage of factor VIII.

Thus it is possible to provide the plasma. The next essential provision concerns staff equipment and accomodation for fractionation. The supply of these facilities depends on priority judgements for the expenditure of public money both nationally and locally. In the provision of fractionation facilities it is absurd to think of factor VIII alone. Fractionation will provide many other valuable plasma components such as albumin and various immune gamma globulins as well as fibrinogen and other coagulation factors. In the future it is very probable that many new components will be found to be useful.

The production of plasma components to meet the needs of various groups of patients (including the haemophiliacs) is possible but it is difficult to know exactly when and how this may be achieved. At present much factor VIII made by commercial companies supplements the National supplies made from volunteer donors in Western Europe. Soon albuminoid fractions will be available commercially. The question of supply and demand in a National organisation is not a simple question of a market place with buyers and sellers of blood. It is a problem for which no entirely satisfactory pattern has as yet been found. This subject is discussed in Chapter 11.

The treatment of patients with factor IX deficiency

Factor IX deficiency is less common than haemophilia. In the United Kingdom 373 were identified between 1969 and 1974. By 1976 493 patients had been identified. It would seem that on average Christmas disease is one fifth to one tenth as common as haemophilia.

Using figures for patients treated in Oxford and the NILH Survey figures fewer doses were given each year to Christmas disease patients than to haemophiliacs. The data is summarised in Table 4.5. The amounts of blood product required to treat patients with factor IX deficiency can be estimated in a way similar to the calculations for haemophilia. The recovery of activity in the patient is given in Table 4.4, where it will be seen that the yield on fractionation is much

Table 4.5. Treatment of factor IX deficient patients in 1973.

	Average values	
	NILH	Oxford
Patients	5,202	42
doses/year/patient	23	11
wt patient	36·6	55·7
units/year/patient	7,136	15,230
units/dose/patient	310	1,384
u/kg/dose	8·46	24·8

higher for factor IX than for factor VIII but that the recovery of activity in the patient is lower. Thus the overall recovery of activity in factor IX deficiency patients given concentrate is about the same as for recovery of high potency factor VIII in haemophilic patients.

The average number of units per dose given to each Oxford patient was about 3 times that given to each haemophilic patient but since only about a third as much of the activity was recovered in the circulation the effective doses were about equivalent in the two conditions. By effective dose is meant the dose required to produce the same plasma concentration of the relevant clotting factor. The NILH figures given in Table 4.5 have not taken into account the low recovery of factor IX activity in the patient's circulation.

Since the factor IX concentrate is made from the same plasma that is fractionated to make factor VIII it is unlikely that there will ever be a shortage of supply of factor IX for the treatment of haemophilia B patients if the need for faetor VIII is met.

References

ALLAIN J.-P. (1976) Management of hemophilia in France. *Thrombosis and Haemostasis,* **35,** 553.
ANDREASSEN M. (1943) *Haemofili i Danmark.* Copenhagen.
BARRAI I., CANN H.M., CAVALLI-SFORZA L.L. & DE NICOLA P. (1968) The effect of parental age on rates of mutation for hemophilia and evidence for differing mutation rates for hemophilia A and B. *American Journal of Human Genetics,* **20,** 175.
BIDWELL E., DIKE G.W.R. & SNAPE T.J. (1976) Therapeutic materials in Biggs, R. (Ed). *Human Blood Coagulation; Haemostasis and Thrombosis,* 2nd edn. Blackwell Scientific Publications, Oxford.
BIGGS R. (1974) Jaundice and antibodies directed against factors VIII and IX in patients treated for haemophilia or Christmas disease in the United Kingdom. *British Journal of Haematology,* **26,** 313.
BIGGS R. (Ed.) (1976) *Human Blood Coagulation, Haemostasis and Thrombosis,* 2nd edn. Blackwell Scientific Publications, Oxford.
BIGGS R., RIZZA C.R., BLACKBURN E.K., CLEGHORN T.E., CUMMING R., DELAMORE I.W., DORMANDY K.M., DOUGLAS A.S., GRANT J., HARDISTY R.M., INGRAM G.I.C., KECKWICK

R.A., MAYCOCK W.D'A. & WALLACE J. (1974) Factor VIII concentrates made in the United Kingdom and the treatment of haemophilia based on studies made during 1969–72. *British Journal of Haematology*, **27**, 391.
BITTER K. (1964) Erhebungen zur Bestimmung der Mutationsrate für Hämophilie A und B in Hamburg. *Zeitschrift for Menschliche Vererbung und Konstititionslehre*, **37**, 251.
BRACKMANN H.-H., HOFMANN P., ETZEL F. & EGLI H. (1976) Home care of haemophilia in West Germany. *Thrombosis and Haemostasis*, **35**, 544.
CASH J.D. (1975) *Factor VIII Concentrates. Transfusion and Immunology.* X. Congress of the World Federation of Hemophilia, Helsinki.
DAVEY M.G. (1976) Vox Sanguinis International Forum on the subject 'Can a national all voluntary blood transfusion service by adequate blood component therapy cover actual and future needs of AHF?' In press.
HALDANE J.B.S. (1935) The rate of spontaneous mutation of a human gene. *Journal of Genetics*, **31**, 317.
HALDANE J.B.S. (1947) The mutation rate of the gene for haemophilia and its segregation ratio in males and females. *Annals of Eugenics*, **13**, 262.
IKKALA E. (1960) Haemophilia: a study of its laboratory, clinical and social aspects based on known haemophiliacs in Finland. *Scandinavian Journal of Clinical and Laboratory Medicine*, **12**, Suppl. 46.
International Forum on the subject 'Can a national all voluntary blood transfusion service by adequate blood component therapy cover actual and future needs of AHF?' (1976) Vox Sanguinis. In press.
JEFFREY H.C. (1976) Blood transfusion and blood products. Problems of supply and demand. *Clinics in Haematology*, Vol. 5, number 1. W. B. Saunders.
LARRAIN C., CONTE G. & GONZALEZ E. (1972) 'El problema Medico y Social de la Hemofilia en Chile'. *Revista Medica de Chile*, **100**, 440.
MANDALAKI T. (1976) Management of haemophilia in Greece. *Thrombosis and Haemostasis*, **35**, 522.
MANNUCCI P.M. & RUGGERI Z.M. (1976) Haemophilia care in Italy. *Thrombosis and Haemostasis*, **35**, 531.
MARTIN-VILLAR J., NAVARRO J.L., ORTEGA F. & YANGUAS J. (1971) The supply and availability of plasma concentrates in the hospital of the Spanish social security. *Proceedings of the 1st European meeting of the World Federation of Haemophilia, Milan.*
MARTIN-VILLAR J., ORTEGA F. & MAGALLON M. (1976) Management of hemophilia in Spain. *Thrombosis and Haemostasis*, **35**, 537.
MASURE R. (1976) Vox Sanguinis International Symposium on the subject: 'Can a national all voluntary blood transfusion service by adequate blood component therapy cover actual and future needs of AHF?' In press.
NATIONAL HAEMOPHILIA FOUNDATION (1971) Michigan Chapter quoted by NILH Survey, volume 3, p. 41.
NATIONAL HEART AND LUNG INSTITUTE BLOOD RESOURCE STUDY (1972).
NILSSON I.M. (1976) Management of haemophilia in Sweden. *Thrombosis and Haemostasis*, **35**, 510.
POOL J.G. & SHANNON A.E. (1965) Production of high-potency concentrates of antihaemophilic globulin in a closed-bag system. *New England Journal of Medicine*, **273**, 1443.
RAINSFORD S.G. & HALL A. (1973) A three-year study of adolescent boys suffering from haemophilia and allied disorders. *British Journal of Haematology*, **24**, 539.
RAMGREN O. (1962) Haemophilia in Sweden. V. Medico-Social aspects. *Acta Medica Scandinavica*, **379**, 37.
ROSENBERG I. (1972) Hemophilia e estados ho Rio Grande do Sul. Frequencia, fisiologia et hevanca. *Brazilian Journal of Medical and Biological Research*, **5**, 287.
SJØLIN K. (1959) *Haemophilic Diseases in Denmark.* Blackwell Scientific Publications, Oxford.

SOULIER J.P. (1976) Vox Sanguinis International Forum on the subject: 'Can a national all voluntary blood transfusion service by adequate blood component therapy cover actual and future needs of AHF?' In press.
SULZ H.A. (1972) *Long-term childhood Illness*. University of Pittsburgh Press.
VOGEL F. VON (1955) Vergleichende Betrachtungen über die mutationsrate der geschlechtsgebunden-rezessiven Hämophilieformen in der Schweiz und in Dänemark Blut, **1,** 91.

Chapter 5. Plasma Concentrations of Factor VIII and Factor IX and Treatment of Patients who do not have Antibodies Directed against these Factors

ROSEMARY BIGGS

In the last twenty years the treatment of haemophilia and Christmas disease has made great advances which may be attributed to the production of larger amounts of more concentrated preparations of clotting factors, to the wide use of more reliable assays of factors VIII and IX and to greater clinical experience gained in large Haemophilia Centres. The general principles that underlie treatment are much the same now as they were ten years ago but since more concentrated preparations have become available it is important that these general principles should be widely understood. The success of treatment is based on giving the correct amounts of the appropriate coagulation factor concentrate to the patient and achieving the desired clotting factor concentrations and maintaining appropriate levels for the necessary time.

The assay of coagulation factor activities is naturally of much importance since these assays are required to assess both the potency of therapeutic materials and the levels of clotting factors in the patients plasma after treatment. Factor VIII may be assayed by one-stage or two-stage methods. These methods are described in more detail elsewhere (Chapter 3 and by Austen & Rhymes, 1975). As with factor VIII, assays of factor IX may be based on one or two-stage methods. The assays have larger experimental errors than the factor VIII assays. Nevertheless careful assays are essential to safe treatment and even assays with rather large errors are useful since the differences in clotting activity produced by treatment are large.

The patient's response to treatment in relation to plasma volume and weight

If the patient's plasma volume is known then it is theoretically very easy to calculate the effect that a given intravenous dose of activity calculated as units should produce. Suppose for example that the patient's plasma volume is 3 000 ml, that his basic level of factor VIII is zero and that he receives a dose of 1,000 units of factor VIII dissolved in 100 ml of diluent. Then his immediate post-infusion plasma concentration of factor VIII should be:

$$\frac{1,000}{3,100} \times 100 = 32\cdot3\% \ (0\cdot323 \ \text{u/ml})$$

It is of course quite impossible to know the plasma volume of every patient at all times but as an approximation the blood volume may be calculated as a proportion of the patient's weight. We have used a formula by which the plasma volume is obtained as follows:

$$\text{Plasma volume (ml)} = \text{wt. kg} \times 41 \ \text{ml.}$$

By this formula a dose of 41 u/kg given in a small fluid volume should produce a factor VIII concentration in the severely affected patient of about 100% of normal.

Table 5.1. Comparison of calculated with observed plasma volume (from van Gastel *et al*, 1973).

Patient	Weight (kg)	Observed plasma volume	Calculated plamsa volume
CK	80	3310	3280
GO	62·3	2710	2554
NA	64·5	3060	2644
KL	30·5	1360	1250
HU	68·8	2860	2821
VE	55·6	2880	2280
MO	60·5	2510	2480
Mean		2670	2473

Van Gastel *et al* (1973) recorded the actual plasma volumes of a number of haemophilic (factor VIII deficient) patients. The authors have kindly sent us the weights of 7 of these patients. The plasma volumes calculated by our method from the patients' weights and the observed plasma volumes were compared (Table 5.1). It will be seen that there is a reasonable general agreement between the two sets of results, though the calculated plasma volumes are somewhat lower than those observed. The relationship between plasma, volume and weight is certainly not exact and does not hold in the same proportion for patients of different ages, and even for the same patient at different times. For example the plasma volume in small children is a larger proportion of the patient's weight than is the plasma volume of adults. It is nevertheless convenient to measure the dose given to a patient as u/kg and to measure the response of the patient as percentage rise in factor VIII/u/kg. On the assumption that the blood volume is 41 ml/kg the maximum expected rise per u/kg dose in 2·44%. The observed response is nearly always less than 2·44%/u/kg and often very much less. The response of children tends to be less than that of adults.

The response of haemophilia A (factor VIII deficient) patients to treatment

A theoretically constructed diagram to represent a patients response to treatment is given in Figure 5.1. In this figure it is assumed that a patient with an initial factor VIII level of zero receives a dose of factor VIII of 16 u/kg daily for four days. The response to be expected from the initial dose is:

$$\frac{16}{41} \times 100\% = 39\%$$

In the diagram is demonstrated the well known fact that the post infusion plasma concentration is not maintained but falls to half in 12 to 14 hours (Biggs & Denson, 1963).

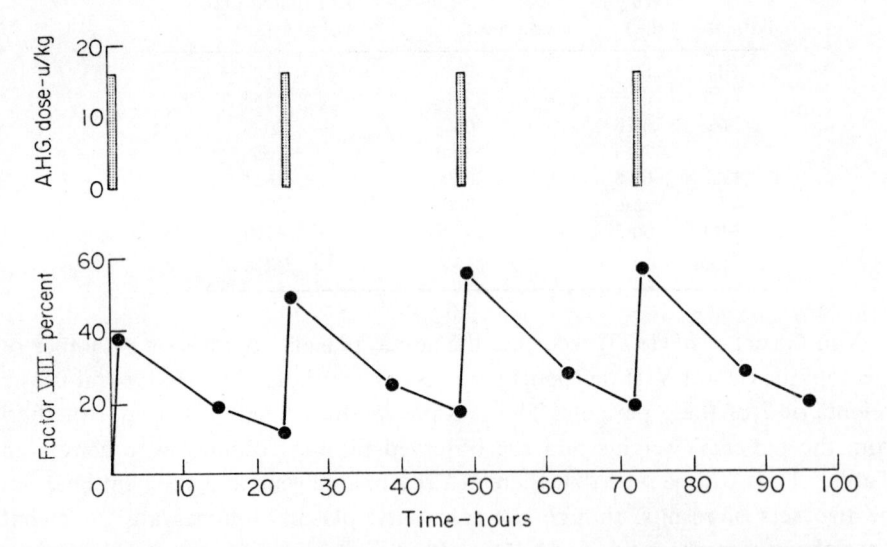

Figure 5.1. The theoretical response of a haemophilic patient receiving a daily dose of antihaemophilic material at a dose of 16 u/kg.

As noted previously the theoretical recovery of activity is seldom achieved. Some patients customarily recover less than the theoretically possible amount of activity in the circulation. When plasma is used as a therapeutic material the plasma volume is substantially increased by the infusion. The therapeutic materials at present available are differently recovered by the 'average' patient.

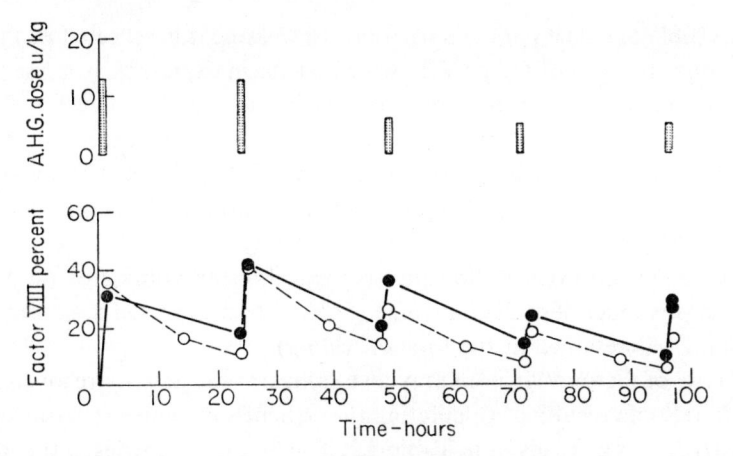

Figure 5.2. The observed and calculated factor VIII concentrations in Case 2 who was treated with daily infusions. The first two days' treatment was with human AHG and for the next 3 days with plasma. The observed response is shown by a continuous line and the theoretical response by a discontinuous line.

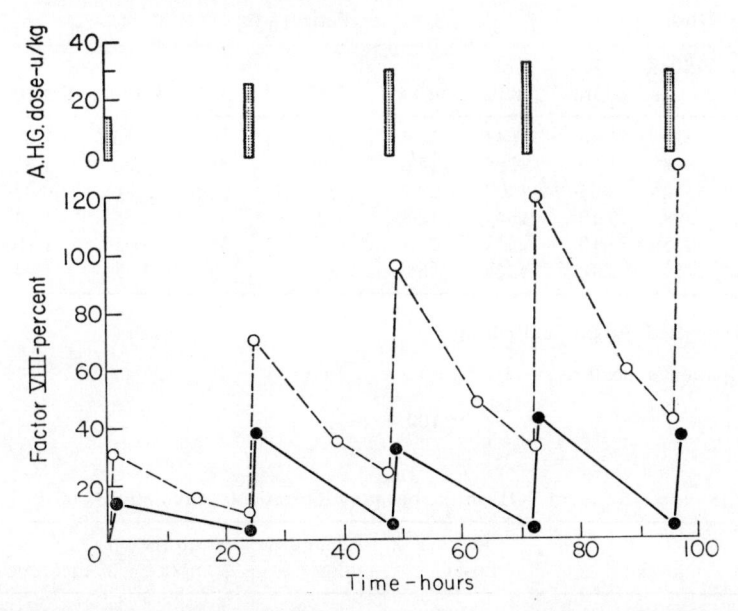

Figure 5.3. The observed and calculated factor VIII concentrations for Case 8 who received daily treatment with human AHG. The observations are shown by a continuous line and the theoretical response by a discontinuous line.

The variation in different patients' responses are illustrated in Figures 5.2 and 5.3 and Tables 5.7, 5.8, 5.9 and 5.10. Using reliable assays for clotting factor activity the dose can be adjusted following an initial assay of response to give the desired post infusion factor VIII concentration. The results of Figure 5.3 are given in detail in Table 5.2. The patient's response to treatment is reflected in the rise in plasma concentration of factor VIII which has been expressed as a rise per u/kg dose. It will be seen that in this case the average rise was 1·13%/u/kg. This gives 46% of the response calculated from the expectation that 41 u/kg should give a rise of 100% or that 1/u/kg should give a rise of 2·44%/u/kg. The response of this patient was less than that which was usual with this particular preparation of factor VIII. In this example the dose volume was not small in relation to the patient's weight but even if allowance is made for the volume of fluid infused the response is much less than average (58% of that expected assuming that all of the fluid was retained at the time of testing).

The type of factor VIII used may also influence the activity recovered in the circulation. Some results of calculating the patient's response in terms of rise in factor VIII %/u/kg are given in Table 5.3. The first three entries in this table are

Table 5.2. The doses given to Case 8 following severe iliacus haematoma. The patient's weight was 47 kg and the material given was human factor VIII concentrate.

	Dose				Patient's reponse			
Day	Volume ml	u/ml	Total units	u/kg	Pre %	Post %	Rise %	Rise/u/kg
1	328	1·96	643	13·6	0	14	14·0	1·03
2	648	1·86	1205	25·6	4·4	38	33·6	1·31
3	552	2·25	1407	29·9	5·4	31·5	25·1	0·87
4	498	3·10	1544	32·8	4·5	45	40·5	1·23
5	435	3·10	1348	28·7	4·5	36	31·5	1·10
6	429	290	1244	26·5	5·2	38	32·5	1·24

The expected rise per unit per kg $= \dfrac{100}{41} = 2\cdot44\%$

The patient's mean rise $= 1\cdot13\%/\text{u/kg}$

% of calculated $= \dfrac{1\cdot13}{2\cdot44} \times 100 = 46\%$

Table 5.3. Recovery of factor VIII in the haemophilic patient's circulation.

Type of material	Number of doses	Mean dose u/kg	Mean rise %/u/kg	% theoretical
Plasma	90	9·29	2·01	82 (96*)
HAHG	183	14·03	1·56	64
Animal factor VIII	59	66·80	1·00	41
Cryoprecipitate (1973)	22	28·04	1·68	69
Oxford factor VIII (1973)	21	5·98	2·31	95
Oxford factor VIII (1974)	70	11·77	1·90	78
Hyland (1973)	34	30·10	2·12	87
Immuno (1973)	14	9·06	1·84	75

* Allowance made for the increase in plasma volume that may have occurred.

derived from data collected before 1966 and the last 5 are based on data collected in 1973 or 1974. In calculating the recovery of activity as percent of theoretical no allowance has been made for the volume of fluid infused except in the case of the plasma infusions. In fact modern concentrated preparations certainly do not cause a measurable increase in plasma volume.

Response of haemophilia B patient's (factor IX deficient patient) to treatment

The response of the factor IX deficient patient may be assessed using the same criteria as for the haemophilic (factor VIII deficient) patients. The response of Christmas disease patients is very variable from one patient to another. Results of tests carried out before 1966 with more recent results are given in Table 5.4. It will be seen that in Christmas disease a relatively small proportion of the dose activity is recovered in the circulation. The dose of factor IX which will achieve haemostasis in Christmas disease must be larger than that of factor VIII in haemophilia. This fact is illustrated in the comparison of doses of factor VIII or IX given to haemophilic or Christmas disease patients before dental extraction (see Tables 6.3 and 6.4).

Table 5.4. Response of Christmas disease patients to treatment.

Therapeutic material	Number of doses	Mean dose u/kg	Mean response %/u/kg	% theoretical
Plasma (pre 1966)	23	16·4	0·54	20
Concentrate (pre 1966)	129	47·1	0·80	33
Concentrate (1973)	15	67·5	0·60	25

The individual variability in response to treatment makes it difficult to compare relative effectiveness of therapeutic material. In five patients who received both plasma and concentrate prior to 1966 there does not seem to be any difference between the two sources of factor IX (Table 5.4).

The half-life of factors VIII and IX following infusion to patients who lack these factors

The effectiveness of treatment with clotting factor preparations depends both on the plasma concentration achieved after infusion and on the length of time for which the factor concentration is achieved.

For haemophilic (factor VIII deficient) patients half of the activity is lost in about 12 to 14 hours (Biggs & Denson, 1963) see also Chapter 6. The rate of loss is quite variable from patient to patient (range 7 to 22 hours) and the rate of loss may be rather more rapid after an initial dose of factor VIII than after the end of a prolonged course of treatment.

For Christmas disease (factor IX deficient patients) the rate of loss of factor IX activity using preparations made before 1966 was rather slower than the loss of factor VIII in haemophilic patients. Half of the infused factor IX activity was lost in 18 to 36 hours. The factor IX made in Oxford (since 1967) by DEAE Sephadex absorption seems to have a rather shorter half-life than the old material made by adsorption onto $Ca_3(PO_4)_2$ (see Chapter 6).

Most preparations of freeze-dried factor VIII or factor IX are presented with reliable estimates of the factor VIII or factor IX activity of the preparation. This means that the preparations can often be used with confidence for patients whose response has been tested without assaying every dose given. For many patients complete data, such as that presented in Figures 5.2 and 5.3, is not available. From incomplete data, when freeze-dried preparations are used, a good deal of information may nevertheless often be extracted. The method by which this can be done is explained using first a hypothetical dose and response graph. It is assumed that the patient's response to treatment is uniform for all doses and that the assay is without error.

Suppose that for the actual time of the operation it is desired to raise the patient's factor VIII to 120% and that after this for 7 days it is required that the level shall not fall below 50%. After this for another 7 days it is desired to keep the factor VIII level above 15%. We then suppose that the patient has a rise of 2% of factor VIII for every 1 u/kg of dose and that the plasma level of factor VIII falls to half in 12 hours after a dose. In this hypothetical example the objectives will be achieved by giving 1 dose of 60 u/kg immediately before operation followed by a dose of 30 u/kg the same evening. Thereafter the patient would receive 25 u/kg morning and evening for the first week and 25 u/kg once daily for a further week. The expected daily record is shown in Figure 5.4a.

In this diagram the observations are plotted to show the highest clotting factor levels achieved in the post-infusion sample, on any particular day (upper line) and the lowest level in that day which occurs at the immediate pre-infusion time. At no time can the patient's plasma factor VIII concentration fall outside the boundaries marked by the two lines. Since it is proposed to use the same style of diagram to illustrate the actual records of surgical cases it is worth considering the effects of various changed conditions on the pattern obtained. Suppose first that when factor VIII is given to a patient the rise in factor VIII level is 1% per unit/kg dose instead of 2% as assumed in Figure 5.4a. In this second case the results would look like those of Figure 5.4b. Considering a patient with this sort

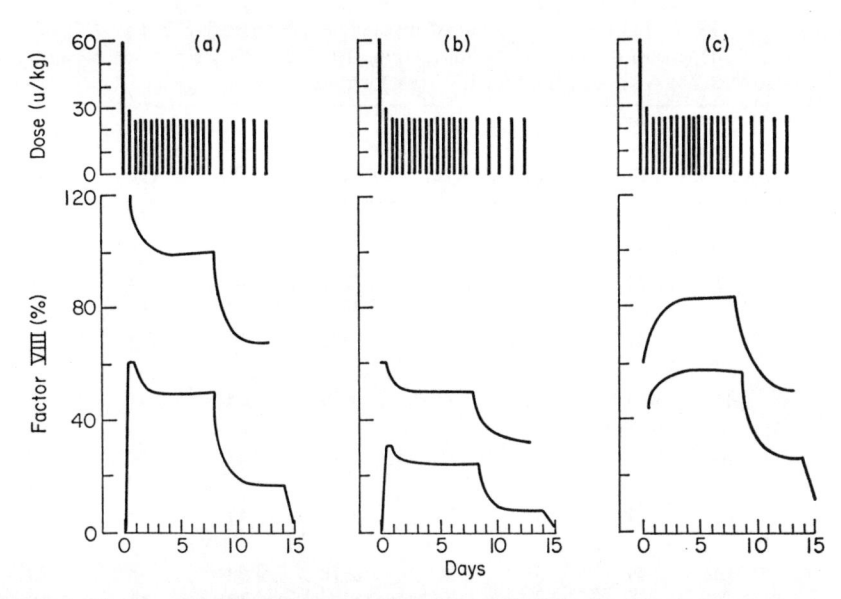

Figure 5.4. Diagrams of the response of supposed haemophilia A patients to therapy assuming a constant dosage scheme (see text) and constant known values for the response to treatment (%/u/kg) and half life of the infused activity. The upper curves in each case represent post-infusion plasma factor VIII and the lower graph the pre-infusion factor VIII. (a) The patient's response to treatment was assumed to be 2%/u/kg and the half-life of infused factor VIII 12 hours. (b) The patient's response to treatment was assumed to be 1%/u/kg and the half life of the infused activity 12 hours. (c) The patient's response to treatment was assumed to be 1%/u/kg and the half life of infused activity 24 hours.

of response one would need to double the dose of factor VIII in order to maintain the factor VIII plasma level between 50 and 100%. Another variable to be taken into account is the duration in the circulation of the infused activity. For Figure 5.4a and b, a half life of 12 hours was assumed. In Figure 5.4c it is assumed that the patient's response was 1%/u/kg (as in Figure 5.4b) but that the half life was 24 hours instead of 12 hours. In this case the objectives set for Figure 5.4a are achieved despite the low response to each dose. Thus individual responses for particular patients must affect the results.

To illustrate the actual case reports one example has been worked out in detail. This patient (Table 5.5 and Figure 5.5) received factor VIII to a total of about 22,000 units in 11 days; he was operated on for the removal of a piece of myositis ossificans. The procedure for analysing the results is carried out in several stages.

1 The first step in analysing the results is to estimate the factor VIII value of the commercial therapeutic material given to the patient. This material was assayed on 6 occasions and the mean of the six results was 265 u/ampoule Since the numbers of ampoules given at each dose was known, the dose expressed as

Table 5.5. Case 178 treated for the removal of myotisis ossificans using factor VIII of average dose value (mean of 8 doses) of 268 u/amp. The patient's weight was 68 kg. The response was 2% u/kg and the half life was 16 hours.

		Observed factor VIII results %				Calculated values		
Day	Dose u/kg	Pre	Post	Rise	Rise/u/kg	Pre	Post	Rise %
1	62	0	110	110	1·77	0	124	124
	3*					73	79	6
2	27	35	100	65	2·40	47	101	54
	16					59	91	32
3	27	42	94	52	1·92	54	108	54
	12					64	88	24
4	23	53	92	39	1·69	52	98	46
	12					58	82	24
5	16					48	80	32
	16					47	79	32
6	16	41	64	23	1·43	47	79	32
	12					47	71	24
7	12	49	75	26	2·16	42	66	24
	8					39	55	16
8	8	42	65	23	2·87	32	48	16
	8					28	44	16
9	8	34	49	15	1·87	26	42	16
	8					25	41	16
10	16					24	56	32
11	16					20	52	32
Mean					2·01			

* NHS factor VIII.

u/kg could be calculated for every day (column 2 of Table 5.5) even if the dose was not assayed on a particular day.

2 Pre- and post-infusion levels of factor VIII were recorded on 8 occasions (columns 3 and 4 of Table 5.5), from these the observed rise in factor VIII level, can be calculated (column 5 of Table 5.5). The observed rise in level in percent may be divided by the dose in u/kg to give the observed rise %/u/kg or response (column 6 of Table 5.5). These 8 observed values can be averaged and in this case it was found that the average response was 2%/u/kg).

3 From the dose in u/kg and the average response the expected (calculated) rise in level of factor VIII for each dose can be calculated (column 9 of Table 5.5.)

4 The rate of fall-off of factor VIII is then *assumed* to be some particular value say a half life of 12 hours. It is then possible to construct a table of calculated pre-and post-infusion factor VIII levels in respect of all of the doses given (columns 7 and 8 of Table 5.5).

Plasma Concentrations of Factor VIII and Factor IX 119

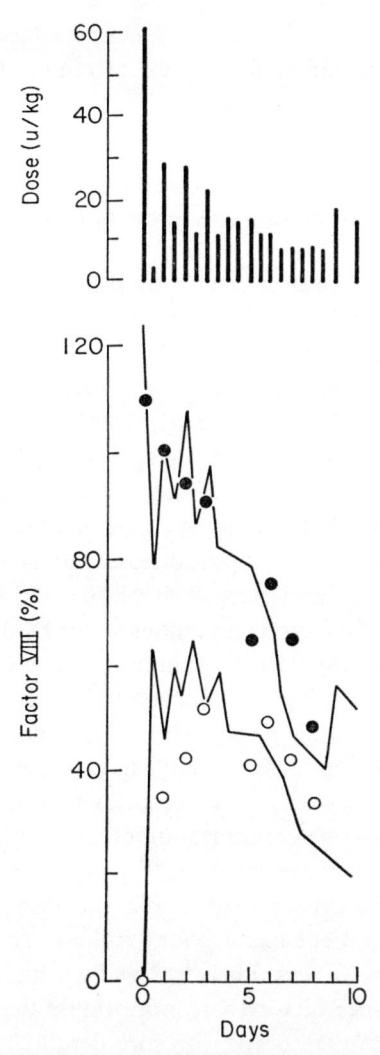

Figure 5.5. The response of Case 178 to treatment (see also Table 5.5). The continuous lines represent the calculated pre and post infusion levels of factor VIII (see Figure 5.4). The solid circles represent observed post-infusion factor VIII levels and the open circles represent the observed pre-infusion factor VIII levels. The patient's response to treatment was 2·01%/u/kg and the half-life of infused activity was 16 hours.

5 The calculated results are then plotted as highest and lowest levels for the day and the observed results are inserted in the correct places (Figure 5.5). Should the observed and calculated results not correspond the calculations under 4 above are repeated assuming a different disappearance rate for infused factor VIII. In the present example the assumption best fitted to the results was a half life of 16 hours and it is the figures derived from this assumption that are

given in columns 7 and 8 of Table 5.5. Diagrams based on this method of computation appear in Chapter 6 and can of course be applied to patients having haemophilia B.

Whole blood or plasma as sources of factor VIII or IX

Whole blood cannot be administered to patients in large quantities and the concentration of factors VIII or IX in the whole blood are low. One or two bottles of whole blood given to a haemophilic patient could never be expected to raise the plasma concentration of factor VIII above 10% of normal and for a Christmas disease patient levels above 5% would be unlikely. Whole blood should be given only to correct anaemia due to acute blood loss. Haemostasis must be achieved using concentrates of factor VIII or IX.

Plasma derived from whole blood by centrifugation is more useful in the treatment of haemophilia and Christmas disease than is whole blood. Assuming the best possible collection and storage of plasma the level of factor VIII is likely to be of the order of 0·6 u/ml and that of factor IX 0·8 u/ml. Because of the risk of overloading the circulation the volume that can be given to a patient at any one time is limited by the high protein content of plasma. In Oxford we have used doses between 15 and 22 ml/kg. Plasma is usually presented in bottles each containing 400 to 450 mls. Thus if the whole bottle is always used the dose expressed as ml/kg will vary very much according to the weight of the patient (Table 5.6). The rise in plasma concentration of factor VIII to be expected from the doses suggested is of the order of 18–26%. Very often of course the response is less because the plasma causes a substantial increase in the patient's plasma volume or because the patient has a poor response. In the case of factor IX deficient patients the dose value is likely to be a little higher than that for factor VIII deficient patients since factor IX is more stable than factor VIII. On the other hand the patient's response is considerably worse than that of haemophilic patients.

Table 5.6. The dose of plasma related to the weight of the patients with haemophilia or Christmas disease and the expected response of factor VIII or factor IX.

Weight of patient kg	Dose volume used	ml/kg	Dose value u/kg VIII	IX	Expected rise in factor VIII %	Expected rise in factor IX %
20–30	450	15–22	9–13	12–17	18–26	6–9
40–60	900	15–22	9–13	12–17	18–26	6–9
70–90	1350	15–19	9–11	12–14	18–22	6–7

The use of plasma therapy for patients with haemophilia and Christmas disease is limited by the volume of this material that can safely be given to the patient. The post infusion plasma concentrations that can be achieved are too low to produce safe haemostasis for both haemophilic and Christmas disease patients. Moreover a proportion of patients with haemophilia and Christmas disease may have serious reactions to plasma infusions as a result of sensitization to plasma components other than factors VIII or IX (see Chapter 9). There is now seldom any reason to use plasma to treat haemophilic patients or those with Christmas disease since safe and reliable concentrates of factors VIII and IX are now widely available.

Concentrated preparations from human plasma used as source of factor VIII

There are now several preparations of factor VIII made from human plasma available for treating patients with haemophilia. The properties of these materials is dealt with in detail in Chapter 4. The characteristics of the preparations that most affect their usefulness for the patient are given in Table 5.7. From the point of view of the doctor giving the infusion the important things are that the dose should be presented in a conveniently small volume and that reconstitution of the dose should be easy and rapid. There are naturally other considerations which affect the choice of material such as availability, economy in the use of blood products and the complications of treatment. These aspects are considered in Chapters 4 and 8.

Probably most doctors would choose the high purity preparations if convenience were the only deciding issue. The materials which should become more generally available in the near future are cryoprecipitate and intermediate purity

Table 5.7. Therapeutic materials available for the treatment of patients having haemophilia

Preparation	Activity u/ml	Protein g/100 ml	Purification	Volume* to give 10% rise	Protein to give 10% rise
Plasma	0.6	6.2	1	417	25.8
Cryoprecipitate (Oxford)	9.6	4.2	16	26	1.1
NHS intermediate purity factor VIII	7.5	3.5	18	33	1.2
NHS high purity factor VIII	15.0	0.9	130	17	0.15
Commercial human factor VIII	25.0	2.7	65	10	0.27

* The volume is calculated to contain 250 units of factor VIII activity which is the amount required to produce a rise of 10% in a patient weighing 50 kg (average patient weight).

Table 5.8. The response of 15 haemophilic patients to cryoprecipitate in 1973.

Case	Number of doses	Mean dose u/kg	Mean rise %	Mean rise %/u/kg*
160	2	21·13	41	2·28
164	4	25·15	43	1·80
9	2	30·34	57	1·92
165	2	35·35	61	1·76
166	2	35·52	37	1·11
154	1	30·03	40	1·33
167	1	39·44	76	1·93
51	1	40·00	68	1·76
26	1	46·67	55	1·18
61	1	20·96	35	1·67
168	1	31·25	34	1·09
169	1	32·25	34	1·53
8	1	11·20	20	1·79
170	1	26·67	74	2·77
171	1	32·46	42	1·29
Mean				1·68

* When more than one dose was given the results are means for the separate values and are not derived by dividing the mean dose by the mean rise in factor VIII.

Table 5.9. Response of 14 haemophilic patients to intermediate purity freeze dried factor VIII 1973.

Patient	Number of doses	Mean dose u/kg	Mean rise %	Mean rise %/u/kg*
91	2	8·97	17	2·03
153	3	5·53	13	2·27
154	2	8·56	25	3·22
63	2	7·36	13	1·84
155	2	5·50	15	2·74
156	1	7·05	8	1·13
157	1	5·10	11	2·16
179	1	3·41	9	2·64
158	1	4·33	10	2·31
159	1	8·29	11	1·33
160	2	3·01	13	4·32
161	1	9·45	19	2·01
162	1	5·80	13	2·24
163	1	6·31	13	2·06
Mean				2·31

* When more than one dose was given the results are means for the separate values and are not derived by dividing the mean dose by the mean rise in factor VIII.

Table 5.10. Response of 10 haemophilic patients to human commercial factor VIII.

Case	Number of doses	Mean dose units	Mean rise %	Mean rise %/u/kg*
94	8	38·2	62	1·43
172	3	27·7	57	2·15
173	1	12·3	34	2·80
174	5	35·9	78	2·25
154	2	28·9	56	1·93
176	3	49·6	74	1·48
177	2	29·7	71	2·65
178	6	25·7	50	2·22
161	2	87·40	70	1·68
Mean				2·12

* When more than one dose was given the results are means for the separate values and are not derived by dividing the mean dose by the mean rise in factor VIII.

factor VIII. When dissolved for use it will be seen that these two preparations have on average about the same general properties. However, the two are far from equally convenient. The cryoprecipitate dose value is not assayed before infusion and may vary very much from one centre to another. The dose must usually be assembled into one container by thawing, dissolving and washing out the contents of 5–30 single plastic bags.

Examples of response to 3 types of human material are given in Tables 5.8, 5.9 and 5.10.

Animal factor VIII in the treatment of haemophilia A.

Before the introduction of cryoprecipitate, factor VIII made from bovine or porcine plasma was used for many patients to protect them during essential major surgical procedures. The treatment was haemostatically very effective but the patients often suffered reactions and they developed resistance to treatment after 7 to 10 days treatment. In addition a retrospective study showed a somewhat higher than expected incidence of factor VIII antibodies in patients previously treated with animal factor VIII. Thus today in countries where human concentrates are available the animal material should not be used for patients who do not have factor VIII antibodies. Where the human material is not available then the animal preparations should still be useful. From Table 5.3 it will be seen that the patient's response to animal factor VIII is less than to human preparations; examples of individual responses to animal factor VIII are in Table 5.11.

Table 5.11. Response of 10 haemophilic patients to porcine factor VIII. Data collected prior to 1966.

Case	Number of doses	Mean dose u/kg	Mean rise %	Mean rise %/u/kg*
9	7	71	85	1·20
10	3	47	40	0·85
7	5	73	62	0·85
11	5	87	64	0·74
12	7	66	67	1·02
13	8	76	55	0·72
14	7	77	95	1·23
15	6	84	63	0·75
2	6	37	49	1·32
16	5	50	68	1·36
Mean				1·004

* When more than one dose was given the results are means for the separate values and are not derived by dividing the mean dose by the mean rise in factor VIII.

Calculation of the dose of factor VIII for haemophilic patients

The dose may be calculated using the relationships established between the rise in plasma concentration of clotting factor and the dose in u/kg. An approximate idea of the dose for haemophilic patients can be derived from the average response of the average patient. As will be seen in Table 5.3 the average response of the average haemophilic patient to human concentrates available in 1973 and 1974 is about 2% per u/kg dose. Thus if the desired rise in concentration of factor VIII is established by clinical judgement then the dose will be:

$$\text{Desired rise in factor VIII \%} = \frac{2 \times \text{units of dose}}{\text{body wt. in kg}}$$

or

Dose units = body weight in kg × 0·5 × desired rise in factor VIII %

In the case of children it is wise to assume a rise of 1·5%/u/kg instead of 2%/u/kg. Thus for children the dose would be:

Body wt. in kg × 0·67 × desired rise in factor VIII %.

The response of factor IX deficient patients to factor IX concentrate and the calculation of the dose of factor IX

The response of factor IX deficient patients to factor IX concentrate is similar to their response to plasma. The concentrates at present available are all uniformly satisfactory and have on average given (in 1973) the response of 0·6% rise per u/kg dose.

The dose may be calculated in exactly the same manner as for factor VIII deficient patients:

$$\text{Desired rise in factor IX \%} = \frac{0\cdot 6 \times \text{units of dose}}{\text{body wt. in kg}}$$

or

$$\text{Dose units} = \text{body weight in kg} \times 1\cdot 7 \times \text{desired rise in factor IX \%}.$$

Conclusion

With available concentrates of factors VIII and IX which have reliably assayed potencies the treatment of patients with haemophilia and Christmas disease is easier. It is easier to obtain the plasma concentration of clotting factor that is desired. In a hospital which is not a haemophilia centre emergency first-aid treatment of a haemophilic patient with freeze-dried concentrate may simply require the intravenous administration of a calculated dose. Cryoprecipitate is less reliable under such circumstances since the dose value in units cannot be predicted before it is given to the patient. It is thus much safer for cryoprecipitate, which must still be used, to be given at haemophilia centres and when the need arises emergency treatment at other hospitals should consist of freeze-dried preparations.

Though the administration of a calculated dose of factor VIII or factor IX is easy, the day to day management of the patients is time consuming and requires much experience, patience, knowledge and tolerance of human nature. Most patients seldom attend hospital, the hospital staff at many clinics are not obliged to be familiar with and good tempered about all of the patients' individual preferences. On the whole patients are expected to tolerate the peculiarities of the hospital staff rather than the other way round. The haemophilic patient is a patient for life and the hospital staff must learn to appreciate each individual patient and must have the time to talk to patients and play with children from which such understanding grows. It is now for this reason mainly that patients should be treated at haemophilia centres.

References

AUSTEN D.E.G. & RHYMES I.L. (1975) *A Laboratory Manual of Blood Coagulation*. Blackwell Scientific Publications, Oxford.

BANGHAM D.E., BIGGS R., BROZEVICH M., DENSON K.W.E. & SKEGG J.L. (1971) A biological standard for measurement of blood coagulation factor VIII activity. *Bulletin of the World Health Organisation,* **45,** 337.

BIGGS R. & DENSON K.W.E. (1963) The fate of prothrombin and factors VIII, IX and X transfused to patients deficient in these factors. *British Journal of Haematology,* **9,** 532.

GASTEL C. VAN., SIXMA J.J., BORST-EILERS E.C.S., LEAUTAUD M., MOES M., PLAS P.M. VAN DER, BOUMA B.N. & SUBESMA J. PH. (1973) Preparation and infusion of cryoprecipitate from exercised donors. *British Journal of Haematology,* **25,** 461.

Chapter 6. The Control of Haemostasis in Haemophilic Patients

ROSEMARY BIGGS &
C. R. RIZZA

Factor VIII and the control of haemostasis is the background to a way of life for the haemophiliac as insulin and the control of carbohydrate metabolism is for the diabetic. The haemophilic patient has a to live and learn to live with certain limitations to his freedom of action. It is the work of the doctor and other haemophilia centre staff to make the limitation as small as possible. As more therapeutic materials become available the role of the doctor is changing. The doctor who cared for the haemophiliac in the past often had a number of very sick haemophilic patients in hospital and was constantly disturbed at night by the need to give emergency treatment to patients having life-endangering episodes of bleeding. Now the doctor administers routine out-patient care to patients who are usually well, and, though night calls remain frequent, the calls are usually for less dangerous bleeding episodes than in the past. Haemophilic bleeding which is treated early does not progress to dangerous complications.

The clinical condition of the population of haemophilic patients is also changing with time. Table 6.1 gives a guide to the probable present status of severely affected haemophilic patients in the United Kingdom. Because of the previous shortage of therapeutic materials one can be certain that the majority of patients who are older than 40 will have severe permanent damage to joints and many patients who would now have been in this age group have died as a result of bleeding episodes which would now be considered to be trivial (e.g. epistaxis, the extraction of one tooth, etc). The patients in the young adult group (20–40) have not died of minor bleeding episodes but passed their early years with severely restricted activity. Most of them had many damaging bleeds into joints and muscles and spent many months in orthopaedic hospitals trying to ameliorate the results of previous bleeding. The patients in the 10 to 20 years age group are in a better state but most of them will have suffered some seriously damaging joint bleeds. Patients in this age group nevertheless have their whole working lives ahead and can learn to live reasonably normal lives and hopefully preserve their musculo-skeletal system from further serious damage. For the patients in the age group 0–10 we can now see over the mountain. It should be

Table 6.1. The probable age distribution of haemophilia A patients in the United Kingdom.

Date of birth	Age in 1974	Probable number of patients	Probable clinical conditions of the patients
1900–1934	40+	618	Most patients have severe crippling deformity of some joints
1935–1954	20–39	1040	Many in this age group have some permanent joint damage
1955–1964	10–19	755	Some patients in this age group have nearly normal joints and muscles
1965–1974	0–9	587	These should all be physically normal

possible to bring these children up without serious joint damage, as normal, if somewhat handicapped members of society.

Treatment of haemophilia will be considered under three main headings:

1 The treatment of episodes of so called spontaneous bleeding. This type of bleeding occurs in the severely affected patient and the bleeding is not preceded by any remembered injury or obvious cause. The commonest sites for such bleeding are muscles and joints but many other sites may be involved.
2 The control of bleeding after dental extraction.
3 The control of bleeding after surgical operations.

Spontaneous bleeding into soft tissues, muscles and joints

The natural history of an untreated bleeding episode into a joint or muscle is as follows: The patient has a sensation of heat or stiffness in the affected part. As time passes the joint or muscle swells and great pain occurs. Joint movement is then prevented by muscle spasm and the limb becomes temporarily useless. The whole process from slight stiffness to an intensely painful, useless limb may take a few hours to several days. If the condition is not relieved the swelling particularly of muscles may affect important structures such as nerves and arteries causing nerve palsies or gangrene. In the long term there may be permanent structural deformity due to contractures of muscles or actual destruction of muscles and bones. Some pictures of the disastrous effects of haemorrhage are shown (Figure 1.6).

The natural progress can be halted at any of the early stages by the administration of suitable amounts of factor VIII. In general the earlier the treatment the quicker the reversal of symptoms and the less the lasting damage and the less factor VIII required for treatment. In the past the pros and cons of aspirating swollen joints in haemophilic patients were discussed. When a joint cavity is swollen and contains enough blood to warrant its removal by aspiration, the joint may be so severely damaged that it may never revert to complete normality; such grossly swollen joints should be aspirated.

The effectiveness of early treatment is illustrated by the fact that in 10 out of 12 bleeds treated at the Treloar College, one infusion was enough to stop the bleeding and little time was spent in the sick bay with disability. The Treloar College is a residential school for boys where those with haemophilia are under constant supervision and treatment is thus always given early. A patient who arrives at hospital with a painful swollen joint may need to spend time in hospital with daily infusions of factor VIII and thereafter may require more infusions to protect him during physiotherapy designed to restore normal movement in convalescence.

The general programme for early treatment is that the patient should receive a dose of factor VIII of between 5–15 u/kg as soon as possible after the onset of bleeding. The size of the dose is adjusted according to the experience of the physician. Some sites of bleeding are more dangerous than others. If the patient is an out-patient who lives a long way away it is important to be sure that a return visit for treatment will not be required within the next day or two. Experience with individual patients will also affect the decision. An older patient with a haemorrhage into a previously damaged joint may require high dosage for every new episode. Some patients without antibodies to factor VIII have a poor response to treatment and may always require high dosage to achieve a good plasma concentration of factor VIII.

In some patients the main complaint may be repeated bleeding into one particular joint. The reason for the localisation of bleeding is not usually obvious. It may be suggested that some particularly damaging bleed has occurred in the past and that inadequate treatment was given for this first occurrence of bleeding. Thereafter the joint developed chronic inflammatory changes which predisposed to future bleeding after every trivial injury. When bleeding recurs frequently in one joint it may be desirable to give a more or less prolonged course of regular infusions to maintain, for a time, nearly normal haemostasis (prophylaxis). For example, in the case of factor VIII deficiency, daily infusions of factor VIII accompanied by progressively vigorous physiotherapy may be given for 1–4 weeks and after this time infusions may be given 3 times a week for some months. It is our experience that a particularly damaged joint may gradually improve with such treatment until bleeds are no more frequent in the one 'bad' joint than in any other joint.

It has been suggested that single chronically inflamed knee joints should be treated by synovectomy and good results have been claimed for this operation

(Storti *et al*, 1970). This operation has been carried out on several of our patients with very chronic knee joint damage and we are still uncertain if any benefit is to be attributed to the operation. It is our opinion that a course of prophylaxis, as outlined above, should always be tried before the operation of synovectomy is even contemplated.

When a hip joint is irretrievably damaged and is causing severe pain and disability the operation of cup arthroplasty or total hip replacement may be undertaken. Fourteen patients have had hip replacement in Oxford and their cases have been reviewed by Duthie (1975). All of these patients have very greatly improved mobility and no complications or failure of this operation have been observed.

It is likely that chronically damaged joints result from inadequate treatment of previous severe haemarthroses. Thus when a patient presents at hospital with a hot, painful, swollen joint it is wise to be certain that recovery from this episode is complete. Several injections of factor VIII may be needed and the doctor should be certain that full power and movement has been restored before supervision is relaxed.

Spontaneous bleeding into specific sites other than joints

Superficial haematomata which are black and blue are seldom dangerous even though they may be very large. These bruises resolve after one or two infusions of clotting factor concentrate. There are some sites of bleeding that are more dangerous.

Haematomata of the scalp are common in small boys and since the scalp is firmly connected to the underlying skull the blood has little opportunity to spread. These bruises may become very lumpy swellings and may even lead to necrosis of the overlying skin; they must always be treated as early as possible and resolution must be seen to be occurring before daily infusions of factor VIII are discontinued. Injuries to the head must in any case be regarded as potentially serious since they may be accompanied by intracranial bleeding.

Haematomata into the floor of the mouth and tongue may often extend into the neck. These haemorrhages are very dangerous. The patient should be brought immediately to hospital. If he is on home therapy he should have twice his normal dose of factor VIII before starting the journey. He should be admitted to hospital and treated to maintain the factor VIII at 50% of normal until swelling subsides. If the swelling is marked on admission he should be seen by an anaesthetist and an ENT specialist in case intubation or tracheotomy should be needed.

Deep muscle haematomata

Deep muscle haematomata are as important if not more important than haemarthroses as a cause of crippling. Haemorrhage into muscle can sometimes be very slow to resolve even with intensive factor VIII or factor IX replacement and may cause irreversible muscle damage muscle scarring and contraction. It is extremely important that muscle haemorrhage be treated quickly with a high dose of factor VIII or factor IX. The peculiar danger of muscle haematomata lies in the fact that the blood is retained within the muscle sheath and results in considerable pressure and pain. Such developed muscle haematomata cause great damage and often permanent crippling deformity. The site of bleeding should be immobilised as completely as possible in the position of comfort since immobility lessens the pain and prevents the continuation of bleeding. Patients who have neglected muscle haematoma may require much hospital care and treatment. The plasma level of factor VIII must be maintained at about 50% of normal for several days until the pain and swelling are much reduced. Thereafter daily infusions and progressive physiotherapy may be needed to restore normal function. If these measures fail to restore normal function it may be necessary, at a late date, to carry out reconstructive surgery such as tendon lengthening or a muscle slide operation. Haematomata into various muscle groups have their own special dangers.

Iliacus haematomata may involve the femoral nerve with loss of sensation on the front of the thigh and loss of power in the quadriceps femoris muscle. In addition haemorrhage into the right iliacus muscle often gives rise to most of the symptoms of appendicitis. Such cases need careful examination bearing in mind the statistical fact that the haemophiliac is much more likely to have an iliacus haematoma than appendicitis. The finding of impaired femoral nerve function of recent onset as well as a falling haemoglobin level and a tender mass in the right iliac fossa support the diagnosis of iliacus haematoma.

Haemorrhage into the forearm muscles may be accompanied by nerve compression and even loss of all use of the hand and ultimately gangrene of the fingers. Haemorrhage into the calf muscles may lead to destruction of muscle, obstruction of the blood and nerve supply to the foot and to contracture.

Massive muscle haematoma at any site which are not treated immediately and continuously until resolution and restoration of function has occurred may progress to form chronic cysts which may cause lasting and progressive destruction of surrounding tissue. Finally muscle haematomas should never be incised or aspirated. The blood in the haematoma infiltrates the muscle tissue and there is no pool of blood to be aspirated or released.

In 1966, when the first edition of this book was written, case histories of patients who had dangerous muscle haematomata were presented. It is hoped that such cases will now seldom be seen.

Other types of spontaneous bleeding

Haematuria, epistaxis and gastro-intestinal bleeding all occur in haemophiliacs but are not encountered so frequently as bleeding into muscles and joints. Haematuria may be very persistent and may require high dosage (25–50 u/kg) to ensure cessation of bleeding. Prednisolone does not in our experience control bleeding when given in association with factor VIII treatment. Neither EACA nor Cyclokapron should be given to patients while they have haematuria. If these antifibrinolytic drugs are given the ureter and calyx of the kidney may become filled with hard rubbery clots which may obstruct the passage of urine.

Gastrointestinal bleeding is usually associated with some lesion of the stomach or duodenum such as a small erosion or ulcer. Aspirin ingestion is an important cause of gastrointestinal haemorrhage. Patients may lose very large amounts of blood into the gastrointestinal tract. Treatment consists in the forbidding of aspirin compounds, the administration of factor VIII and if required, transfusion of whole blood. Persistent or recurrent bleeding may have to be treated by the standard operation for gastric or duodenal ulcer.

The treatment of the spontaneous type of bleeding in patients who have Christmas disease (factor IX) deficiency

The treatment of the 'spontaneous' type of bleeding in Christmas disease patients is the same as that given for haemophilic patients with the exception that about twice the dose of factor IX, expressed as u/kg is required. Thus if 8 u/kg of factor VIII would be considered to be adequate for a haemophilic patient then 16 u/kg would be needed for an equivalent lesion in a Christmas disease patient.

The administration of factor VIII or factor IX to the patient

The average number of infusions of factor VIII given annually to a haemophilic patient depend on the amount of material available and on the policy of a particular clinic. These two factors are closely linked. Poor supplies promote a careful parsimonious attitude in the doctor and sometimes even the fixed belief that it is better for the patient not to be treated too often. In Oxford the average number of infusions given to each patient every year has been steadily increasing since 1970 (Table 10.1) from 9–11 prior to 1970 to 24·4 in 1974. The NIHL (1972) survey of haemophilia treatment in the USA showed about 30 infusions annually given to each severely affected adult during the years 1970 and 1971 and substantially more frequent doses were given to children and adolescents. At the Treloar College at Alton the boys resident at the school would have received about 32·5 infusions annually had the rate of infusions given during school terms been continued over the holiday periods (Rainsford & Hall, 1973). We are far from certain that there is any 'optimum' average number of infusions to be given to each patient but the higher rate of infusions in recent years is certainly due to the fact that progressively more and more treatment has been given for spontaneous bleeding into joints and muscles (see also Chapter 4).

At this stage it may be worth considering the situation of a family of mother and father and two small children one of whom is a haemophiliac and less than 10 years old. If the child has on average 18 occasions on which he needs treatment every year then approximately every three weeks he will have to be taken to hospital. Were it possible to predict and plan for this hospital visit the family could usually make arrangements quite easily. But the need arises at random at any hour of any day or night. In the day time mother must make sudden arrangements for the normal child and husband, she must drive or arrange transport for the haemophilic child, she must notify the hospital that she is coming and she must reckon that 3–4 hours will be so spent.

One may consider the actual probable time intervals that may occur between visits in a period of 10 years calculated from the Poisson series (Table 6.2). It will be seen that taken over a 10 year period of time, intervals between visits of one week or less will occur on 50 occasions and at the other hand there will be 12 time intervals exceeding two months free of visits to hospital.

The disruption and insecurity occasioned by this random occurrence of bleeding is easy to see. The family must live as near to a haemophilia centre as possible and the father cannot envisage frequent moves to improve his situation

Table 6.2. Distribution of time intervals of 1 week between visits to hospital over a 10 year period for a patient who on average needs to visit hospital once every 3 weeks.

Time interval in weeks between visits	Number of visits with the given time interval during 10 years
0–1	50·4
1–2	37·8
2–3	25·2
3–4	18·0
4–5	9·0
5–6	7·2
6–7	5·4
8+	12·6
Total	180·0

in life; he also cannot easily take a post in a distant part of the world. Holidays must be planned in advance and may, and usually will, be disturbed by attempts to obtain treatment at a strange hospital. Schooling is interrupted and the child may not be admitted to an ordinary school and must make what progress he can with a few hours of home tuition every week. Above all every day that passes is lived with the knowledge that at any particular second in time the need may arise to drop everything and make a visit to hospital.

It is easy to see that there must be occasions and circumstances when patients delay a visit to hospital. In the evening for example, the parents may go out and leave the children with a baby sitter. Then no decision about a hospital visit will be taken until the parents return home. Many children dread visits to hospital and for such children there will always be a tendency to let a few hours elapse to see if the bleeding will stop without treatment. If the Haemophilia Centre is at a considerable distance from the patient's home this will also cause delay in obtaining treatment.

Home therapy and prophylaxis

The difficulties of treating every episode of bleeding in hospital has convinced many doctors and patients that the only way to an easier and safer life for patients lies in home therapy. For this form of therapy the patient, or a relative, is instructed in the art of intravenous therapy and a supply of suitable factor VIII or factor IX is kept in the home. This form of therapy has many advantages but involves a special course of instruction for patients; an organisation by which a close link is maintained for consultation between doctor and patient at all times and a willingness on the part of the doctor to relinquish some of his or her medical authority to the patient. Home therapy is so important that a special chapter has been devoted to the subject.

The maintenance at all times of normal haemostasis by frequent regular doses of factor VIII or IX, would presumably prevent all abnormal bleeding and enable the patient having haemophilia A or B to lead a normal life. There are several reasons why such prophylactic treatment has not been applied to large numbers of haemophiliacs. The infused activity lasts for such a short duration in the circulation that infusions would need to be given daily or at least on alternative days to be effective for haemophilia A patients (Aronstam *et al,* 1976). Since even severely affected patients bleed so irregularly and sometimes have periods of 3–4 weeks and more with no bleeding, prophylaxis would be wasteful of therapeutic material and in any case there is not enough material for such treatment of all patients to be feasible. In addition infusion therapy has complications such as hepatitis, antibodies to coagulation factor etc. (see Chapter 9), which are dangerous and it seems wise at present to give the least amount of treatment compatible with prevention of crippling and the promotion of reasonably normal activities. It is our opinion that regular treatment should be restricted to circumscribed periods of time and directed for the care of particularly intransigent types of bleeding.

The dental care of patients having haemophilia or Christmas disease

In addition to restriction of sweets and starch in the diet the care of teeth in the normal population involves regular teeth cleaning with fluoride toothpaste, the regular scaling of teeth to prevent periodontal disease and regular inspection of the teeth for dental caries and the filling of the carious teeth to prevent the need for their extraction and the carrying out of orthodontic treatment to ensure that cleaning remains effective. Such care based on six-monthly visits to a dentist runs into difficulties in the case of haemophilic patients. One problem is that there may not be enough dentists in a particular area to cater for all the patients. The second difficulty is that many patients dread visiting the dentist because they fear the pain and discomfort of the drill. The dentist may also be reluctant to carry out even the simplest orthodontic procedure because the patient has haemophilia. It is a reasonable aspiration for normal people and for haemophiliacs to retain useful natural teeth into old age. The knowledge of the role of fluoride in early childhood in protecting against caries, the great improvements in orthodontic technique and the increased numbers of dentists all make this objective realisable. Dental extraction will always be a hazard (though a decreasing one) to a haemophilic patient and this makes conservation of teeth particularly desirable for these patients.

If fillings become necessary these should, if possible, be carried out without local anaesthesia. If the patient will not tolerate fillings without local anaesthetics, then papillary infiltration for front teeth is in our experience quite safe. If injections are required for filling molar teeth the haemophilia specialist should be informed by the dentist so that an infusion of factor VIII or factor IX can be given just prior to the dental appointment.

The most important aspect of this conservative care is the co-operation arranged between the dentist and haemophilia specialist so that individual plans may be made for each patient.

Dental extraction in haemophilia A patients

The amount of factor VIII treatment required to control any particular episode of haemophilic bleeding depends very much on the trauma which caused the bleeding. Although so called spontaneous bleeding is the commonest and most important type of bleeding in haemophilic patients the defect in the vessel walls through which blood escapes is small and each such episode of spontaneous bleeding requires a relatively low dosage of clotting factor for its control. The trauma caused by dental extraction is considerable and healing is relatively slow; a higher level of clotting factor is required to control bleeding after a dental extraction than is required for an episode of spontaneous bleeding.

Before 1950 dental extraction was a dangerous painful experience for the patient with haemophilia. In one patient treated in Oxford from 1940 to 1950 it took numerous sessions of dental extraction over a period of 10 years to remove all of his decayed and infected teeth. Each of these episodes of extraction required the administration of 5–15 pints of whole blood.

So predictable was the excessive bleeding after dental extraction that we have, in the past, used the operation as an index of therapeutic effectiveness of different preparations containing factor VIII. The effectiveness of animal factor VIII was first established by its ability to control bleeding after dental extraction. During the years 1963–65 human factor VIII was tested on patients having dental extraction. At that time there was a great shortage of all therapeutic materials and an attempt was made to define the minimum amounts of factor VIII required to prevent dangerous bleeding. Of the 34 severely affected patients treated during that period 18 bled excessively and 10 required whole blood transfusion. The total volume of blood lost by the patients in that series was proportional to the number of teeth removed, the more teeth removed the more blood was lost. None of these patients had very high post-infusion factor VIII levels. The results of pre- and post-infusion factor VIII levels were recorded and in 27 of the 34 cases the average post-infusion factor VIII levels were less than 30% of average normal. It should be emphasised that the amount of blood lost by these patients was substantial and this degree of bleeding would be unacceptable today. During that time a total of about 6,000 units of factor VIII were given to each patient undergoing dental extraction and on average each patient received 8·3 doses of factor VIII (Table 6.3).

During the period 1965–1969 much more factor VIII was given for each episode of extractions, 14,443 units being the average amount given in an average of 11·5 doses (Table 6.3). During this time 7 of the 20 patients bled, none were transfused and the amounts of blood lost were much less.

In 1969 and 1970 a controlled trial was made of the antifibrinolytic agent Epsilon amino caproic acid (EACA) in conjunction with factor VIII treatment in the control of bleeding after dental extraction (Walsh *et al,* 1971). In the trial period patients were allocated at random to the control or trial group. All patients (trial or control) received enough concentrated clotting factor (VIII or IX), to raise the level of clotting factor in their blood immediately before

Table 6.3. Dental extraction in haemophilic patients. Records made at different times.

Measurement	Pre 1966	1966–68 No EACA	1969 EACA	Controlled trial 1969–70 EACA	1969–70 Controls	1970–73
No. patients	34	20	18	9	9	56
Mean age	—	28·6	24·8	33·3	28·6	31
Severity (preoperative factor VIII)	0	3·4	4·2	2·3	2·4	3·8
No. teeth per patient (mean)	8·5	10·9	4·0	8·5	6·4	5·9
Bleeding	18*	7	7	1	8	17
% all cases	53	35	39	11	89	30
Post infusion factor VIII	mostly less than 30%	—	—	41	65	54
Therapeutic material u/patient (mean)	5998	14,443	2212	1990	4667	2641
Doses/patient	8·26	11·5	2·1	1·1	5·0	1·6

* 10 patients transfused.

operation to 50% of normal. All patients received 600,000 units of penicillin orally 4 times a day. The trial patients received EACA 6 g intravenously just before operation and thereafter received 6 g EACA 4 times daily by mouth for 10 days. The control group received a placebo instead of EACA. The results of this trial showed conclusively that the patients receiving EACA bled less than those who did not receive EACA and required less factor VIII replacement.

During the clinical trial period the immediate pre-operative (post-infusion) levels of clotting factors was relatively high and post-operative sepsis was controlled in all cases. It will be noted (Table 6.3) that although 8 of the 9 patients in the control group bled in the post-operative period none was transfused and less therapeutic material was used than in the era before 1966. It is unwise to make comparisons between patients treated at different times since so many things can change with time. The patients become less frightened, the doctors and nurses more confident, the therapeutic materials better tolerated and the teeth less infected and decayed at the time of operation. Nevertheless it is possible that for safe dental extraction a high initial clotting factor dose at the time of operation may be very important. The last column of Table 6.3 shows the results for haemophilic patients treated since the clinical trial. It will be seen that the mean dosage per patient has been about 2,500 units.

Dental extraction in haemophilia B patients

The results for Christmas disease patients treated in recent years are similar to those for haemophilia. Because of the poor recovery of factor IX in the circulation the dose required to attain a level of 50% of this factor was higher than that of factor VIII in haemophilia (Table 6.4).

Table 6.4. Dental extraction in Christmas disease patients.

	1969–70 trial		
Measurement	Control	EACA	1970–73
Number of patients	3	2	15
Mean age	32	26·5	31
Severity (preoperative factor IX)	4·5	2·5	2·4
Bleeding	2	None	4
% all cases	66	0	25
Post infusion factor IX	53	57	41
Therapeutic material u/patient	8558	3900	5572
Doses per patient	1·7	1·0	1·75

It might well be thought that some distinction could usefully be made between severely and mildly affected patients, in that mildly affected patients might require less treatment with concentrates. In fact our data cannot be used to test this assumption. In Table 6.5 the patients treated from 1970 to 1973 have been divided into severely and mildly affected. On the whole the mildly affected patients bled less than those who were severely affected and they received somewhat smaller doses of concentrates. On the other hand fewer teeth were removed from the mildly affected patients than from those who were severely affected.

Bleeding which has occurred in patients following dental extraction in recent years has been much less severe than in the early cases. Bleeding when it did occur was most common either on the first post-operative day or 7 to 10 days after the extraction.

Before 1970 local measures were taken to minimise bleeding after dental extraction by applying an acrylic plate to cover the extraction site during healing. Since 1970 these plates have not been applied. This change in policy has advantages, the plates are a considerable work to make. They may fit well initially but as the tissues shrink in the post-operative period they become loose and may rub against the socket to cause bleeding, and if food gets under the plate this may promote sepsis.

Table 6.5. Dental extraction in haemophilic and Christmas disease patients considered according to the severity of the coagulation defect 1970–1973.

Measurement	Severe 1% or less	Mild 2% or more	All cases
Haemophilia			
No. patients	25	31	56
Dose pre op. (u/kg)	34·96	29·05	31·68
Dose post op. (u/kg)	12·42	9·32	10·70
No. teeth removed	7·0	5·0	5·89
No. episodes of bleeding per patient	0·80	0·48	0·63
Christmas			
No. patients	8	8	16
Dose pre op. (u/kg)	77·2	57·65	67·5
Dose post op. (u/kg)	24·4	19·3	21·8
No. teeth removed	8·9	3·25	5·5
No. episodes of bleeding per patient	1·6	0·5	1·06

A suggested regime for dental extraction in haemophilic patients

A detailed time-table of procedure for dental extraction will now be considered. It is supposed that a patient from another area has been referred to the Oxford Haemophilia Centre for dental extraction. The first step will depend a good deal on the distance from the Haemophilia Centre at which the patient resides. If this is within 100 miles it is usual for the patient to come for an out-patient visit.

At this out-patient visit the patient is seen by the oral surgeon who carries out a clinical examination, takes X-rays and decides how many teeth should be extracted, and if there are any particular problems for that patient. The patient is also seen by the haemophilia specialist who considers the severity of the defect and takes blood tests to confirm the diagnosis and to exclude the presence of antibodies directed against clotting factors. The patient is then given an appointment to come to hospital for dental extraction at a later date. The delay before extraction varies from patient to patient according to the urgency.

The patient comes to hospital on the day before operation. He is weighed and the dose of factor VIII calculated according to the formula previously described (Chapter 5) as follows:

(a) For haemophilic patients:
    Dose in units = weight in kg × 50 × 0·5 = wt. kg × 25
(b) For Christmas disease patients:
    Dose in units = wt. kg × 50

If factor VIII concentrate is to be used then the number of units contained in the bottle is indicated on the label and this is used to calculate the number of bottles needed. If cryoprecipitate is to be the source of factor VIII then the average assayed value of recent doses may be used to assess the probable value of the dose and the amount adjusted upwards to the nearest whole number of cryoprecipitates.

On the day of operation, the patient is prepared for general anaesthesia and is given, immediately before operation, the calculated dose of factor VIII and 1 gm cyclokapron intravenously. The operation is carried out and the patient rests for the day. Cyclokapron is preferred to EACA since cyclokapron produces fewer side effects.

For 10 days post-operatively the patient receives 1 g cyclokapron 4 times a day if his weight is more than 40 kg. For smaller patients the dose is halved. In addition all patients receive 250 mg phenoxy-methyl penicillin 3 times a day unless they are allergic to penicillin in which case they are given erythromycin. A diagrammatic representation of this treatment is given in Figure 6.1.

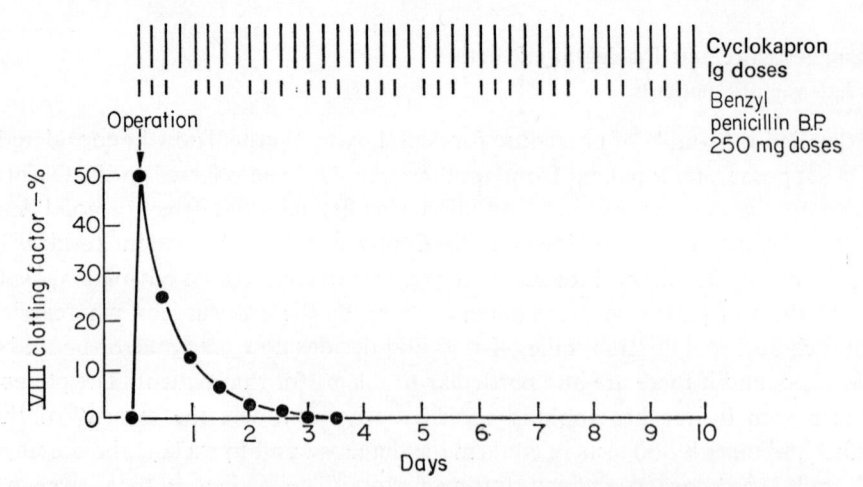

Figure 6.1. A diagrammatic representation of the treatment of a haemophilic patient for dental extraction. On day 1 enough factor VIII is given to raise the patient's factor VIII level to 50% of normal. It is assumed that this factor VIII has a half-life of 12 hours. Cyclokapron in 1 g doses is given 4 times a day and Benzyl Penicillin 3 times a day.

If bleeding should occur during the healing period then a further dose of factor VIII should be given to haemophilic patients or of factor IX to patients having Christmas disease.

In some cases healing is promoted by stitching the sockets after extraction. This is particularly the case following extraction of molar teeth. As mentioned earlier plates are not now used to cover tooth sockets. The practice of stitching the tooth sockets is the result of greater confidence in Oxford about the effectiveness of treatment and 20 years experience of dental extraction. If there is any doubt whatsoever about the effectiveness of the therapeutic material being used then the sockets should not be sutured. If haemorrhage occurs into a sutured socket the blood tends to track into deep tissues of the neck where it may do much damage and indeed endanger life.

The patient should remain in hospital at least 3 days if he lives near the hospital and for 7 days if he lives at a distance. During the healing period the patient's diet should consist of soft food and fluids.

CAUTIONS

Dental extraction is a dangerous operation even with care and experience. Although on average each case has required about 2,500 units of factor VIII or 5,000 units of factor IX, no operation should be undertaken unless 10 times these amounts are in stock or easily available. Accidents may occur; a small artery or arteriole may be torn at operation; the patient may develop an antibody directed against factor VIII or factor IX during the healing period; the patient may be involved in an accident, fall out of bed, attend a football match, take part in a fight, etc. Some of these contingencies may seem far fetched but they do occur and there should be sufficient reserve stock to deal with any emergency.

There are reports of cases where no factor VIII has been given to patients having dental extraction. Caution must be exercised in assessing these reports. Some cases recorded in the past have done well because in fact, they did not have haemophilia. In other cases the process of 'doing well' has been assessed against low standards of expectation. In our opinion no patient need suffer sleep disturbing haemorrhage following dental extraction. A patient may bleed heavily from 1 or 2 sockets without requiring transfusion. In some instances at least patients said to 'do well' have in fact bled quite heavily.

EACA did sometimes produce undesirable side effects such as nausea, vomiting, diarrhoea, postural hypotension, etc. The symptoms are seldom encountered using cyclokapron and for this reason cyclokapron is preferred. Presumably these antifibrinolytic drugs act by making the clots formed at the time of operation into more permanent structures than is usual in normal healing wounds. It is supposed that a normal wound is dry during healing because clots in the wound area lyse and then reform. In the haemophilic lysis would normally be accompanied by bleeding since no new clot would form unless more factor VIII were given. Since antifibrinolytic drugs should not be given to patients with haematuria it is desirable to postpone dental extraction if the patient has haematuria.

The control of haemorrhage following major surgery

Members of the general population who have no particular haemostatic defects do not require numerous major surgical operations. We have assumed (Biggs et al, 1973) that each haemophilic patient may expect to need one major operation in his lifetime. This may be an underestimate since at present about half of the operations required by patients with haemophilia are for orthopaedic deformities caused by previous undertreatment, such operations clearly would not be needed by normal people. The types of surgical operations undertaken for haemophilics at the Oxford Haemophilia Centre in the years 1972–1973 are shown in Table 6.6.

Table 6.6. Major surgical operations carried out for haemophilic (factor VIII deficient) patients at the Oxford Haemophilia Centre during 1972 and 1973.

	Year		
Operation	1972	1973	Total
Orthopaedic	11	9	20
Gastro-intestinal	3	2	5
Prostatectomy	2	0	2
Haemorrhoidectomy	3	0	3
Nephrectomy	1	0	1
Hernia	0	2	2
Miscellaneous	2	8	10
Total	22	21	43
Total factor VIII units used for surgery	331,245	414,815	746,060
Average units of factor VIII per operation	15,057	19,753	17,350
Factor VIII units used for surgery as a percentage of all factor VIII used	18	19	18·5

Twenty years ago nearly all of the concentrated factor VIII that was made was used to treat patients who had serious accidents or who needed emergency surgery. The dramatic success of this early surgical treatment was the initial stimulus which prompted the production of much more therapeutic material so that patients having spontaneous bleeding could receive treatment. At present in Oxford less than 20% of all factor VIII concentrate is used for major surgery (Table 6.6) and at other centres the proportion is probably less. There should now never be any shortage of factor VIII for the treatment of patients requiring surgery.

It should be noted that patients who have haemophilia and require surgery require more special skills than the provision and correct use of factor VIII preparations important though these may be. There must be proper co-ordination between surgeons, nurses, physiotherapists and haemophilia specialists. This co-ordination of diverse specialists in the care of a patient is not easy to achieve or maintain and requires patient and continuing attention. No rules seem to apply to all situations. There are still some very dangerous things that can happen to patients with haemophilia and related conditions and the only real rule is always to consult before acting.

It may be wise to illustrate some difficulties that may arise. The mildly affected patient is always in danger if he is injured or needs surgery. The patient is so normal in everyday life that it is difficult to realise that he may be at great risk following trauma. For all surgical procedures the mildly affected patient will need just as much treatment as a severely affected patient. If the patient has a blow on the head followed by headache he should be taken as an emergency to a haemophilia centre.

A patient having factor VIII antibodies always needs careful management for all episodes of bleeding. Any lesion that could need surgical treatment has a grave prognosis and the patient should always be admitted to a haemophilia centre in such an emergency. The haemophilic patient having surgery should have his blood tested pre-operatively to exclude the presence of antibodies and during surgery the infusion therapy should be controlled by specific factor assays. These laboratory tests are not reliable unless carried out in laboratories where many such tests are done. The treatment of patients having factor VIII antibodies is considered in Chapter 9.

There are so many details of laboratory skill, nursing practice, physiotherapy and medical experience that it is certain that operations should not be undertaken at hospitals where haemophilic patients do not normally attend.

The factor VIII treatment of
haemophilia A patients who require surgery

Treatment following surgery is very important since the bleeding in an incorrectly treated patient may endanger life. Obviously the amount and duration of treatment required by a particular patient having a particular operation will depend on many factors. In addition to the patient's response to treatment and the half-life of infused factor VIII activity, the amount and duration of treatment will depend on the severity of the operation, on the time taken to heal and on the extent to which the wound site can be immobilised.

The control of haemostasis in patients requiring surgery is now technically quite straightforward. The detailed results of factor VIII assays for one patient

144   *Chapter 6*

during operation and the post-operative period are given in Table 5.5. In Chapter 5 it was emphasised that the two considerations which affect the doses of factor VIII (or factor IX) are the response to treatment (%/u/kg) and the half-life of infused material. Usually neither of these will be known when the patient presents for treatment.

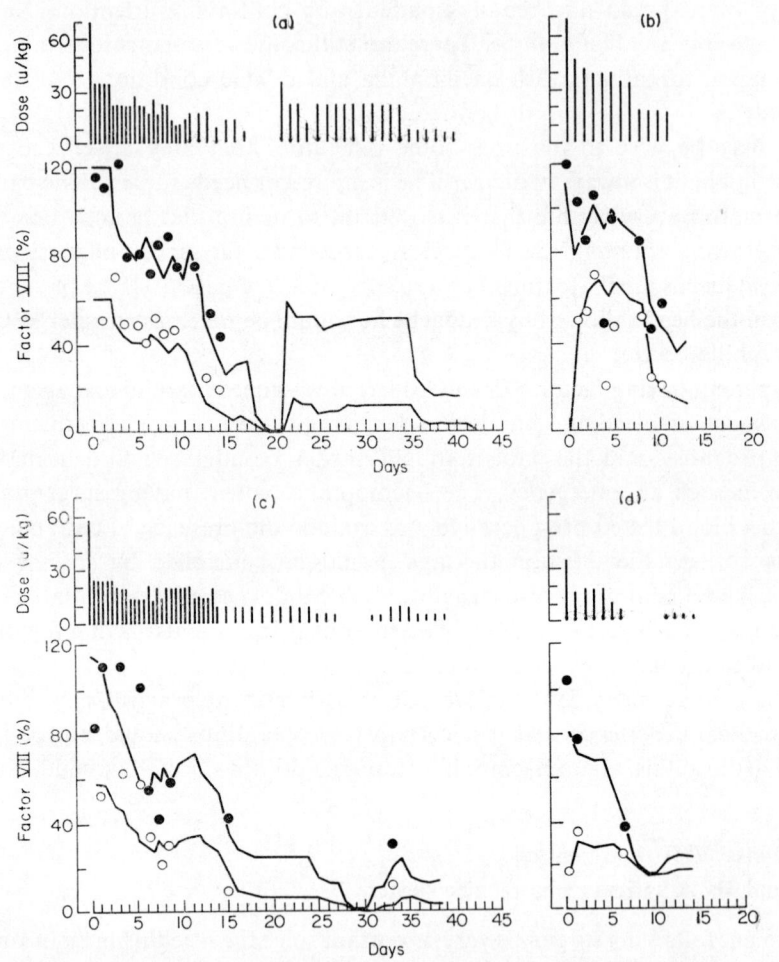

Figure 6.2. Factor VIII levels in haemophilia A patients having major surgical operations. The upper line (●) indicates post infusion levels and the lower line (○) indicates pre-infusion levels of factor VIII:

(a) Case 176 was severely affected and operated on for total hip replacement; wt. 75 kg.
(b) Case 188 was severely affected and operated on for duodenal ulcer; wt. 75 kg.
(c) Case 161 was severely affected and operated on for hip replacement; wt. 51 kg.
(d) Case 162 was mildly affected with a pre-infusion factor VIII level of 14–16%. He had a hernia operation wt. 82 kg.
(e) Case 174 was severely affected and had an operation for duodenal ulcer; wt. 74 kg.
(f) Case 187 was severely affected and operated on for arthrodesis of the knee.

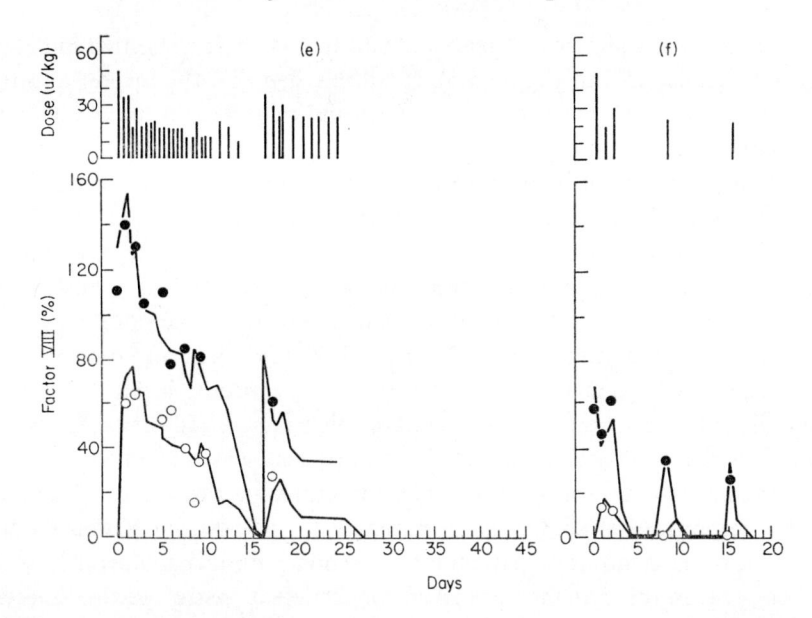

The Control of Haemostasis in Haemophilic Patients

A sensible course of action for haemophilia A patients is to give immediate pre-operative factor VIII dose of 50 u/kg and, on the evening of operation, a second dose of 25 u/kg. The pre- and post-infusion factor VIII levels should be measured for the first dose. On the second day 25 u/kg should be given in the morning and pre- and post-infusion factor VIII levels should be measured. A dose of 25 u/kg is given on the evening of the second day. Thereafter twice daily infusions will be continued for 7–10 days. A safe objective is to keep the post infusion factor VIII near 100% and the pre-infusion level near 50% for the first week.

As time passes less frequent assays may be done (e.g. Saturday and Sunday assays may be omitted). The duration of treatment will depend on the magnitude of the operation and the anticipated duration of healing. After 7–10 days it is usually safe to reduce the frequency of doses from twice to once daily.

During treatment the rise in factor VIII level will establish the mean response to treatment. The comparison of the immediate pre-infusion level with the level immediately after the previous infusion will establish the rate of fall-off of factor VIII or its half-life. As explained in Chapter 5, the half-life can be calculated restrospectively from consideration of the observations on any particular case, but in general low pre-infusion factor VIII levels indicate a short half-life and a short half-life can be treated by more frequent doses.

The factor VIII levels for 6 haemophilia A patients who had surgical operations are given in Figure 6.2. Table 6.8 shows the response to treatment and half-life of infused factor VIII activity for 7 patients. These seven patients are the six whose responses are shown in Figure 6.2 and the one case presented in detail in Chapter 5 (Table 5.5 and Figure 5.5). It will be seen that the response to treatment varied from 1·42%/u/kg to 2·28%/u/kg and that the half-life of factor VIII varied from 12 to 18 hours.

There is now very little purpose in describing individual operation cases in detail. The operations can be carried out exactly as for haemostatically normal people. Treatment of each individual patient depends on the extent of the trauma caused by the operative procedure, the time that healing is likely to take and the extent to which the traumatised area can be immobilised. A few special points may be made in relation to Figure 6.2. Figures 6.2a and c provide data about patients who had total hip replacement operations, it will be seen that twice daily infusions were used to maintain high factor VIII levels for the first 10 and 14 days. The later treatment in each patient was related to removal of plasters and rehabilitation. After the initial treatment periods it was felt that the patient's response was so well known that very little assaying was required. Figure 6.2e is the record for a patient operated on for duodenal ulcer. The second series of doses in this patient were given for recurrent gastrointestinal bleeding. The patient whose record appears as Figure 6.2b was also operated on for duodenal ulcer. The results obtained on day 5 are much lower than should be expected from the dose given, the patient's clinical state or the response to all other doses. Some error was probably involved in these assays. Even in the best regulated establishments errors of this sort occur and must be correctly interpreted and allowed for by the clinician. The record in Figure 6.2d is that of a very mildly affected patient. It will be seen that quite high factor VIII doses were required to maintain adequate factor VIII levels. Small doses, as would be expected, had virtually no effect on the patient's basic factor VIII level (note particularly the last 4 doses). Figure 6.2f is the record for a patient having arthrodesis of the knee. In this case the use of EACA and immobilisation meant that relatively few doses of factor VIII were needed to achieve safe haemostasis.

The factor IX treatment of Christmas disease patients who required surgery

The principles which apply to patients with haemophilia can be used in considering the treatment of patients having Christmas disease. From our previous observations the response of Christmas disease patients to factor IX (%/u/kg) tends to be rather less than half the response of haemophilic patients to factor VIII. Thus larger initial doses are required. From 1961 to 1963 observations on Christmas disease patients suggested a longer half-life for infused factor IX than was at that time observed for factor VIII. Biggs & Denson (1963) calculated half lives for factor IX of 18 to 30 hours with a mean of 24 hours. These calculations

The Control of Haemostasis in Haemophilic Patients

Table 6.7. The response to treatment (%/u/kg) and half-life in hours of factors VIII and IX given to haemophilic and Christmas disease patients who had surgical operations in 1972 and 1973. In the case of Christmas disease patients calculations have also been made for patients treated between 1961 and 1963.

Diagnosis and date	Case number	Operation	Response %/u/kg	Half-life in hours
Haemophilia A	178	Removal of bone from muscle	2·00	16
1972–73	176 (a)	Hip replacement	1·70	12
(Figure 6.2)	188 (b)	Duodenal ulcer	1·61	18
	161 (c)	Hip replacement	1·85	12
	162 (d)	Hernia	2·15	12
	174 (e)	Duodenal ulcer	2·28	12
	187 (f)	Arthrodesis	1·42	12
Mean			1·85	13·4
Christmas	184 (a)	Hernia repair	0·39	18
disease	183 (b)	Adenoidectomy	0·56	8
1972–1973	185 (c)	Wedge tarsectomy	0·81	12
(Figure 6.3)	185 (d)	Hip replacement	1·0	8
	186 (e)	Laparotomy	0·83	12
	182 (f)	Gastrectomy	1·75	8
	189	Lengthen tendo achilles	0·77	12
	190	Skin graft	0·72	18
Mean			0·85	12
Christmas	106 (a)	Haemorrhoidectomy	0·95	18
disease	104 (b)	Dental extraction	1·07	12
1961–1963	103 (c)	Dental extraction	1·04	12
(Figure 6.4)	109 (d)	Pneumonectomy	0·46	24
	108 (e)	Evacuation of clot from knee	0·77	18
	100 (f)	Dental extraction	1·57	16
	114	Dental extraction	0·86	24
Mean			0·96	17·8

were based on the observation of disappearance of factor IX at the end of courses of treatment lasting 5–10 days. After a single dose or after a first dose in a series, factor IX tends to disappear from the circulation rather faster than at the end of a course of treatment. The method of calculating the half-life presented here takes all doses from the first to the last into account and thus the method might be expected to give a shorter value for the half-life than observations on the disappearance of the last dose in a series. In recently studied cases (Table 6.7, 1972–73) infused factor IX had a substantially shorter half-life in different patients than we observed previously. In one operation for hip replacement the half-life of 8 hours meant that 3 infusions of factor IX per day were required to maintain adequate factor IX concentrations in the early stages of treatment

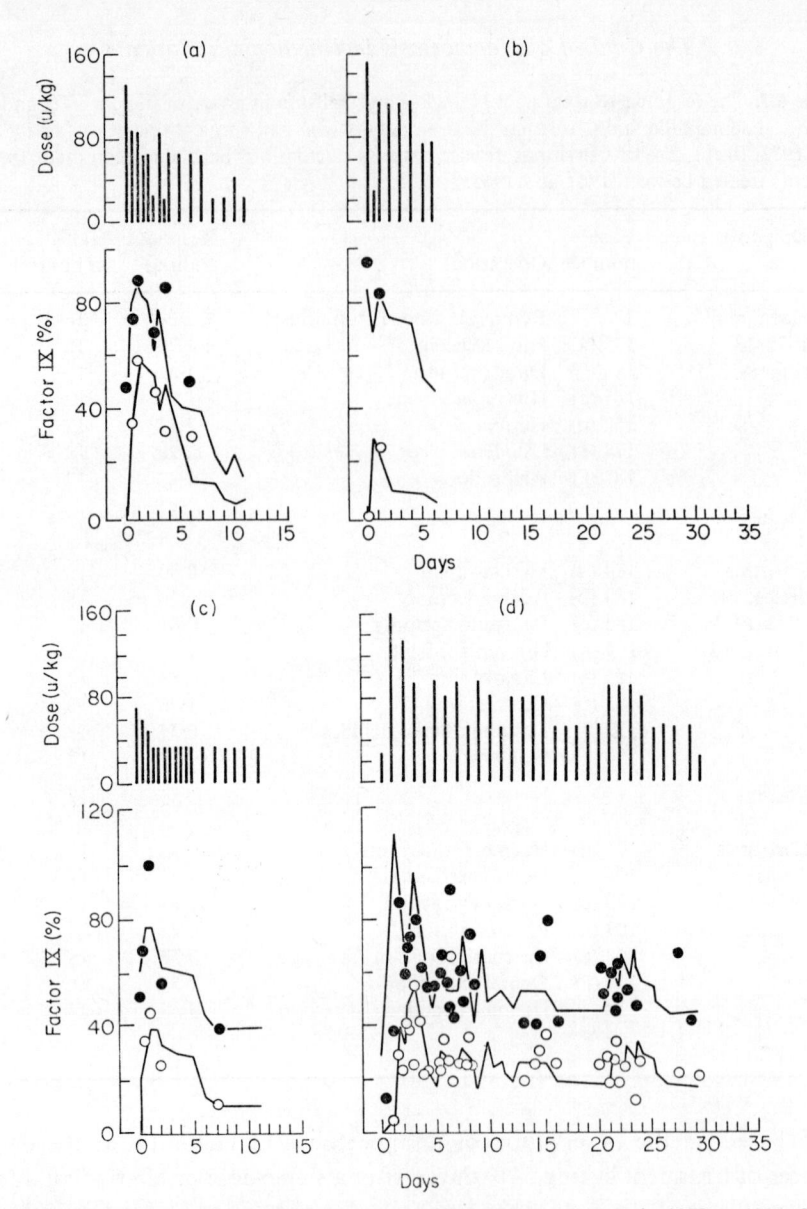

Figure 6.3. Factor IX levels of Haemophilia B patients operated upon in 1972 or 1973. See Figure 6.2.

(a) Case 184 was severely affected and was operated upon for hernia; wt. 45 kg.

(b) Case 183 a severely affected child who had adenoidectomy; wt. 22 kg.

(c) Case 185 a severely affected patient who had wedge tarsectomy; wt. 66 kg.

(d) Case 185 a severely affected patient who was operated on for total hip replacement; wt. 66 kg.

(e) Case 186 mildly affected pre-operative factor IX 10% operated on for abdominal pain; wt. 79·5 kg.

(f) Case 182 a mildly affected patient with pre-operative factor IX of 5–10% operated on for gastrectomy; wt. 80 kg.

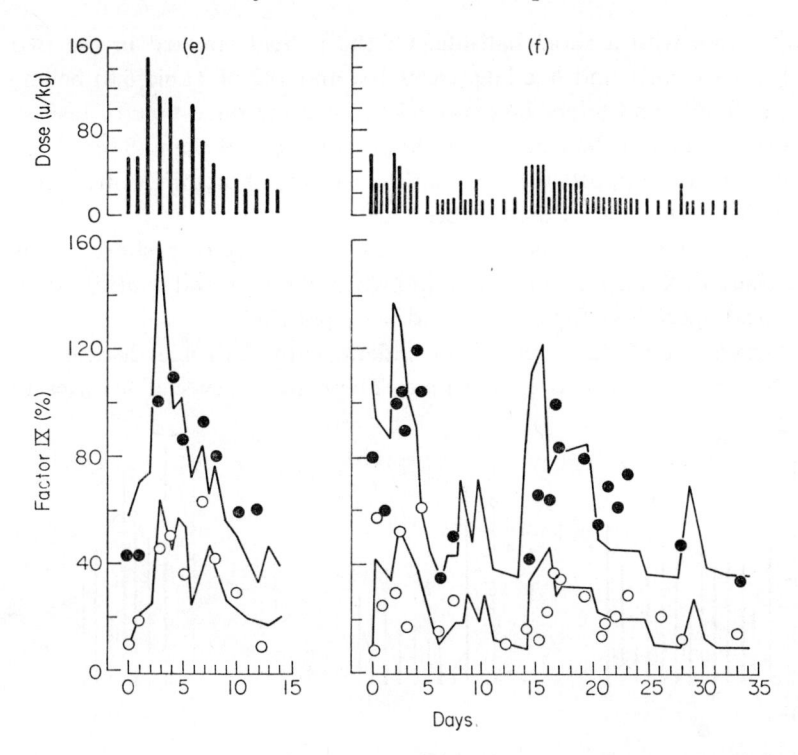

The Control of Haemostasis in Haemophilic Patients

(Figure 6.3f). To make a valid comparison between recently and previously treated patients, calculations were made from the records of 7 patients treated between 1961 and 1963 using exactly the method of the present study (see Chapter 5). A half-life of about 18 hours was found for the cases treated from 1961 to 1963 (Table 6.7).

None of the Christmas disease patients treated from 1961 to 1963 and none of those treated from 1972–1973 showed any adverse reactions or any evidence of thrombosis. There are a number of possible differences between patients treated at the two times. One difference is that the material used in the earlier period was heparinised and prepared by adsorption onto and elution from tricalcium phosphate. The material used in 1972–73 was prepared by adsorption onto DEAE sephadex. Another difference is that by 1972–73 all the patients had received much treatment whereas in 1961 to 1963 little treatment was available; it is possible that patients are now more resistant to treatment. Another possible factor is chance since Christmas disease is so very rarely encountered. Our data in 1961–1963 was based on very few patients. Similarly the recent observations include only 7 patients. It is not beyond the realm of chance that the patients treated at both times were not representative. Those treated from 1961–1963 could represent those with a long half-life of factor IX and those treated more recently those with a short half-life. Of the patients treated in the two time periods 2 (one early and one late, cases 100 and 182 of Table 6.8) belonged to the same family and might be expected to have the same type of response. In these two patients the half-life was 16 hours for 1961–1963 and 8 for 1972–1973. This observation supports the idea that the half-life of factor IX after infusion is now really shorter than it used to be.

Whatever the cause it is noted that the possibility of a short half-life for infused factor IX must be borne in mind when planning and controlling therapy for surgical operations for Christmas disease patients.

Figures 6.3 and 6.4 give records of patients with Christmas disease who were operated upon at the two eras in time. There are no special features to note

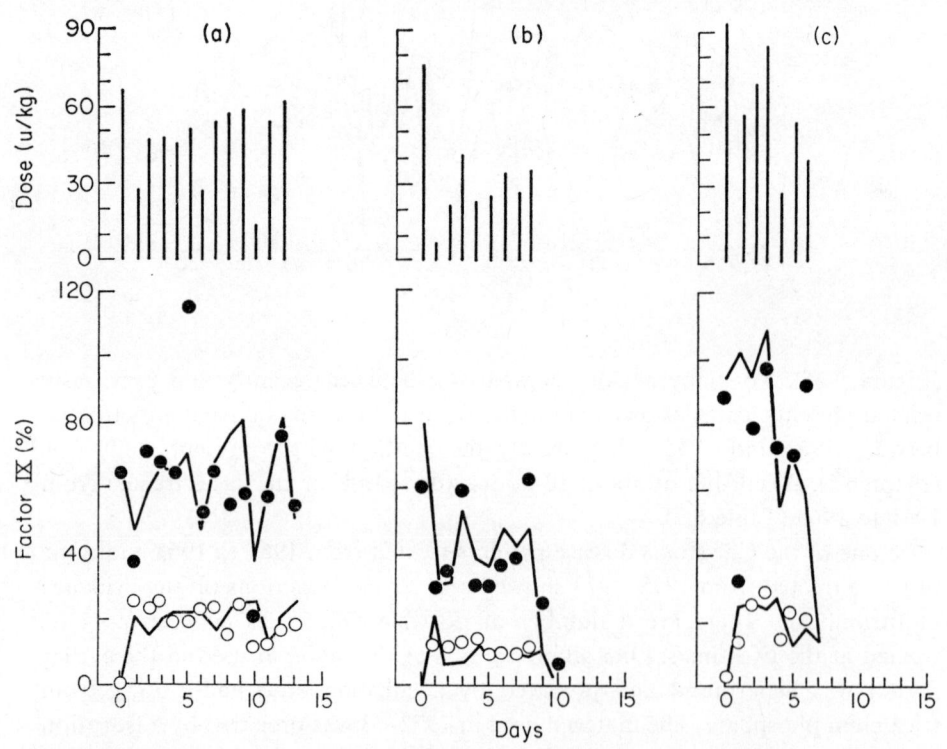

Figure 6.4. Factor IX levels in haemophilia B patients operated on from 1961 to 1963. See Figure 6.2.

(a) Case 106 severely affected patient who was operated on for haemorrhoidectomy; wt. 74 kg.

(b) Case 104 severely affected patient who had dental extraction; wt. 65 kg.

(c) Case 103 a severely affected patient who had dental extraction; wt. 51 kg.

(d) Case 109 a severely affected patient who had pneumonectomy; wt. 46 kg.

(e) Case 108 a severely affected patient who had an open operation for removal of clot from the knee joint; wt. 52 kg.

(f) Case 100 a mildly affected patient who had dental extraction; wt. 98 kg.

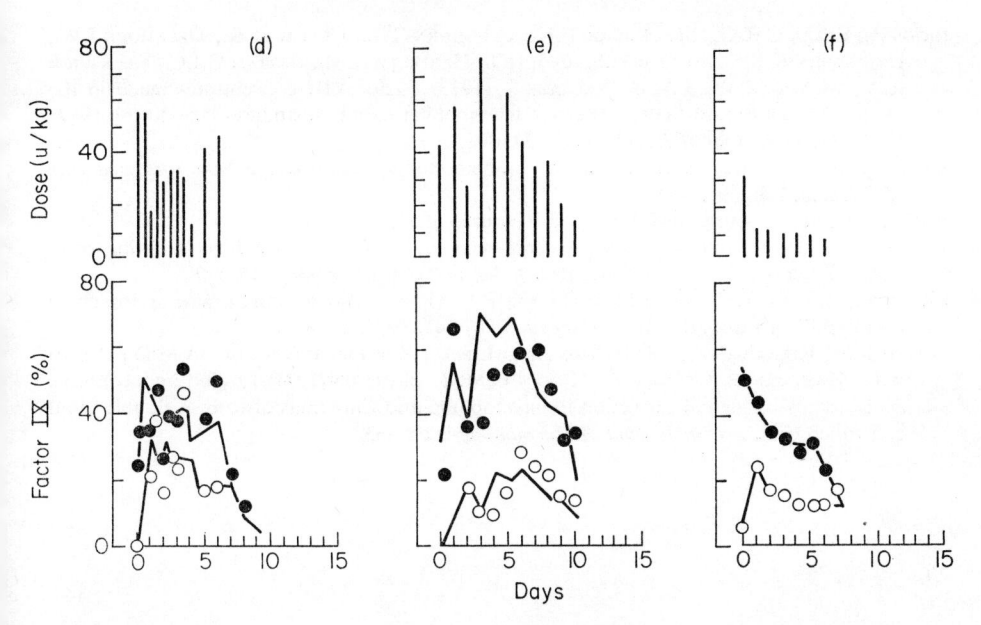

except that on the whole the random scatter of observed factor IX levels was rather larger than the scatter in factor VIII levels seen in haemophilic patients' records. This observation reflects the greater reliability of the factor VIII assay in our laboratory.

Conclusion

The safe administration of factor VIII or IX to haemophilic or Christmas disease patients and the selection of the dose need not now be a very major worry to the staff of the Haemophilia Centre. With modern concentrates the dosage required is predictable and the response easily observable and thereafter consistent. The problems of the Haemophilia Specialist now concern the proper organisation of the Centre, the provision of staff to train patients and to administer doses, public relations with other departments and attempting to obtain a reasonable financial allocation for the provision of adequate amounts of treatment.

References

Aronstam A., Arblaster P.G., Rainsford S.G., Turk P., Slattery M., Alderson M.R., Hall D.E. & Kirk P.J. (1976) Prophylaxis in haemophilia a double-blind controlled trial. *British Journal of Haematology*, **33**, 81.

Biggs R. & Denson K.W.E. (1963) The fate of prothrombin and factors VIII, IX and X transfused to patients deficient in these factors. *British Journal of Haematology*, **9**, 532.

Biggs R., Rizza C.R.C., Blackburn E.K., Cleghorn T.E., Cumming R., Delamore I.W., Dormandy K.M., Douglas A.S., Grant J., Hardisty R.M., Ingram G.I.C., Keckwick R.A., Maycock W. d'A. & Wallace J. (1973) Factor VIII concentrates made in the United Kingdom and the treatment of haemophilia based on studies made during 1969–1972. *British Journal of Haematology*, **27**, 391.

Duthie R.B. (1975) Reconstructive surgery in hemophilia. *Annals of the New York Academy of Sciences*, **240**, 295.

National Heart and Lung Institute Blood Resource Study 1972.

Rainsford S.G. & Hall A. (1973) A three-year study of adolescent boys suffering from haemophilia and allied disorders. *British Journal of Haematology*, **24**, 539.

Storti E., Traldi A., Tosatti E. & Davoli P.G. (1969) Synovectomy, a new approach to haemophilic arthropathy. *Acta Haematologica*, **41**, 193.

Walsh P.N., Rizza C.R.C., Matthews J.M., Eipe J., Kernoff P.B.A., Coles M.D., Bloom A.L., Kaufman B.A., Beck P., Hanan C.M. & Biggs R. (1971) Epsilon aminocaproic acid therapy for dental extraction in haemophilia and Christmas disease. A double blind controlled trial. *British Journal of Haematology*, **20**, 463.

Chapter 7. Home Therapy

C. R. RIZZA, ROSEMARY BIGGS & ROSEMARY SPOONER

It is now widely acknowledged that haemophilia A or B patients should receive early treatment for every episode of bleeding however trivial. In the past patients themselves have assessed degrees of severity of bleeding and chosen whether or not to come to hospital for treatment. For example Hermens (1975) says that his life was altogether changed by the introduction of cryoprecipitate in about 1967 and that after this time he had relatively infrequent hospital admissions and received outpatient treatment once or twice a month. He goes on to say:

'I continue to sustain frequent minor bleedings mainly in the joints for which I do not judge it necessary to obtain cryoprecipitates and from which it usually takes about 3 days to recover.'

A mental attitude of this sort was usual in haemophilic patients particularly in those who lived at some distance from a Haemophilia Centre and particularly in older patients who had become accustomed to invalidity. The change, made possible by cryoprecipitate, from the selective treatment of severe haemarthroses to an attempt to treat all, even minor, episodes of bleeding caused a massive increase in the work of those who care for haemophilic patients in hospital. The number of infusions given to patients in Oxford in 1967 was about 1,500 per year whereas in 1975 nearly 6,000 infusions were given (see Table 10.1).

Two separate but related difficulties arose in the new era of frequent treatment. One difficulty was that patients had to make increasingly frequent visits to hospital or to exercise discretion about hospital visits in the way so clearly described by Hermens (1975). To say that the frequent hospital visits were inconvenient is a gross understatement. For a family having a haemophilic son hospital visiting can become a way of life to which everything else is subordinated. As Robert and Suzanne Massie said 'For eighteen years haemophilia has dominated our lives. It has moulded our relationships with people and our attitude towards the world.'

At the hospital, staff and space to treat haemophilic patients did not increase in proportion to the increased work. Moreover 15–20% of all treatments were and are given out of office hours (Chapter 10) and it is difficult for limited numbers of staff to give a 24 hour service to large numbers of patients when such an appreciable proportion of treatment is at night. It thus became very important for both doctors and patients in Oxford to consider home therapy and home therapy was started in 1971.

The criteria for admitting patients to the Home Therapy Programme

In the first year of home therapy in Oxford very little therapeutic material was available and the nine patients who had the most frequent bleeding episodes were started on home treatment. Eight of these patients have been studied carefully and information about them is given in Table 7.1. As the years have passed other patients who bleed less frequently have been included. By December 1975 56 severely affected haemophilia A patients, 7 severely affected haemophilia B patients were receiving regular home therapy from the Oxford Haemophilia Centre. Over the 6 year period the criteria for inclusion have slowly changed. Throughout the time frequency of bleeding episodes remained an important criterion for inclusion.

Table 7.1. The amount of factor VIII given to 8 haemophilia A patients who commenced home treatment in 1971.

Time	Patient-months on treatment	Units of factor VIII used	Average per patient per month Doses	Average per patient per month Units of factor VIII
Before home therapy	237	474,085	7	2,000
1971	45	171,690	12	3,815
1972	96	249,230	7	2,596
1973	96	199,981	6	2,083
1974	96	208,950	6½	2,177
1975	96	208,886	8½	2,176
Total on HT & mean	429	1,038,737	8	2,421

The distance from the Centre at which the patient lives has also been a criterion for selection. The 56 haemophilia A patients who, in December 1975 were attached to the Oxford Haemophilia Centre to receive home therapy live on average 43 miles away from the Centre. Since the patients so far selected for home therapy need treatment on average 2 to 8 times a month the amount of travelling saved by home therapy is quite considerable in the majority of cases ranging between 2,000 and 8,000 miles a year per patient (total range 96–19,000 miles).

Another essential requirement for home therapy is that the patient, his parents and his general practitioner shall wish to have home therapy and that someone shall be willing, competent and responsible for organising and giving the treatment. These are very individual requirements. For example if the patient has difficult veins it may be impractical to arrange home therapy. If a child has frequent disagreements with his parents it may not be possible for infusions to be given by a parent. It is also essential for patients to keep proper records of the material used and the reasons for each infusion.

In general patients who have anti-factor VIII antibodies are not given home therapy but 4 patients who have low titre antibodies have had home therapy for short periods of time in special circumstances.

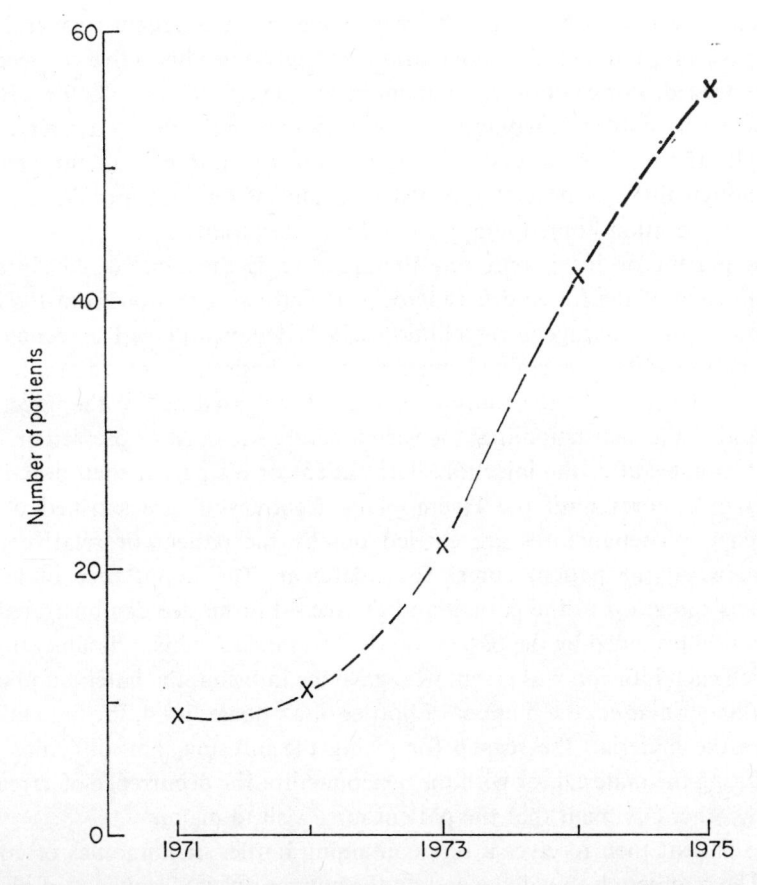

Figure 7.1. Cumulative total of haemophilia A patients on home therapy at the Oxford Haemophilia Centre.

At first many patients were excluded from home therapy by these criteria and by the shortage of factor VIII but as time has passed more and more patients have been included. The change has been brought about by increasing willingness of patients to take part in the programme and by increased amounts of therapeutic material mainly provided by commercial companies. The commercial factor VIII has been used for operation cases and this has freed NHS factor VIII for home therapy. The general trend in home therapy is illustrated in Figure 7.1 which shows the numbers of the haemophilia A patients introduced to home treatment from 1971 to 1975.

The introduction of a patient to home therapy

Once a patient has expressed the wish to have home therapy and the therapy has been shown on discussion to be reasonable then the patient's general practitioner is contacted and his co-operation is sought since his active co-operation may be needed. For example if a patient has made up a dose of factor VIII and then has been unable to carry out a venepuncture then the G.P.'s assistance may be sought. If a reaction occurs the G.P. might be called to give an antihistamine drug though this has never happened with any of our patients. Without the G.P.'s co-operation home therapy should not be started.

The patient or his parent or other relative is then instructed. First the reconstitution of the freeze dried factor VIII and its extraction from the bottle or ampoule into a syringe using a filter needle is demonstrated. The technique of venepuncture is then explained, particular emphasis is given to aseptic techniques, to the fact that the tourniquet must be released before the injection is made and to the instruction that the venepuncture site must be pressed on firmly for 3–4 minutes after the injection. The patient or his parent then practise the various procedures until the Haemophilia Centre staff are satisfied of their proficiency. Venepunctures are carried out by the patient or relative at the hospital when the patient comes for treatment. The importance of keeping records is explained to the patient and the record forms are demonstrated. The information provided by the patient on the form include: his full name, the date on which each infusion was given, who gave the infusion, the batch number and type of material used, the number of bottles or ampoules used, the time taken to dissolve the material, the reason for giving the infusion, any difficulty in reconstituting the material, or with the venepuncture, the occurrence of a reaction and any other comment that the patient may wish to make.

The patient then receives a box containing bottles or ampoules of concentrate. The number given will depend on the patient's usual frequency of bleeding episodes and the distance of his home from the Centre. It is explained that the material may be kept in an ordinary refrigerator but will come to no harm if kept at room temperature for many hours. The box also contains the bottles of 'distilled water for injection' to make up the concentrate; the patient is told that once a bottle of distilled water has been opened it must be discarded if not used. A supply of filter needles for making up the doses and 'steret' swabs and sterile cotton wool balls are also included. The dose is drawn into disposable syringes and the venepuncture is carried out using 'Butterfly' needles (Abbott) size 21 or 23 gauge, both of these are in the supply box. A special bag is provided into which used needles and syringes must be put for return to the hospital and safe disposal in hospital waste. In the box are also micropore adhesive strips to cover the venepuncture sites, a tourniquet and the home treatment record forms in an envelope.

During the training period the criteria for deciding to give an infusion are discussed with the patient and/or his parents. It is explained that some sites of bleeding are more important than others and that in the case of some types of bleeding the patient must always be brought to hospital. The most dangerous types of bleeding are those into the floor of the mouth or neck; knocks on the head followed by headache; abdominal pain or any laceration sufficiently large to require stitching. Care is taken to make sure that the patient understands that he should not take aspirin for headaches and joint pains; other suitable analgesics such as Panadol are recommended.

It is explained to the patient that treatment should be given as soon as possible after the onset of bleeding. In general we do not advise haemophilia A patients to take regular doses with the intent to prevent the onset of bleeding (prophylaxis). Short periods of regular treatment are given to some haemophilia A patients in specific individual circumstances. For example a knee may recover full movement faster after a severe bleed if regular treatment is given for a few days or weeks after the bleeding has stopped. It is our experience that stress may increase the frequency of bleeding and thus patients are advised to have a prophylactic infusion every day during school examinations, before interviews, when starting a new job or for other special occasions.

The haemophilia B patients on the other hand are nearly all advised to have a prophylactic dose once a week or once a fortnight since we find that prophylactic treatment greatly reduces the frequency of bleeding. About 40% of all treatment for haemophilia B patients was in the form of prophylaxis.

During the instruction period the patient's attention is drawn to any publications about haemophilia treatment which are considered suitable. The DHSS booklet entitled *Notes on the Care of Patients with Hereditary Haemorrhagic States* and Dr Jones' book entitled *Living with Haemophilia* are at present available and it is to be hoped that other books will appear as time passes.

The time taken to complete the home treatment training varies from 1 to 3 months. A good deal depends on the number of episodes of bleeding experienced by the patient during the training period. A patient is normally not permitted to take home treatment supplies for the first time until he or his relatives have given him 6 doses under supervison at the Centre without encountering problems. When the training is complete it is explained to the patient that home therapy should not cut him off from the Haemophilia Centre. He is free to drop in at any time as in the past and can telephone at any time when in doubt about symptoms or the advisability of giving a dose. He should always telephone if a reaction occurs. We do not give antihistamine pills or injections to patients on home therapy since the therapeutic materials that we issue for home therapy rarely cause reactions. Before starting home therapy the patient receives 'on demand' treatment at the Oxford Centre and during this time the type of therapeutic material best suited to the particular patient is selected. So far no patients on home therapy have had a reaction to material given at home.

The patient is given an instruction sheet which provides reminders about venepuncture technique and some notes about particular types of bleeding. An appointment is then made for him to attend a follow-up clinic in case he does not come to the centre sooner. The G.P. is informed immediately that the patient has left the hospital with a supply of home therapy material. The patient is asked to telephone when he needs further supplies so that a new box can be made ready for collection. Most patients collect their home treatment supplies from the Centre but alternative arrangements can also be made for the convenience of patients. For example a set of supplies may be sent by the Blood Transfusion Service Transport to an Associate Haemophilia Centre. At the Associate Centre the patient may also obtain help and advice in an emergency. The supplies may be sent by train for collection from the patient's local railway station or supplies may be left in a safe place at the Churchill Hospital for collection at the patient's convenience outside office hours.

We expect the patients to consult the doctors and the nursing sister at the Haemophilia Centre quite frequently both during the training period and later. It is a little important for the patient to absorb information and to gain experience at a reasonable rate. It is quite easy to try to give the patient too much information all at once. There are very many subjects that will arise as the boy grows up. These include: the choice of toys; the activities which should be encouraged or discouraged; the choice of schools and a proper procedure for introducing the boy to his school teacher so that the school teacher will understand his special problems. As time passes various immunisation procedures will need to be considered. This last problem is one which is important to school medical officers and general practitioners as well as to the patients. Our advice about immunisation is that oral vaccine may be given for polyomyelitis.

Subcutaneous or intracutaneous procedures carry little risk. Thus immunisation against yellow fever, common cold, tuberculosis and smallpox vaccination are unlikely to cause excessive bleeding. Intramuscular injections such as those for diphtheria, tetanus, whooping cough, typhoid, paratyphoid A and B may cause a haematoma at the injection site and, should undue pain or swelling occur after the injection a dose of factor VIII should be given.

Very many other problems will arise and it is most reassuring to the patients to know that they can ask a doctor or nursing sister at their next visit without making any special appointment.

The dosage of factors VIII and IX for home therapy patients

When a patient comes to hospital to be treated for a bleed into a joint or muscle he receives a dose of factor VIII of about 10 u/kg or factor IX of about 20 u/kg. In individual circumstances the dose may vary from 5 to 15 u/kg of factor VIII or 10 to 30 u/kg of factor IX. When the patient is on home therapy the dose tends to be given early after the onset of bleeding and quite small doses are usually effective. We adjust the dose for each patient according to his weight and according to his experience about the effectiveness of each single dose. Usually we recommend one ampoule of commercial factor VIII or one bottle of NHS factor VIII for each dose. Each ampoule or bottle contains about 250 units of factor VIII. For factor IX the usual dose is one bottle of NHS factor IX which contains about 600 units of factor IX. Large adults may need two bottles of factor VIII or factor IX for a dose.

If a patient on home therapy takes a prophylactic dose of factor VIII or IX then the dose is the same as that used for therapy.

Observations on Oxford home therapy patients

In all, 56 haemophilia A and 7 haemophilia B patients were on home therapy from the Oxford Haemophilia Centre at 31 December 1975. Of these 36 reside in the Oxford Regional Health Authority region, 15 reside outside the Region but in the territory allocated to the Oxford Haemophilia Centre (see Chapter 10) and 12 reside in other parts of the United Kingdom. The age distribution of patients who started home therapy in Oxford is given in Table 7.2. Twenty-one patients give the treatment to themselves (33% of all patients). Of the remaining patients 30 are treated by relatives and for 12 special arrangements have been made for infusions to be given by the general practitioner or at a local hospital. The youngest of our patients to infuse himself is aged 14.

Table 7.2. Age when haemophilia (A) and Christmas disease (B) patients started home treatment.

	Number of patients	
Age (years)	A	B
<5	2	—
5–9	12	—
10–14	10	1
15–19	10	3
20–29	11	1
30–39	4	—
40–49	3	—
50–59	12	—
60+	2	2
Total	56	7

Average age for starting home treatment:
Haemophilia = $20\frac{1}{2}$
Christmas disease = $31\frac{1}{2}$

Table 7.3. The reasons haemophilia and Christmas disease patients received home treatment doses during 1971–1975.

Reason for treatment	Haemophilic patients Total no. HT doses recorded	% all HT doses	Christmas disease patients Total no. HT doses recorded	% all HT doses
Knee haemarthroses	1857	33	104	25
Elbow haemarthroses	1131	20	58	14
Ankle haemarthroses	582	10	25	6
Shoulder haemarthroses	580	10	9	2
Prophylactic doses	196	4	165	40
Hip	149	3	21	5
Thigh	136	2	5	1
Feet	126	2	4	1
Hands	94	2	3	0·72
Wrists	101	2	—	—
Accidents	67	1	2	0·48
Calf	64	1	2	0·48
Haematuria	56	1	1	0·24
G.I. bleeds	22	0 (0·40)	3	0·72
Epistaxis	10	0 (0·18)	—	—
Other reasons	510	9	12	3
Total	5581	100 (0·58)	414	99·64

Home Therapy

Table 7.4. The reasons 33 out of 56 haemophilic patients on regular home treatment required admission to hospital.

Reason for admission	No. admissions	No. patients	No. doses
Operations (including dental extractions)	20	16	239
Haemarthroses	48	18	207
Haematoma	10	5	47
Iliopsoas	5	3	9
Gastro-intestinal and stomach	6	3	28
Haematuria	2	2	Nil
Accidents	8	5	38
Several reasons	1	1	4
Jaundice	2	2	11*
Miscellaneous	2	2	4
Total	104	33	87

* For haemarthroses while in hospital.

The reasons for giving home treatment doses are analysed in Table 7.3. During the period of home treatment, from 1971 to 1975, 33 of the 56 haemophilia A patients have been admitted to hospital for various reasons given in Table 7.4. The most usual reason was for operation or dental extraction but the proportion of all therapeutic material received by home therapy patients for operation and dental extraction was small, about 4% for operations and 1% for dental extraction. The figures for operation and dental extraction for all Oxford patients include many patients who came to Oxford especially to have dental extractions and operations. The 18·5% of material used for operations noted in Chapter 6 was mainly used for these patients who were referred to the Oxford Centre from elsewhere and who received day to day treatment for haemarthroses at other centres. The small proportion of the concentrate used for surgery in the home therapy cases is probably a fair estimate of the use for this purpose in the United Kingdom as a whole. The 8 operations carried out on haemophilia A patients on the home therapy programme were: circumcision, synovectomy, patellectomy and synovectomy, elongation of achilles tendon, appendicectomy, post-traumatic splenectomy, injection of haemorrhoids and removal of a cyst from an eyelid.

In addition to admission to hospital for operations and other serious bleeding episodes, patients on home therapy continue to have a proportion of all infusions as outpatients at the hospital. Quite often patients wait till a bleed occurs before visiting hospital to collect new home treatment material. On such a visit treatment is given at the Centre.

Chapter 7

The amounts and types of therapeutic material used for home therapy at the Oxford Haemophilia Centre

Of those patients on home treatment supervised by the Oxford Centre in 1975, 37 received no material other than NHS freeze-dried factor VIII. Ten patients received one variety of commercial factor VIII and 9 received both NHS and commercial factor VIII. Cryoprecipitate is not used at the Oxford Centre for home treatment. Cryoprecipitate cannot be used for this purpose in Oxford since this material is no longer available except in small amounts and for special cases. Most of the fresh plasma separated by the Oxford Regional Transfusion Service is sent for fractionation. Were cryoprecipitate available we should nevertheless prefer to use a freeze dried preparation.

The choice of therapeutic material must at present be decided mainly by the types of therapeutic material that are available. Enquiry to 39 United Kingdom Centres which had home therapy programmes early in 1976 showed that cryoprecipitate was used at 13 and that at 4 no preparation other than cryoprecipitate was used (Jones, 1976). Other Centres used a variety of preparations and of these commercial factor VIII was the one most commonly used.

At the Oxford Haemophilia Centre about half of the factor VIII used for all patients in hospital and for home therapy is made at the Oxford Plasma Fractionation Laboratory and about half is commercial in origin. Since more than half of the 56 haemophilia A patients on home therapy are under the age of 20 we reserve as much as possible of the locally made NHS factor VIII for home therapy. As far as we know, the NHS factor VIII is rather less likely to cause jaundice than is the commercial factor VIII and it is therefore preferred for young patients and for others who may not have any immunity to hepatitis. Thirty-eight per cent of all NHS factor VIII used at the Centre in 1975 was given to home therapy patients. The commercial factor VIII used in 1975 was in the main used to treat patients undergoing surgery and only 16% of the commercial factor VIII used was given to home therapy patients. All of the patients who regularly receive commercial factor VIII for home therapy are HB_sAg or HB_sAb positive and of these 9 are included in a special study of the use of commercial factor VIII for home therapy. The proportion of all factor VIII used in Oxford that is used for home therapy is shown in Table 7.5. It will be seen that by 1975, 27% of all material used at the Oxford Haemophilia Centre was used for home therapy.

The patients who receive home therapy have been selected from among those who bled most frequently, it is thus to be expected that they will need on the whole more factor VIII than is recorded as the average for all patients. Figure 7.2 is an attempt to compare the use of factor VIII by home therapy patients with

Table 7.5. Amount of material used to treat haemophilic patients under the care of Oxford Haemophilia Centre during 1971–1975, showing the proportion of the material used for home treatment.

Reason for treatment	1971 Factor VIII units	% total	1972 Factor VIII units	% total	1973 Factor VIII units	% total	1974 Factor VIII units	% total	1975** Factor VIII units	% total
Surgery	97,430	6·51	359,875	18·13	414,815	18·52	714,503	28·99	511,515	20·89
Dental extractions	81,270	5·43	50,675	2·55	43,590	1·95	47,830	1·94	36,484	1·49
Used at hospitals for other reasons	1,208,480	80·80	1,352,235	68·13	1,443,240	64·42	1,061,252	43·07	1,237,277	50·53
Supplied for home therapy*	108,540	7·26	222,000	11·19	338,550	15·11	640,700	26·00	663,250	27·09
Total	1,495,720	100·00	1,984,785	100·00	2,240,195	100·00	2,464,285	100·00	2,448,526	100·00

* Including holiday issues.
** International units: 1 International unit = 1·2 old units, therefore 2,448,526 units in 1975 would correspond to 2,938,231 units in 1974.

the use by all patients at the Oxford Centre. The use of factor VIII is expressed as the average number of units of factor VIII given to each patient each month. The month was used as the unit of time since patients entered the programme at various times in the year.

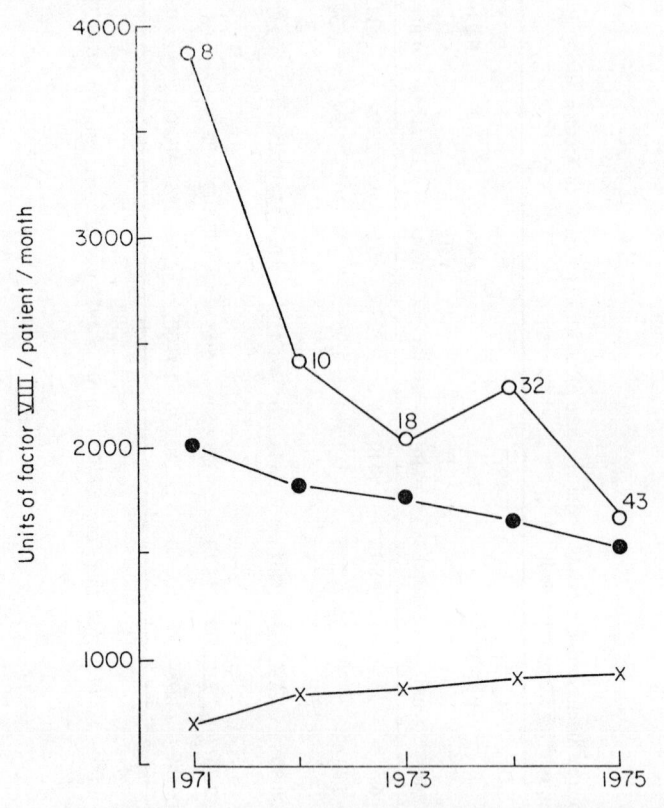

Figure 7.2. The amounts of therapeutic material used to treat haemophilia A patients in Oxford from 1971 to 1975. (×) All patients; (●) patients before starting home therapy; (○) patients after home therapy. The numbers on the upper graph indicate the total number of patients included in the home therapy programme. The data includes those patients on home therapy for whom complete information is available.

The lowest line in Figure 7.2 represents the average monthly use of factor VIII by all patients attending the Oxford Haemophilia Centre from 1971 to 1975. The number of units of factor VIII used per patient per month increased from 696 in 1971 to 923 in 1975. The upper two lines in Figure 7.2 express the number of units of factor VIII used by home therapy patients before and after they started home therapy. The data expressed in this diagram includes those patients for whom we have reliable evidence about the treatment received before home therapy was started. Thus each year a small number of patients have been omitted from the statistics because we have no data about their treatment before starting home therapy. The middle line of Figure 7.2 represents the average units of factor VIII per haemophilic patient per month prior to the starting of home therapy. In 1971 the 8 patients included received on average 2,000 units of factor VIII per month; this was about 3 times the average for all patients at this time. In 1972 2 patients were added to the home therapy programme and the average units of factor VIII for these two patients before starting home therapy together with the 8 for the previous year was 1,781 units per patient per month. Similarly for subsequent years the treatment received by newly admitted home therapy patients was added to previous totals. This line gives a general idea of the severity of bleeding in the patients who have been included in the home therapy programme. As time has passed patients who bled less frequently were admitted. The top line represents the treatment received by home therapy patients after starting home therapy. It will be seen that those on home therapy have used more factor VIII than they used before starting treatment but that the difference has reduced with the passage of time. In fact Figure 7.2 gives an insufficiently detailed picture of the use of factor VIII by home therapy patients. Reference to Table 7.1 shows that the 8 patients who entered the programme in 1971 used nearly twice as much factor VIII in their first year on home therapy as they used before starting home treatment. As the years have passed the level of use has tended to settle at about 15% higher than that used before home therapy was started. A very similar phenomenon was observed with most of the other patients admitted to the home treatment programme. Maximum use of factor VIII occurred during the first year or two following the start of home therapy and the amount used tended to decrease thereafter.

Home therapy for haemophilia B patients

All of the 7 haemophilia B patients who are on home therapy receive NHS factor IX concentrate. The amounts of material given to them are listed in Table 7.6. As with factor VIII deficient patients there was often an initial rise in the amount of factor IX used per patient but after the first year the amounts used tended to decrease again. As with haemophilia A patients most of the treatments were given for knee or elbow haemarthroses. As previously noted about 40% of treatment for haemophilia B patients is given as regular prophylactic doses.

Table 7.6. Treatment received by Christmas disease patients receiving home therapy.

Date	No. of patients included	Patient months on treatment during the year	Total factor IX units	Factor IX per patient per month
Pre home treatment**	6	317	929,273	2931
1972	2	8	38,000	4750
1973	3	28	80,000	2886
1974	4	42	103,200	2457
1975	7	80	440,000	5500

** No information about treatment before home therapy for 1 patient.

Home therapy for special occasions

There are 29 patients attached to the Oxford Haemophilia Centre who have received home therapy occasionally or for part of each year. Four boys attended a local boarding school in Oxford and while at the school received 'home' therapy under the supervision of the School Medical Officer. All of these boys were trained in self infusion while at the school. Four haemophiliacs who had anti-factor VIII antibodies have had doses to be given at home for short periods of time and under very close supervision by the general practitioners and in close co-operation with the Haemophilia Centre doctors. Twenty-five patients (18 haemophilia A and 7 haemophilia B) have been given material to take on holiday on 57 occasions. For these patients careful individual arrangements were made for the infusions to be given by a general practitioner or by a doctor at a hospital near to the holiday resort.

Complications of treatment

Three of the haemophilia A patients receiving home therapy became jaundiced. Of these, 2 were admitted to hospital for observation. One patient had 2 episodes of jaundice. Of the 4 episodes of jaundice, in 2 cases NHS factor VIII was the only material given prior to the onset of jaundice. One of the other two episodes was preceded by the use of commercial factor VIII only and in the second the jaundice was preceded by NHS and commercial factor VIII. None of the patients were seriously ill. No haemophilia B patients developed jaundice.

There have been 5 recorded occasions when difficulty in venepuncture obliged the patient to visit the Haemophilia Centre.

The assessment of the benefits of treatment

Very few patients who have started home therapy training have reverted to regular reliance on the hospital. One or two patients who live or work very near to the hospital did not at first think it worth while to learn the technique and take responsibility for their own treatment but several of these are now receiving home therapy. One little boy has periods of time when he prefers not to be venepunctured by his mother. With these exceptions patients and their parents say that home therapy has made a great deal of difference to their lives. The most usual comment is that the episodes of bleeding are resolved more rapidly with prompt home therapy than following painful journeys to hospital. There is also a general feeling that less time is lost from school or work though there are instances when children stay home from school unnecessarily because the mother does not feel able to decide about the safety of going to school. This problem is usually most common in the early days of home therapy. There are also remarks from parents and adult patients about the greater peace and security of home life and being able to arrange safe holidays.

On the medical side there is a greater feeling of co-operation and confidence between haemophilia centre doctors and the patient. A vivid picture of the life of a haemophilic schoolboy is given by the home infusion diary of one boy who receives home therapy from Oxford (see below). We feel that this record and some comments that patients have made when writing to the doctors at the Centre may give very clear evidence about the benefits of treatment. The parents in letters have referred to their sons by name. We have changed the name on each occasion to 'our son'.

A year in the life of a haemophilic schoolboy

6.1　Stiff in part of body at top of leg where it joins onto trunk. Said he had felt it 2 days earlier but it 'wasn't bad and stayed the same but now it hurts a bit'.

8.1　Sudden and severe pain back (left side) and tummy. After consultation with Haemophilia Centre gave dose and took him to local hospital for examination also blood/urine tests.

14.1　Elbow joint bleed.

21.1　Knee—apparently spontaneous.

23.1　Knee.

29.1　Knee bleed after clonking on desk.

4.2　Arm and elbow bleeds.

9.2　Haematuria.

17.2	Knee swollen, stiff and puffy. No apparent cause (but first day back at school after ½-term—roughness?).
24.2	Ankle bleed (not joint). Was kicked in a crowd at school and bruise was spreading right over ankle and foot swollen and sore. Rather than 'wait and see' and perhaps miss another few days at school, gave dose.
28.2	At school twisted ankle walking round the playground and slipped into a rut.
3.3	No dose since 28.2. Disastrous economy attempt. Aware of dwindling stocks and distance from Oxford. Result back to square one.
13.6	Twisted ankle at school.
18.6	Peppered all over with bruises in particular one on thumb joint and one in arm muscle.
23.6	Bleed into thigh muscle.
29.6	Swollen knee.
7.7	Strange pain in top of thigh.
23.7	Bruise across toe joints making it impossible to walk normally.
26.7	Foot bleed bad again. Also large bruise on thigh.
4.8	Calf bleed following much exercise.
7.8	Toe stubbed on rock painful and spreading making him walk badly when only just over a calf bleed.
15.8	Bleed in elbow swelling rapidly no reason given.
18.8	Stubbed toe getting out of swimming pool 2 days ago. This was not mentioned until yesterday. We were getting low on bottles so we gave no dose which was a mistake as he was soon unable to walk.
28.8	Painful bleed over ankle and right across foot causing severe restriction of movement and too painful even to hobble painful at rest.
30.8	Bleed smothering foot again.
2.9	Ankle bleed.
14.9	Massive arm and thigh bruises
16.9	Knee bleed.
18.9	Mobilisation for knee bleed.
24.9	Accident at school caused nose bleed and swelling, may be nose broken.
27.9	Bad knee bleed puffy and swollen.
30.9	Bleed smothering foot again.
12.10	Clonked on the head. Did not wait to find out whether a dose was necessary after the last head bleed. Complained of headache.
30.10	Calf muscle bleed also bruises on hand and fingers.
7.11	Slipped coming upstairs and somehow clonked the side of his knee. He said that it hurt and that he could feel it spreading. Dose within 45 minutes of injury.

8.11	Booster for yesterday's knee injury as he is not too happy about it. Says it is still painful and 'twangs'.
19.11	Knocked knee.
27.11	Bleeds into both upper arm and thigh muscles.
10.12	Tummy pains, uncomfortable to walk and has to bend over.
15.12	Elbow bleed arm fast stiffening.
17.12	Swollen painful knee which cannot be bent or straightened.
18.12	Knee still painful.

In addition to this full record the patient had 37 doses of factor VIII for which there are no recorded diary notes; of these 14 were given in April and May. The patient thus had 79 doses for 73 known bleeds. This patient has more than average bleeding frequency for a severely affected patient and even with home therapy his parents clearly had a worrying time supervising his treatment.

Comments by haemophilic patients and their parents on the benefits of home therapy

1 Comments from the parents of the boy whose diary is reproduced above:

'Every possible advantage. Treatment can be given promptly, obviously lessening the extent of injury and pain. A great benefit to the entire family, giving far greater freedom of movement and much less disruption. Highly uncomfortable and time-consuming journeys to and from hospital are avoided. There is also now only very occasional need for our son to take up a hospital bed, which must save the NHS a small fortune considering the cost of this. For example, one year he spent several *months* in hospital. missing $1\frac{1}{2}$ *whole terms* at school, before home therapy. HT makes all the difference to life and the thought of life without it is now intolerable. We are occasionally reminded of the "bad old days" when we do have to take our son to hospital—the accompanying pain and inevitable delays making any situation so much worse. Obviously the entire family benefit from HT and surely quick home treatment means less treatment and therefore less financial burden on the Health Service. It simply seems such a modern, sensible, obviously practical way of dealing with haemophilia and is surely an enterprising scheme which could certainly benefit future sufferers.'

2 Comments from a mother of 2 haemophilic sons.

'(a) Avoidance of problem when or if to take our youngest son to Oxford. (b) Home treatment being more prompt seems to put him on his feet again more quickly and helps his confidence. (c) If he goes away the medicine can go with him. Comment: There were times with our eldest son when an elbow, say would blow up quickly and he would actually find it too painful to go up to Oxford (from Surrey) by car and prefer to let the bleed take its own course.'

3 Comment by a mother of a haemophilic son.

'(a) School absences cut by 2/3rds. (b) Saving on petrol in first six months—£30. (c) Time factor, treatment within 1 hour, previously up to 4 hours, consequently bleeds not so severe and back to normal almost immediately. (d) Family life tensions and upsets as far as having a haemophiliac virtually removed. (e) Since home treatment able to plan holidays abroad etc. without fear of last minute cancellations.'

4 Comment by a mother of a haemophilic son.

'(a) Prompt treatment is avoiding lengthy painful bleeding episodes. (b) Only minimum amount of schooling is lost. (c) Definite psychological advantage for our son knowing treatment is close at hand. (d) Less travelling expenses for parents—saving of £5 a week.'

5 Agreed comment of a teenager with haemophilia B and his parents.

'We have found the home treatment particularly advantageous financially as we were travelling down to Oxford every fortnight with our son. From the patient's point of view it has been considerably more helpful in that it has averted serious bleeds developing because he has been able to dose himself with factor IX immediately there has been any sign of trouble as well as once fortnightly prophylactic treatment. This in turn has meant that our son has been able to lead a much more normal way of life and has been able to attend school much more regularly.'

6 Comment by the parents of a haemophilic boy.

'Due to being able to give our son treatment as soon as it is needed we find that there is now no need for him to retain a wheelchair at home. We are, therefore, arranging for this to be returned for a more needy case.'

7 Comments from the parents of 2 haemophilic boys.

'Our eldest son used to have a terrible fear of staying in hospital. Now with home treatment the bleeds can be checked much quicker and there is less chance of a stay in hospital. This has made a big difference to him and he has certainly accepted now that he has haemophilia.

Our younger boy has very much less time off school. The bleed can be stopped almost as soon as it starts, without having to travel to Oxford, which although it only takes $1\frac{1}{4}$ hours to get there is a whole day by ambulance.

Before I did home treatment I used to dread waking up in case it was "another journey to Oxford", but if our youngest boy has a bleed in the morning he very often goes off to school after his injection.'

8 Comment from the mother of a haemophilic son.

'I am able to get our son treated right at the start of a bleed, which means that he has far less pain, and therefore he now tells me as soon as he has a bleed. Before he was very upset at having to go to hospital and would say nothing, which made it worse.'

9 Comments from a number of adult patients.

(i) No problems; why didn't I apply years ago for home treatment. Happiness is a fridge full of AHG.

(ii) Early treatment eliminates pain, reduces muscle wastage, allows joints to settle and enables me to lead a more active and full life.

(iii) Home treatment has changed my life immeasurably. I can now keep a job and my employer can rely on me. I can now lead a normal life.

(iv) (a) Less time off work. (b) Able to enjoy an active life. (c) Less trouble for parents and yourself. (d) Able to keep a job for a good length of time.

(v) Home treatment is a tremendous help in stopping or minimising bleeds quickly—it should ideally be extended to all haemophiliacs.

(vi) It is impossible to estimate the great advantages of early and speedy treatment with consequent quick recovery—I am extremely grateful.

(vii) Because treatment is immediately available, haemophilia is becoming less of a day-to-day burden than arthritis. It is the latter which is making earning a living increasingly difficult. Living only 30 minutes away from the Centre, I have always (in recent years) been lucky enough to get very prompt treatment anyway. The great advantage is peace of mind (e.g. being able to take away material on holiday).

In conclusion we feel that the introduction of home therapy has opened a new era in the treatment of haemophilia. The concept is as a parent has said, 'such a sensible and obviously practical way of dealing with haemophilia'. The system recognises the fact that there are not infinite resources for the care of patients under the NHS. The cost to the NHS were truly equivalent treatment available in hospital would be enormous. We have every reason to believe that as the years pass patients will tend to use less factor VIII rather than more for several reasons. Their muscular development will improve from the regular moderate exercise that patients now take. Chronically inflamed joints will occur less frequently since early treatment will become the rule. The earlier treatment is given, the smaller will be the dose that will be needed to control the bleeding.

References

HERSENS W.TH. (1975) The haemophilic way of life, in Brinkhous K.M. & Hemker H.C. *Handbook of Haemophilia.* Exerpta Medica, Amsterdam.
JONES P. (1974) *Living with Haemophilia.* MTP Medical and Technical Publishing Company, Lancaster.
JONES P. (1976) Personal communication.
MASSIE R. & MASSIE S. (1975) *Journey.* Alfred Knopf, New York.
RAINSFORD S.G. & HALL A. (1973) A three-year study of adolescent boys suffering from haemophilia and allied disorders. *British Journal of Haematology,* **24,** 539.

Chapter 8. Von Willebrand's Disease

C. R. RIZZA

This disease was described by von Willebrand in 1931 amongst the Aaland Islanders in the Gulf of Bothnia. The condition is inherited as an autosomal dominant, affects males and females and is characterised clinically by bleeding from the mucous membranes of the gastrointestinal tract, menorrhagia and bleeding from superficial injury of the skin. The bleeding time is prolonged but the whole blood clotting time and platelet count are usually normal.

Nature of the disease

Though most of the usual blood clotting tests are normal it is now known that many patients with von Willebrand's disease have a reduced level of factor VIII activity in their blood (Alexander & Goldstein, 1953; Larrieu & Soulier, 1953; Nilsson et al, 1957a). Another interesting observation made by Nilsson and her colleagues (1957b) and by Cornu et al (1963) was that the factor VIII response following transfusion is different in patients with von Willebrand's disease compared to that seen in haemophiliacs; in the patients with von Willebrand's disease the level of factor VIII in their blood rises higher than would be expected from the amount of factor VIII transfused and the level remains raised for 2–3 days sometimes (Figure 8.1). Also the transfusion of haemophilic plasma, containing no factor VIII activity, produces a prolonged rise of the factor VIII in the patients with von Willebrand's disease (Cornu et al, 1963). The transfusion of von Willebrand's plasma into a haemophiliac has no such effect. The correction of the bleeding time in von Willebrand's disease following transfusion is variable and it may not be corrected, even although high levels of factor VIII activity have been achieved, or the bleeding time may be corrected for a few hours only.

Clinical features

Apart from the fact that von Willebrand's disease may affect both males and females and the inheritance is autosomal dominant, the condition is different from haemophilia in its clinical manifestations. Whereas in haemophilia bleeding takes place typically into joints and muscles, in von Willebrand's disease

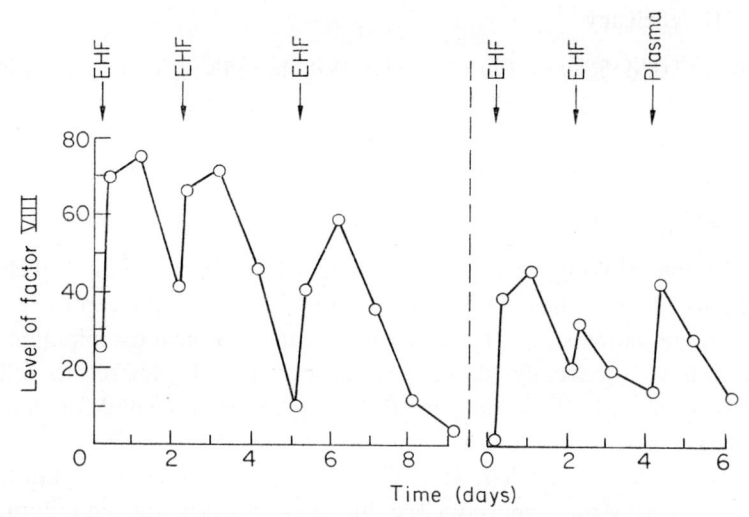

Figure 8.1. The blood levels of factor VIII observed in Case 132. The doses of EHF (human factor VIII) were in order of administration 200 ml, 100 ml, 200 ml, 200 ml, 100 ml; 500 ml of plasma was also given. Time is in days after operation.

bleeding is from mucous membranes, epistaxis, gastrointestinal bleeding and menorrhagia being the commonest forms of bleeding. Bleeding from the skin can occasionally be troublesome and bruising is common. Haemarthroses, so common in haemophilia, are very rarely seen in von Willebrand's disease even in the patients with no circulating factor VIII. If joint swelling does occur it is important to consider and exclude the other possible causes of joint swelling for example rheumatoid arthritis, before making a diagnosis of haemarthrosis. It may very occasionally be necessary to aspirate the joint and demonstrate the presence of blood in order to arrive at a more certain diagnosis.

The defects of von Willebrand's disease

Bleeding time

A prolongation of the bleeding time has always been one of the most important and consistent features of severe von Willebrand's disease and there are many who hold that the diagnosis should not be made unless the bleeding time is prolonged.

The bleeding time is technically a test of considerable inaccuracy; the Ivy method, with or without a template is probably the most reproducible method available.

Factor VIII deficiency

The factor VIII deficiency found in von Willebrand's disease is usually mild ranging from 10–50% of normal, but levels lower than 5% are found in which case the patient is usually severely affected.

Capillary and platelet defects

Because of the prolongation of the skin bleeding time in von Willebrand's disease many attempts have been made to find a defect in the capillaries or the platelets. Some patients have been shown on microscopical examination of the nail-bed to have abnormally shaped capillaries which do not retract following injury (Macfarlane, 1941) but in general the capillaries of the nail-fold have been found to be normal in most cases.

With regard to the platelets, several defects have been described but the two which are probably most reproducible and easy to study are the failure of the platelets to adhere to glass beads (Salzman, 1963; O'Brien & Heywood, 1967; Murphy & Salzman, 1972) and the failure of the platelets to be aggregated by the antibiotic ristocetin (Howard & Firkin, 1971; Dowling *et al,* 1975; Ekert *et al,* 1976). Both those phenomena have been widely studied in recent years and although the results depend on the method used those studies have provided some insight into the possible nature of the von Willebrand's defect or defects.

Adhesion of platelets to glass beads

There is no doubt that the platelets of some patients with von Willebrand's disease do not adhere to glass as readily as do normal platelets but the tests for platelet adhesiveness are not easy to standardise and give extremely variable results in normal people. The difference between normal people and those having von Willebrand's disease with respect of platelet adhesiveness is a statistical difference and little reliance can be placed on platelet adhesiveness tests in reaching a diagnosis of von Willebrand's disease in individual patients. It is also not certain that reduced adhesion to glass is a defect limited to von Willebrand's disease patients (Walsh, 1972).

The aggregation of platelets in the presence of ristocetin

Ristocetin is an antibiotic which was withdrawn from clinical use because it caused thrombocytopenia and precipitation of fibrinogen in haemostatically normal recipients. The aggregation of platelets caused by ristocetin is mediated by a plasma factor and the majority of patients with von Willebrand's disease so far tested have had low levels of this factor in their plasma.

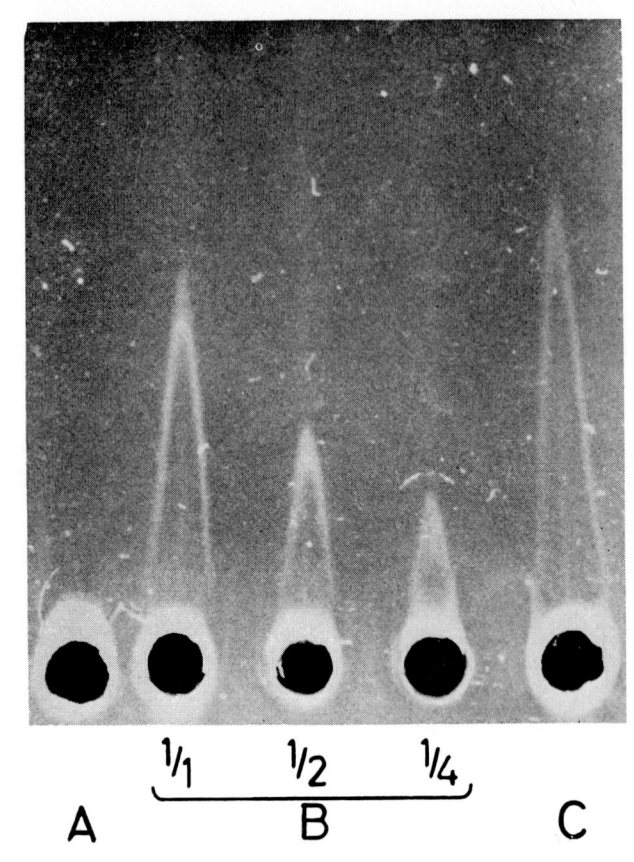

Figure 8.2. Electroimmunoassay (Laurell) carried out on
A: Plasma from patient with von Willebrand's disease
B: Doubling dilution of normal plasma
C: Plasma from a haemophiliac

Factor-VIII-related antigen

Immunological studies have led to the recognition of an antigen present in normal plasma and haemophilic plasma but reduced or absent in von Willebrand's disease.

The most striking results have been obtained using the Laurell (1966) electroimmune assay (Figure 8.2) employing heterologous rabbit antibody produced by injection of semi-purified factor VIII (Zimmerman et al, 1971). This antigen has been called cross reactive material (CRM) factor-VIII-related protein, or factor-VIII-related antigen. The latter term is the one more widely used although the relationship of the antigen to factor VIII activity is not fully understood.

Transfusion studies in von Willebrand's disease

When therapeutic material containing factor VIII activity is transfused into a haemophiliac the transfused factor VIII activity disappears from the circulation with a half disappearance time (half-life) of approximately 12 hours. The course of events following transfusion of factor VIII is different in patient's with von Willebrand's disease; immediately after transfusion the patient's factor VIII level rises to the level expected from the dose given but instead of falling off steadily over the next 24 hours back to the pre infusion level, there is an initial fall in the factor VIII level followed by a secondary rise some hours after the transfusion. This is generally agreed to be the case with most cases of von Willebrand's disease (Figure 8.3). When one comes to consider the behaviour of factor-VIII-related antigen in the patient's circulation after transfusion the results have been variable. Some workers have found that the factor VIII-related antigen shows a fall-off pattern similar to factor VIII clotting activity (Kernoff et al, 1974) (Figure 8.3). Whereas others have found that the level of factor-VIII-related antigen falls very quickly back to the pre-infusion level so that the level of factor VIII activity some hours after transfusion is often found to be much higher than the level of factor-VIII-related antigen (Bennett et al, 1972).

Following the infusion of plasma and plasma fractions containing factor VIII the bleeding time may be reduced towards the normal range (Nilsson et al, 1957b; Nilsson & Blombäck, 1962; Biggs & Matthews, 1963). The reduction in bleeding time may be short lived and not into the normal range. The characteristics of this 'bleeding time' factor have not been well defined but it is presumed that a plasma 'factor' is responsible for the alteration in bleeding time.

It is now generally accepted that the plasma of patients with classical von Willebrand's disease lacks at least six 'factors' or activities:

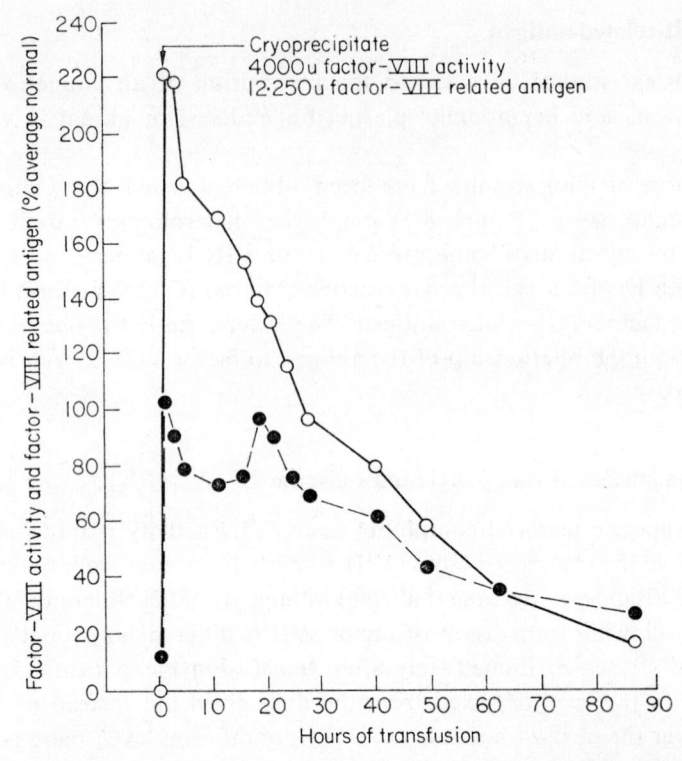

Figure 8.3. Response to transfusion of cryoprecipitate in case 191. ●, factor VIII activity; ○, factor VIII-related antigen.

1 a bleeding time factor;
2 factor VIII clotting activity;
3 a factor stimulating release or production of factor VIII clotting activity;
4 a factor necessary for adhesion of platelets to glass beads;
5 factor-VIII-related antigen;
6 a factor necessary for aggregation of platelets by the antibiotic ristocetin.

Some of the properties of those factors are shown in Table 8.1.

It is not known to what extent the different activities represent different molecular entities but it seems unlikely that all six activities represent six different molecules. Recent work suggests that the ristocetin co-factor, factor-VIII-related antigen and the factor promoting adhesion of platelets to glass beads are all functions of the same molecule.

The diagnosis of von Willebrand's disease

The diagnosis of the disease in the severely affected patient is rarely difficult. The clinical feature of dominant inheritance, epistaxis, menorrhagia and bleeding

Table 8.1. The properties associated with factors or activities (other than factor VIII clotting activity) which may be lacking from the plasma of patients with von Willebrand's disease.

Activity or factor	Properties
Plasma factor which controls the aggregation of platelets by Ristocetin	Heat labile. Neutralised by rabbit antibodies directed against factor-VIII-related antigen. Present in haemophilic plasma
Factor-VIII-related antigen	Heat stable, present in serum, stable on storage. Measured by Laurell technique using rabbit antibody. Present in haemophilic plasma. Not absorbed by Al(OH)$_3$ precipitated by 33% (NH$_4$)$_2$SO$_4$ and in Cohn fraction 1
Factor which causes the delayed rise in plasma factor VIII	Stable on storage. Present in normal serum and in haemophilic plasma. Duration of effect 24–48 hours. Present in haemophilic plasma and in cryoprecipitate and Cohn fraction 1
Factor which shortens the bleeding time	May be labile on storage. The effect is of a few hours duration. May be present in haemophilic plasma. Present in cryoprecipitate and Cohn fraction 1. Absent from purified fibrinogen
Factor which promotes adhesion to glass	Heat labile. Neutralised by rabbit antibody directed against factor-VIII-related antigen. Present in haemophilic plasma

from the gastro-intestinal tract along with the laboratory findings of a prolonged Ivy bleeding time, a reduced level of factor-VIII activity and a reduced level of factor-VIII-related antigen are characteristic.

Diagnosis of the mildly affected patients however, can be sometimes difficult especially if there is only a slight prolongation of the bleeding time and nearly normal levels of factor VIII activity and factor-VIII-related antigen. In some cases a diagnosis may be rendered more probable by assaying the patient's factor VIII activity level at intervals after a transfusion of factor VIII to see if the infusion gives rise to a prolonged elevation of plasma factor VIII (Figure 8.1). Also studies of adhesion of platelets to glass beads and aggregation of platelets by ristocetin may give some useful additional information.

The diagnosis in these mild cases may be almost a matter of opinion. The disease does not seem to have one clearly defined cause though in time one such primary cause may be identified. At present some physicians reserve the diagnosis of von Willebrand's disease for the severely affected cases whereas others would classify as von Willebrand's disease all patients who had abnormal platelet aggregation in the presence of ristocetin. The problem of diagnosis in these cases is also discussed in Chapter 3.

The management of patients with von Willebrand's disease

It is our experience that haemorrhage in von Willebrand's disease is usually controlled by giving transfusions of factor VIII-containing material even although these transfusions may not correct the skin bleeding time as measured by the Ivy method or may correct it for only a short time (Biggs & Matthews, 1963).

The principles of replacement therapy are much the same as in the management of haemophilia, that is the level of factor VIII in the patient's blood should be raised to a haemostatic level and maintained there until healing is well advanced.

In addition to transfusions of factor VIII, it is important, especially during abdominal surgery, to ensure that local haemostasis is achieved at the time of operation by packing the wound and applying local pressure.

Von Willebrand's is in general a much less severe disease than haemophilia; and bleeding is usually the consequence of accidents or surgical operations.

Epistaxis

The less severe bouts of nose bleeding are often controlled by simply pinching the nostrils for 5–10 minutes providing the site of haemorrhage is low down in the nose. Failing this it may be necessary to pack the nose with ribbon gauze soaked in saline or Russell's viper venom. Care must be taken to see that the pack extends all the way to the back of the nose and includes the bleeding point. A dose of factor VIII sufficient to raise the patient's plasma factor VIII level to 30–40% of normal should also be given. With this treatment the majority of epistaxes can be controlled. It is undesirable to leave the nasal pack in place for more than 24–36 hours for fear of encouraging infection in the nose or para-nasal sinuses. A dose of factor VIII should be given a short time before the pack is removed. We have rarely found it necessary to carry out cautery of the nose to control nose bleeding. In the few instances in which we have employed it the results have been disappointing and after a short period of days or weeks when the treatment was apparently successful, the epistaxes recurred.

Dental extraction

The regime of treatment used for dental extraction is the same as that used in haemophiliacs. A dose of factor VIII sufficient to raise the patient's factor VIII level to 50% of normal is given immediately before operation along with a dose of Cyclokapron intravenously in a dose of 1 g. Thereafter no more factor VIII is given unless haemorrhage occurs but Cyclokapron is given daily for 7 days in a dosage of 1 g four times a day. Penicillin is also given by mouth during the same post-operative period (Chapter 6).

Menorrhagia

Menorrhagia is a common feature of von Willebrand's disease and may be severe enough to require the patient to have blood transfusions to correct anaemia. Dilatation and curettage of the uterus should not be carried out unless there is a strong suspicion that there is some important underlying pathology causing the bleeding. The operation of dilatation and curettage may make the bleeding worse. If D and C is to be carried out the patient should be given a dose of factor VIII to raise her factor VIII level to 60–80% of normal. A second dose of factor VIII should be given 24 to 48 hours later depending on the patient's factor VIII level. Menorrhagia in von Willebrand's disease especially in younger women may often be diminished by the taking of the contraceptive pill.

Major surgery

Factor VIII replacement therapy is necessary for the control of post-operative haemorrhage in von Willebrand's disease. The levels of factor VIII required for haemostasis is the same as that required in haemophilia. Because of the prolonged rise of factor VIII in the patient's plasma after transfusion of the first dose subsequent doses need not be given as frequently as in haemophilia. In addition to achieving a haemostatic level of factor VIII in the blood, it is important at the time of operation to be sure that all capillary bleeding has been controlled before closing the wound.

References

ALEXANDER B. & GOLDSTEIN R. (1953) Dual haemostatic defect in pseudohemophilia. *Journal of Clinical Investigation*, **32**, 551.

BENNETT B., RATNOFF O.D. & LEVIN J. (1972) Immunologic studies in von Willebrand's disease. Evidence that antihaemophilia factor (AHF) produced after transfusion lacks an antigen associated with normal AHF and the inactive material produced by patients with classic hemophilia. *Journal of Clinical Investigation*, **51**, 2597.

BIGGS R. & MATTHEWS J.M. (1963) The treatment of haemorrhage in von Willebrand's disease and the blood level of factor VIII (AHF). *British Journal of Haematology*, **9**, 203.

CORNU P., LARRIEU M.J., CAEN J. & BERNARD J. (1963) Transfusion studies in von Willebrand's disease: effect on bleeding time and factor VIII assay. *British Journal of Haematology*, **9**, 189.

DOWLING S.V., MUNTZ R.H., D'SOUZA S. & EKERT H. (1975) Ristocetin in the diagnosis of von Willebrand's disease. A comparison of rated per cent of aggregation with levels of plasma factor(s) necessary for ristocetin aggregation. *Thrombosis et Diathesis Haemorrhagica*, **34**, 465.

EKERT H., ANANTHAKRISHNAN R., MUNTZ R.H., DOWLING S. & D'SOUZA S. (1976) Family studies of patients with reduced ristocetin aggregation and abnormal factor VIII and/or platelet function. *Thrombosis and Haemostasis*, **36,** 78.

HOWARD M.A. & FIRKIN B.G. (1971) Ristocetin a new tool in the investigation of platelet aggregation. *Thrombosis et Diathesis Haemorrhagica*, **26,** 362.

KERNOFF P.B.A., RIZZA C.R. & KAELIN A.C. (1974) Transfusion and gel filtration studies in von Willebrand's disease. *British Journal of Haematology*, **28,** 357.

LARRIEU M.J. & SOULIER J.P. (1953) Déficit en facteur antihémophilique A chez une fille associé à un trouble du saignement. *Revue d'hématologie*, **8,** 361.

LAURELL C.-B. (1966) Quantitative estimation of proteins by electrophoresis in agarose gel containing antibodies. *Analytical Biochemistry*, **15,** 45.

MACFARLANE R.G. (1941) Critical Review: the mechanism of haemostasis. *Quarterly Journal of Medicine*, **33,** 1.

MURPHY A.E. & SALZMAN E.W. (1972) Platelet adhesiveness in von Willebrand's disease. A co-operative study. *Thrombosis et Diathesis Haemorrhagica*. Supplement, **51,** 341.

NILSSON I.M. & BLOMBÄCK M. (1962) Von Willebrand's disease in Sweden, occurence, pathogenesis and treatment. *Thrombosis et Diathesis Haemorrhagica*. Supplement 2 to volume 9, 103.

NILSSON I.M., BLOMBÄCK M. & VON FRANKEN I. (1957a) On an inherited autosomal hemorrhagic diathesis with antihemophilic globulin (AHG) deficiency and prolonged bleeding time. *Acta Medica Scandinavica*, **159,** 35.

NILSSON I.M., BLOMBÄCK M., JORPES E., BLOMBÄCK B. & JOHANSSON S.A. (1975b) Von Willebrand's disease and its correction with human plasma fraction 1–0. *Acta Medica Scandinavica*, **159,** 179.

O'BRIEN J.R. & HEYWOOD J.B. (1967) Some interactions between human platelets and glass. Von Willebrand's disease compared with normal. *Journal of Clinical Pathology*, **20,** 56.

SALZMAN E.W. (1963) Measurement of platelet adhesiveness. A simple *in vitro* technique demonstrating an abnormality in von Willebrand's disease. *Journal of Laboratory and Clinical Investigation*, **62,** 724.

VON WILLEBRAND E.A. (1931) Über hereditare Pseudohämophilie. *Acta Medica Scandinavica*, **76,** 52.

WALSH P.N. (1972) Platelet coagulant activities in thrombasthenia. *British Journal of Haematology*, **23,** 553.

ZIMMERMAN T.S., RATNOFF O.D. & POWELL A.E. (1971) Immunologic differentiation of classic hemophilia and von Willebrand's disease. *Journal of Clinical Investigation*, **50,** 244.

Chapter 9. Complications of Treatment

ROSEMARY BIGGS

The complications that arise from the treatment of patients with plasma fractions are of four main types:

1   The transmission to the patient of an infective organism contained in the fraction in particular the agents causing hepatitis.
2   Pyrogenic and other adverse reactions to infusion therapy.
3   Thrombosis.
4   The development of antibodies against coagulation factors and particularly against factor VIII.

Transmission of diseases contained in the fractions

Hepatitis

There are several types of virus that can transmit hepatitis when given by injection. One is called hepatitis virus A or infective hepatitis. The second is hepatitis virus B or serum hepatitis. The disease caused by virus A has an incubation period of 15–40 days whereas that caused by hepatitis virus B has an incubation period of 60–160 days. Virus A has been demonstrated in faeces whereas virus B has been found in blood only. Early experiments on volunteers showed that virus A could be transmitted by oral and parenteral routes whereas virus B was only infective parenterally. More recent studies have in fact found that the B virus can also be transmitted orally (Krugman & Giles, 1970; Giles & Krugman, 1972). Both viruses can also be transmitted by blood sucking insects (Metselaar *et al*, 1973) and this may account for the high incidence of hepatitis B found in the populations of malarial areas.

The earlier observations concerned the occurence of hepatitis in patients receiving adult serum as a prophylactic against measles or yellow fever vaccine containing some normal serum. In 1964 Blumberg found an unusual antibody in the serum of a transfused haemophiliac which reacted with the serum of Australian Aborigines. This same antibody was found in the blood of a proportion of patients having viral hepatitis and the antigen was called the Australia antigen. It was later found that the antigen was associated with the long incubation type of virus hepatitis infection and the antigen is now often called HB_sAg and the antibody, HB_sAb.

The reported incidence of HB_sAg positive samples in the normal blood donor population varies considerably. In the United Kingdom the incidence was reported as 1 in 1,200 to 1 in 1,500 donor samples. In the United States of America the incidence is similar for blood collected from volunteer donors but may be as high as 1 in 50 to 1 in 100 for commercial donors (Maycock, 1972). In both the United Kingdom and in the United States of America, donor blood is tested for HB_sAg and positive samples are excluded. There are difficulties in these testing procedures (Prince *et al,* 1974). Some tests detect smaller amounts of virus than others and thus give a more sensitive indication of infectivity. For example the counter electrophoresis (CEP) method detects one tenth of the amount of virus that is detected by the immunodiffusion technique. The Radio Immuno Assay (RIA) detects virus at a concentration of 1 in 100 of that detected by CEP. If one or other of these tests were entirely reliable the exclusion of positive donors would eliminate one source of blood transmitted hepatitis. In fact using the immune diffusion method to detect virus it was found that transfusion of positive blood to 42 recipients was followed by 22 cases (52%) of hepatitis whereas the transfusion of negative blood to 126 recipients resulted in 8 cases (6%) of hepatitis. Using CEP tested blood 3·7 per 1000 recipients of negative blood (0·37%) developed hepatitis B. These statistics show marked progressive reduction in hepatitis following the testing donors for hepatitis B antigen and the exclusion of positive donors. The RIA test, though much more sensitive than CEP test in detecting small amounts of virus, gives an undefined proportion of positive results in samples that apparently do *not* contain virus. For example the blood of guinea-pig handlers had a high incidence of positive tests which was attributed to non-specific antibody to guinea-pig protein and not to the presence of hepatitis virus. Donor testing is important but at present no testing procedure will eliminate all samples infected with hepatitis B virus. The very high incidence of HB_sAg in the blood of commercial donors means that even when the known positive samples are excluded, the blood products made from commercial donor blood are liable to be more infective than similar products made from volunteer donor blood.

A rather high proportion of haemophilic patients who develop hepatitis have no serological evidence of hepatitis B virus infection. These patients may have hepatitis A for which no serological tests are at present available. They may also have long incubation type hepatitis the causative agents for which have as yet not been identified. They may even develop jaundice for other reasons, for example haemolytic response to the infusion of blood group antibodies.

When considering the infectivity of plasma fractions it is clear that, whatever virus types may contaminate donor blood, the pooling of blood from many donors will increase the probability of including a sample containing some virus. It is obvious that volunteer donors and small pool fractionation methods will result in the safest plasma fractions. While these conclusions are not disputed it must be said that small pools of volunteer donor plasma cannot easily be reconciled with commercial fractionation practice and that the voluntary and national organisations, which can work with small pools of volunteer donor plasma, have not so far developed efficient fractionation programmes from which sufficient amounts of fractions are prepared.

The discussion up to this point favours fractionation procedures using small pools of donor plasma but the development of disease may be related to the amount of virus administered. Thus fractions made of large pools may be more likely to contain some virus to which all patients receiving the fractions will be exposed, but a patient who receives a single whole infected donation may be more liable to contract hepatitis than one who receives pooled material in which the virus is much diluted. This idea is supported by the early studies on volunteers (Barker et al, 1970) and by observations made in a United Kingdom study of haemophilia (Biggs, 1974). In the study of haemophilic patients a comparison was made between the patients treated wholly with cryoprecipitate and those treated with both cryoprecipitate and concentrate. The patients treated with cryoprecipitate were each exposed to relatively few different donations of blood but when a patient received a donation containing hepatitis virus he received the whole donation. Patients treated with concentrate on the other hand would receive pooled material and thus be exposed to much larger numbers of blood donations and each patient had a greater chance of receiving some infected material than those exposed to cryoprecipitate alone but in each exposed patient the dose would be smaller. The incidence of clinical jaundice in the two groups was similar, a finding which suggested that the lower rate of exposure to virus of the cryoprecipitate-treated patients was counter-balanced by a higher incidence of disease as a result of exposure. If the incidence of disease is related to amount of virus received then there could also be some argument against the use of cryoprecipitate and against reserving small batches of NHS concentrate for individual patients.

The diagnosis of hepatitis

In the MRC Survey (1974) of hepatitis in normal people following transfusions it was found that, of 768 cases carefully studied and followed up, 158 showed some abnormalities of liver function tests (alanine transaminase ALT). Of these 8 (1%) were diagnosed definitely as having contracted transfusion transmitted hepatitis. The diagnosis was confirmed by other clinical evidence of hepatitis and the presence of HB$_s$Ag in two patients and by liver biopsy in 6 patients. Of the 150 other patients with raised ALT 35 had sustained prolonged rise and thus could have had hepatitis but the diagnosis was not confirmed though 4 of these cases had positive HB$_s$Ag tests. Anaesthetics, drugs or alcohol seemed likely causes of the abnormal liver function tests in 17 cases. 'Acceptable' reasons for the abnormal results were reported in 27 patients. The remaining 71 patients had no 'acceptable' known cause for the ALT abnormality. These details are reported to show some of the difficulties that may occur in trying to decide which ratients have contracted hepatitis. In this MRC Survey the whole of the evidence as it concerned each patient was taken into account. The greatest reliance was placed on liver biopsy which is, of course, contra-indicated in haemophilic patients. In the MRC study of haemophilic patients Biggs (1974) the diagnosis was based on occurrence of clinical illness with jaundice. This limitation will certainly have excluded a number of cases of true an-icteric hepatitis.

The susceptibility of patients to infection with hepatitis

When blood known to be HB$_s$Ag positive is given to recipients not previously transfused about 50% of them develop clinical hepatitis and a further 25% develop a positive HB$_s$Ag or HB$_s$Ab test. The studies from which these conclusions are drawn concern the administration of blood to volunteers (Murray, 1955 and Barker *et al*, 1970) or to studies on normal recipients who inadvertently received HB$_s$Ag positive blood (Gocke, 1970). These receipients were previously untransfused and must be presumed to be susceptible to virus. In the early studies using volunteers (Murray, 1955) it was found that a large dose favoured disease and a small dose a subclinical or negative response.

The dangers of transfusion of infected blood are undoubtedly large. It has been estimated that there may be 30,000 cases of transfusion hepatitis in the USA annually and that 5 to 10% of these patients die of the disease (Maycock, 1972). It is thus of major importance to do everything possible to improve the safety of transfusion blood and of the products that are made from blood. Most receipients of blood have not previously been transfused and are thus not immunised to hepatitis by repeated eposure to virus.

In considering the haemophilic population the issue is less clearly defined though the hope is for blood products with low incidence of hepatitis virus contamination. The severely affected haemophilic patient is transfused usually many times a year from early childhood. There is some evidence that the presence of HB$_s$Ab may protect the patient against infection (Krugman *et al*, 1971a, b). The effects produced by virus on recipients are very diverse. There may be no effect, there may be positive test for **HB$_s$Ag** or **HB$_s$Ab** and no clinical effects. There may be positive liver function test and no clinical effect. There may be all grades of clinical illness from a mild influenzal syndrome to fulminant liver necrosis and death. The recovery from illness may be rapid or delayed and the illness may go on to a stage of chronic cirrhosis and ultimate liver failure.

From the number of different donations to which haemophilic patients are exposed in the United Kingdom one can calculate that more than half probably receive virus infected material at some time in the year. With the use of commercial human factor VIII derived from commercial donors it may not be long before every haemophilic patient receives some virus infected material every year. From the virologist's point of view the situation of the haemophiliac is frightening and unacceptable. The virologist has a natural aversion to the use of a therapeutic material which may contain viral agents, but the virologist does not understand the choice which faces haemophiliacs. For the haemophilic patient the present choice is not between a treatment of marginal effectiveness and no treatment at all. The treatment given to haemophiliacs is for saving life, for the prevention of crippling. The danger of getting hepatitis is a risk that must at present be taken and the problems are to assess how great is the current risk and how the risk may best be reduced. An analysis of the reported incidence of jaundice in Oxford cases and in those reported from other United Kingdom Haemophilia Centres for the years 1969–1975 are presented in Table 9.1 (Biggs & Spooner, 1977). It will be seen that the incidence of jaundice up to 1973 remained remarkably constant both in Oxford and at the other Centres. The incidence is low when it is considered that more than half the patients must have been given virus contaminated material at some time in each year. The increased use of commercial factor VIII concentrate in 1973 and 1974 will certainly have increased the proportion of patients exposed to virus and may have produced an increased incidence of disease (see Table 9.1).

We can say that illness associated with jaundice probably occurs in 4 to 6% of haemophilic patients who are exposed to virus. This incidence is to be compared to a 50–75% infection rate in normal people who receive transfusions. The reason for the difference is almost certainly that haemophilic patients as a class are immunised to viral hepatitis whereas normal people are not. Tests for HB_sAg and HB_sAb show that 30–50% of haemophilic patients are HB_sAb positive at any one time. A much lower proportion, about 3%, are HB_sAg positive. There has been some belief that concentrated preparations of factor IX are more liable to cause hepatitis than preparations of factor VIII made from similar sized pools of plasma. This belief is not well founded. Factor IX has been given to many patients who have not been much transfused in the past (e.g. liver disease patients, patients on coumarin anticoagulants and premature infants) and those patients are more susceptible to hepatitis than are Christmas disease patients who have received many previous infusions. The Christmas disease patients treated in the United Kingdom had a lower incidence of hepatitis than haemophilic patients (Table 9.1).

Table 9.1. The incidence of jaundice in patients having haemophilia A and B observed at Haemophilia Centres in the United Kingdom from 1969 to 1974. From Biggs & Spooner, 1977.

	All cases			Oxford		
Year	Number of patient treatment years	Number of incidents of jaundice per year	%	Number of patient treatment years	Number of incidents of jaundice per year	%
	Haemophilia A					
1969	1022	20*	1·96	174	4	2·30
1970	1111	26	2·34	166	5	3·01
1971	1154	16	1·39	179	8	4·47
1972	1234	18	1·46	207	3	1·45
1973	1434	26*	1·81	217	8	3·69
1974	1634	85**	5·20	219	16	7·30
Mean	1265	31	2·45	194	7·3	3·70
	Haemophilia B					
1969	142	2	1·40	37	1	2·70
1970	131	0	0	35	0	0
1971	132	2	1·51	25	2	8·00
1972	171	4	2·34	38	1	2·63
1973	190	2	1·05	43	0	0
1974	200	5	2·50	35	0	0
Mean	162	2·50	1·47	35·5	0·67	2·22

* One patient was jaundiced twice in the year.
** Five patients were jaundiced twice in the year.

At the present time no very clear decision can be reached about this problem but a number of interim suggestions can be made which may influence policy for a particular patient.

1 Mildly affected patients who have never been transfused or have been only infrequently transfused should not receive large pool commercial concentrates. These patients are more liable to develop hepatitis than those who are frequently transfused and should be given cryoprecipitate or small pool concentrates.

2 Severely affected patients who have positive test for HB_sAb can in general safely receive large pool commercial concentrates.

3   Treatment should not be withheld from the severely affected patient because of the danger of hepatitis. The danger of death from haemorrhage and crippling are of more immediate importance.

The need for future observations for the prevention of hepatitis

There are two urgent problems which need solution, one concerns the production of virus free fractions, and it is to be hoped that progress will be made in testing plasma submitted to fractionation procedures to eliminate virus. The second important line of study concerns the fate of virus and clinical disease in patients. In this latter problem it is important to know the liver function of patients who receive frequent dosage of factors VIII or IX and the relationships of liver function to tests for HB_sAg or HB_sAb. It is only by keeping the most meticulous records of individual cases that progress can be made in assessing the long term danger to patients of repeated infusions of virus contaminated materials. So far our attention has centred on clinical illness associated with jaundice but it will be necessary to assess the significances of various abnormalities in liver function tests and of alterations in the results of tests for HB_sAg on the patient's general health over a long period of time.

An attempt to analyse the source of hepatitis in patients during 1974 in Oxford

During 1974 sixteen patients developed some evidence of hepatitis. During 6 months prior to the development of illness the sixteen patients had received 40 different batches of NHS concentrate each batch being made from pools of plasma each derived from 400 donors. In addition 5 different batches of commercial human factor VIII had been used, each of these batches being made of pools from more than 2,500 different donations. Four of the NHS batches received by some of the patients were reported as HB_sAg positive a long time after all of the material had been given to the patients. A survey was made of all the different batches of concentrate used and those batches which had been received by three or more of the patients who developed jaundice were selected as probable sources of virus infection. The patients were then divided into those who had had a change from negative to positive of either HB_sAg or Hb_sAb at the time of developing jaundice and those whose plasma showed no change in this respect. This separation is shown in Table 9.2. For the patient with a positive change in HB_sAg or HB_sAb a long incubation period for jaundice is to be anticipated. Six batches (5 NHS and one commercial) are disclosed as possibly causing infection. Of the NHS batches which may have been implicated 2 were not tested by RIA, 2 were tested by RIA and recorded as positive and one was

Table 9.2. Cases of hepatitis in Oxford (1974 treatment year).

Cases	Material given to patients NHS	Commercial	Probable donor exposure
5	1	2	5400
81	12	–	4800
208	7	3	10,300
49**	9	1	6100
180**	3	1	3700
204	3	1	3700
205	4	1	4100
72	1	–	400
168**	3	2	6200
197	4	2	6600
206	2	–	800
22	2	–	800
207*	—	2	5000
64	3	2	6200
192*	—	1	2500
34	9	1	6100

Cases 1 to 9 showed some change of Hb_sAb or Hb_sAg at the time of developing hepatitis, patients from 10 to 16 had no change in Hb_sAb or Hb_sAg.

* The patients received only commercial concentrate but one patient developed jaundice while actually receiving the material.

** By careful analysis hepatitis in these patients could have been due to one batch of commercial concentrate but two of them also received suspect batches of NHS concentrate.

tested and found to be negative. It should be noted that eleven other NHS batches were recorded as positive by RIA long after they had been given to patients and none of these preparations gave rise to jaundice in the recipients. The patients who had no change in HB_sAg or HB_sAb may be suspected of having virus A and it is not easy to be sure which batches should be considered to be responsible. There are also other possible explanations which might account for jaundice in some of these cases.

Other diseases transmitted by whole blood plasma or other fractions

One or two patients have in the past received whole blood or plasma containing malarial parasites and have developed malaria. Two such cases are recorded by

Vartan (1967) and Dike (1970). Patients could also develop cryptomegalovirus infection but to the best of our knowledge this has not been recorded in haemophiliacs.

Pyrogenic and other adverse reactions to infusion therapy

In the past patients were usually infused with whole blood or plasma rather than with concentrates of clotting factors. To achieve safe haemostatic levels of factor VIII using plasma infusions it was often necessary to give the largest volume of plasma that could safely be administered without overloading the circulation. Most of the patients who were treated were young and had normal cardiovascular systems and thus seldom showed evidence of circulatory overloading. Nevertheless the need to give the largest safe volume must occasionally lead to a patient suffering from hypervolaemia when plasma is used.

A small proportion of patients developed reactions to plasma infusions. The least dangerous type of reaction involved urticaria but pyrexia, bronchospasm and pulmonary congestion and even death have been reported (Kernoff et al, 1972). The reactions have been attributed to white cell antibodies or to anti Gm(l) precipitins in the donor plasma. Patients who have ever had reactions to plasma should always be given coagulation factor concentrates since these seldom give rise to this type of reaction.

Injections of crude concentrates of animal factor VIII commonly caused pyrogenic reactions and rigors in the early days of specific coagulation factor therapy. These reactions were probably due to materials extracted from rubber tubing and possibly to reactions between the factor VIII and the patients' platelets.

Patients who receive large amounts of plasma do occasionally develop haemolytic reactions from infused anti-A or anti-B antibodies which react with then lyse the patients own red cells (Mollison, 1972). Some preparations of factor VIII contain blood group isoagglutinins. Such preparations given in small doses do not cause haemolysis. Sometimes the large doses needed by patients undergoing operations or by patients having factor VIII antibodies do cause haemolysis (Rosati et al, 1970; Seeler, 1972 and Tamagnini et al, 1975). We have seen one patient with factor VIII antibody who required surgery who developed haemolysis due to anti-B isoagglutinin from the very high dosage of Hemofil required to assure haemostasis. Study of the cases recorded in Table 9.2 who were jaundiced but had no change in HB_sAg or HB_sAb reveals two patients who both had factor VIII antibodies and received large doses of factor VIII. It seems possible that haemolysis could have been a factor in producing icterus in these patients. This is particularly likely for one of them who developed icterus in the middle of a course of factor VIII treatment.

Thrombosis and the administration of clotting factor concentrates

As far as is known modern human factor VIII concentrates have not caused thrombosis in haemophilic patients. Concentrates of animal factor VIII, used in the early days of coagulation factor therapy, were often given through indwelling intravenous catheters that remained in the vein for several days. The veins treated in this way were often used by anaesthetists to administer Pentothal and other drugs. These ill-treated veins very often thrombosed. As a result of this experience, indwelling catheters are not used by us except in very special circumstances. Infusions are given through small needles that are removed from the vein immediately after completing the infusion. It is probable that the administration of concentrated coagulants into injured and possibly infected veins is always liable to promote thrombosis. In recent years and with recent preparations and modern techniques of venepuncture no problems with venous thrombosis have arisen in treating haemophiliacs (factor VIII deficient patients) in Oxford.

Factor IX concentrates which contain also factor II and X and sometimes also factor VII were developed for the treatment of patients having Christmas disease (factor IX deficiency); these concentrates have also been used to treat patients with other coagulation defects such as those with liver disease and vitamin K deficiency and patients who have received overdosage of coumarin type coagulants. When given to Christmas disease patients it is usual for the prothrombin level to rise to between 200 and 600% of normal (Figure 9.1). No adverse consequences of the high prothrombin level have been reported.

The evidence for the occurrence of intravascular coagulation as a result of treatment with factor IX concentrates consists in the observation of altered laboratory results on plasma samples and the occurence of clinical thrombosis. The observations have been made on Christmas disease patients and on those suffering from other diseases.

The laboratory evidence consists of a rapid rate of disappearance of the infused activity suggesting that the material infused might have been partly activated and of various alterations in clotting factor activity suggestive of intravascular clotting such as reduced platelet count, fall in the levels of clotting factors V and VIII, decrease in antithrombin or antifactor Xa and the appearance of fibrinogen degradation products. The significance of these laboratory results must be considered in relation to the total situation of the patient. For example Lane *et al* (1975) reported the results of laboratory tests on Christmas disease patients treated with concentrate in Oxford from 1970 to 1975. Of 72 patients treated none had any clinical evidence of thrombosis. A detailed study

Complications of Treatment

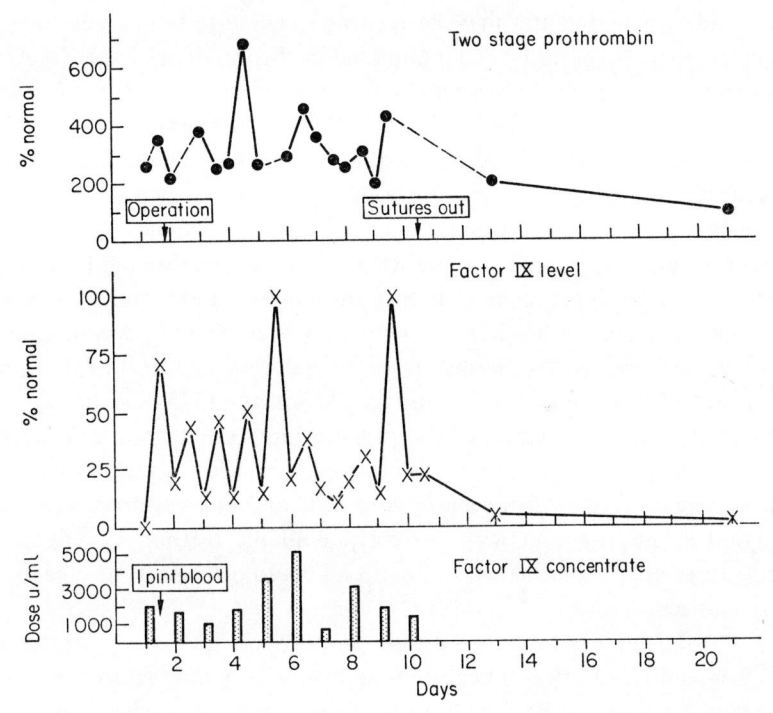

Figure 9.1. The response of a factor IX deficient patient to factor IX concentrate. The prothrombin level rose to more than 600% but no ill effects were observed.

of laboratory tests was made in some of these patients and in particular of one patient undergoing continuous high dose therapy for more than two months following surgery. There was a significant fall in antithrombin level in the patient on continuous high dosage therapy and small doubtfully significant alterations in factors V, VIII and platelets. Such finding cannot be taken as evidence of abnormal intravascular coagulation. Reports of laboratory evidence of consumption of clotting factors together with evidence of venous thrombosis and pulmonary embolism in patients having factor IX deficiency have been recorded by Edson, 1974; Steinbert & Dreiling (1973), Marchesi & Burney (1974). Kaspar (1973, 1974 and 1975) has reported incidents of thrombosis in six patients having factor IX deficiency.

For patients having factor IX deficiency it seems probable that some factor IX preparations are safer and less liable to cause thrombosis than others. It is important to be able, by laboratory testing, to distinguish 'safe' from 'unsafe' preparations from point of view of tendency to produce thrombosis in patients. Simple tests for coagulants have been used to screen therapeutic preparations. For example the concentrate may be added to fibrinogen and the occurrence of a clot is observed or the concentrate may be added to plasma and the clotting time on the addition of calcium may be recorded. These tests have excluded from clinical use some preparations contaminated by thrombin or factor Xa. Attempts to make the test systems more scientific by devising specific tests for factor Xa or factor IXa have not so far proved practically useful. These test systems are not easy to standardise or interpret. In fact such narrowly directed tests have little connection with reality since important therapeutic concentrates contain several clotting factors any one of which might or might not be activated.

Another approach concerns the association of certain simple non-specific laboratory tests with tendency to induce thrombosis in experimental animals or man. Such a test system has been developed by Wessler and his colleagues (1955 and 1959) and applied to the testing of coagulation factor II, VII, IX and X concentrates by Kingdon Veltkamp & Aronson (1975). From the results presented it seems that many of the preparations tested produced thrombi in rabbits when given in doses that could easily be used for Christmas disease patients. The correlation between *in vitro* tests and *in vivo* thrombosis was not very good suggesting that with currently available methods it might not be possible to predict which batches of material could be dangerous when given to human subjects.

This unsatisfactory situation clearly requires further study before a universally agreed set of safety precautions and rules for manufacture and testing of factor concentrates can be drawn up. In fact some authors feel that, until this problem of defining dangerous preparations can be solved factor IX preparations should not be used for the day to day treatment of patients having congenital factor IX deficiency (Roberts & Blatt, 1975). In Europe this extreme view is unlikely to gain much support for the simple reason that concentrates of factor IX made in Paris have been used with complete safety for nearly 20 years and concentrates made in Oxford have been used for 15 years with no record of thrombosis or defibrination in any single factor IX deficient patient. The methods of manufacture of the Paris material (PBSB) and the two Oxford preparations are clearly described and the methods are available for use at other fractionation laboratories. The danger of thrombotic complications concerns the use of one or two commercial factor IX concentrates. It should surely be possible for the commercial preparations to be made with the same care and attention to detail given to the French and English preparations.

These last remarks concern the use of factor IX concentrates for patients having congenital factor IX deficiency (Christmas disease). Used for conditions other than Christmas disease it must be remembered that it may be dangerous to use powerful coagulants for patients whose natural balancing inhibitory systems are defective. In England the Oxford concentrate was given to patients with acute toxic liver necrosis with adverse effects (Gazzard *et al*, 1973). In France on the other hand the Paris concentrate has been given to many patients with chronic liver disease without ill effects. Clearly a certain caution is required in the selection of liver disease patients to whom these concentrates may be given. In England no adverse effects have been seen in the use of factor IX concentrate for the rapid reversal of the oral anticoagulant defect.

The occurrence of antibodies directed against factor VIII or factor IX

Patients who have no factor VIII or no factor IX may have an immune system to which the proteins carrying these activities may be regarded foreign and against which antibodies may be directed. The production of specific antibody is rare in patients having factor IX deficiency but occurs in about 6% of patients having haemophilia (Brinkhous, Roberts & Weiss, 1972). A similar incidence of factor VIII antibodies was reported by Biggs (1974) and Biggs & Spooner (1977). The United Kingdom data concerned the observed incidence of antibodies to factor VIII reported by Haemophilia Centre Directors during 1969 to 1974. The data is included in Table 9.3, and it will be seen that incidence of anti-factor VIII antibodies in the United Kingdom has remained remarkably constant. Since the amount of treatment given to patients has increased with the passage of time one might have expected the incidence of antibodies to increase. It is reassuring that this has not happened.

It has been felt for some time that patients who develop factor VIII antibodies may differ in some respect from patients who do not. It was postulated for example that patients who developed antibodies might be totally lacking in

Table 9.3. The incidence of factor VIII or factor IX antibodies in patients having haemophilia A or B. From Biggs & Spooner, 1977.

Year	Haemophilia A Cumulative total number patients in survey	Cumulative number with factor VIII antibody	%	New cases detected	Haemophilia B Cumulative total number patients in survey	Cumulative number with factor VIII antibody	%	New cases detected
1969	1050	79	7·52	21	142	4	2·82	0
1970	1418	97	6·84	18	185	5	2·70	1
1971	1703	113	6·64	17	223	5	2·24	0
1972	1977	131	6·63	17	276	5	1·81	0
1973	2281	150	6·58	19	322	5	1·55	0
1974	2600	166	6·38	15	388	5	1·29	0
Mean			6·75					

the factor VIII protein whereas those who failed to become immunised had an abnormal protein which differed too little from the normal for the patient's immune system to react to administered factor VIII by making a specific antibody. Attempts to make such a distinction have been made by seeking to discover whether or not haemophilic plasma contains a protein which can absorb and neutralise factor VIII antibody. The results of such studies have been astonishingly variable. The variability was probably due to the use of various different types of anti-factor VIII antibodies and various methods for measuring antibody. This topic is also discussed in Chapter 3; in the present context it is fair to say that no certain connection has been found between tendency to produce antibody and the presence or absence of any particular protein in the patient's plasma.

The presence of antibodies might be related to the type of factor VIII used for treatment. The retrospective report of Brinkhous *et al* (1972) does not suggest that patients who have received concentrates of factor VIII are more liable to develop anti-factor VIII antibodies than those who have only received plasma. The development of factor VIII antibodies might have some undefined familial tendency. The studies of Brinkhous *et al* (1972) and Biggs (1974) could find no such familial tendency.

At the present time we can discover no way of distinguishing patients who will develop antibodies to factor VIII from those who do not. The low incidence could have several causes. Factor VIII is known to be at very low concentration in normal plasma thus the dose of potential immunogen is probably low in terms of mg/ml of protein. In addition the factor VIII activity is rapidly eliminated from the circulation following infusion. There may also be genetic factors which influence response to immunisation which are in no way linked to the haemophilia gene. Thus one haemophilic patient in a family could be more susceptible to immunisation by any foreign protein than a related haemophiliac.

The method of measuring anti-factor VIII antibody is discussed in Chapter 3, Using the method described we find that a dose of factor VIII of about 20 u/kg is required to neutralise 1 u/ml antibody in the patient.

Antibodies to factor IX

Antibodies to factor IX occur in patients having factor IX deficiency but these antibodies are very rare. Of 388 haemophilia B patients observed in the United Kingdom from 1969 to 1974, 5 patients (1·34%) had antibodies to factor IX (Table 9.3).

The antibody to factor IX usually destroys factor IX very rapidly. The antibody may be measured by a system similar to that used for factor VIII antibody.

The treatment of patients who have factor VIII antibodies

There are probably 150 to 200 patients in the United Kingdom who have antibodies directed against factor VIII. From the study of more than 40 patients having factor VIII antibodies it is our conviction that these patients bleed no worse than patients who do not have this complication. The number of occasions on which the patients present with haemorrhages is no more frequent than for severely affected patients who do not have antibodies. The major difficulty concerns the decision about treatment for each individual patient who has factor VIII antibody and on each occasion that bleeding occurs. There are a number of reasonably definable criteria which will influence the decision. These include the potency of antibody in the patient at the time of proposed treatment and experience of the effect of treatment on antibody potency in the particular patient in past episodes of treatment. The potential danger to the patient of each particular bleeding episode will also naturally influence the doctor's decision. Although it is not possible to enunciate absolute rules about treatment it is possible to illustrate certain categories of treatment situations.

THE TREATMENT OF PATIENTS WITH LOW TITRE ANTIBODIES OR THOSE WHOSE ANTIBODIES HAVE TEMPORARILY DISAPPEARED

When a patient who has antibody to factor VIII remains without factor VIII treatment the antibody titre falls to a low level and in a number of patients a state may be reached where no antibody can be detected. In these patients it can be predicted that factor VIII treatment will, over the short term, be as effective or almost as effective as treatment for a patient who has no antibody. The response of 9 such patients to treatment on various occasions is presented in Table 9.4.

One patient studied in detail was observed without treatment for a year and retained factor VIII antibody during this time of 1–2 u/ml. He required an operation for the removal of a locally invasive tumour of the parotid gland, his case has been recorded by Gibson, Matthews & Rizza (1976). A record of treatment is given in Figure 9.2. It will be seen that after the first day of treatment the antibody titre was reduced to zero. The half-life of factor VIII infused was about 10 hours, the rise in factor VIII level per u/kg dose approached 2%/u/kg dose which was the usual response when the material with which he was treated was given to other patients. During the second to fifth days of treatment the doses of factor VIII were similar to those required by patients who do not have antibodies and good levels of factor VIII were maintained. After the fifth day and anti-factor VIII antibody increased in titre and both the half-life of infused factor VIII and the rise %/u/kg fell rapidly. The patient had no post-operative bleeding. Experience with other patients who have low titre antibodies and who received

Table 9.4. Response of 9 haemophilic patients who had no detectable antibody to factor VIII at the time of testing (from Rizza & Biggs, 1973).

			Factor VIII activities				
Patient	Date	Wt. (kg)	Pre % average normal	Post % average normal	Dose Units	Dose u/kg	Rise in factor VIII %/u/kg
56	15.10.68	20	0	47	535	27	1·74
9	22.5.68	62	3	18	980	16	0·94
	18.5.70		10	50	1400	22	1·82
	19.5.70		9	50	1400	22	1·86
	20.5.70		12	46	1200	20	1·70
	21.5.70		10	40	1440	23	1·30
	7.9.70		12	81	2100	33	2·09
	8.9.70		18	48	1100	17·5	1·71
	9.9.70		10	—	—	—	—
	8.12.70		0	33	1800	20	1·65
192	20.3.70	73	0	30	1080	14·5	2·07
193	24.5.70	73	0	22	850	11·5	1·91
194	24.6.70	47	0	8	230	4·8	1·67
64	30.11.70	56	0	16	500	8·8	1·82
	30.8.71		13	45	900	16	2·00
195	21.8.70	73	0	40	2000	27	1·48
	22.8.70		3	34	2100	29	1·06
196	4.6.68	51	15	37	750	15	1·47
	15.7.69		0	23	1250	25	1·09
	4.4.71		0	46	2280	45	1·02
	5.4.71		4	62	3136	61	0·95
	6.4.71		9	105	4900	96	1·00
	7.4.71		22	80	1680	33	1·76
	8.4.71		25	100	3380	67	1·12
197	12.9.68	27	0	36	1000	37	0·97
	13.9.68		4	18	360	13·4	1·04
Mean							1·48

daily injections show a similar pattern of response. After an initial loading dose effective plasma concentrations of factor VIII following treatment can be achieved for 4–6 days.

Patients who have low titre antibodies and who require single doses of factor VIII need much higher than usual doses of factor VIII to overcome the existing antibody and to leave a residual amount of measurable factor VIII. It is probable that patients having 2 u/ml antibody will require at least twice the dose of factor VIII that would usually be given to a patient without antibody and who required treatment for a similar lesion. Higher antibody levels will suggest greater dosage. The results of infusions to 9 patients having low titre antibodies are given in Table 9.5.

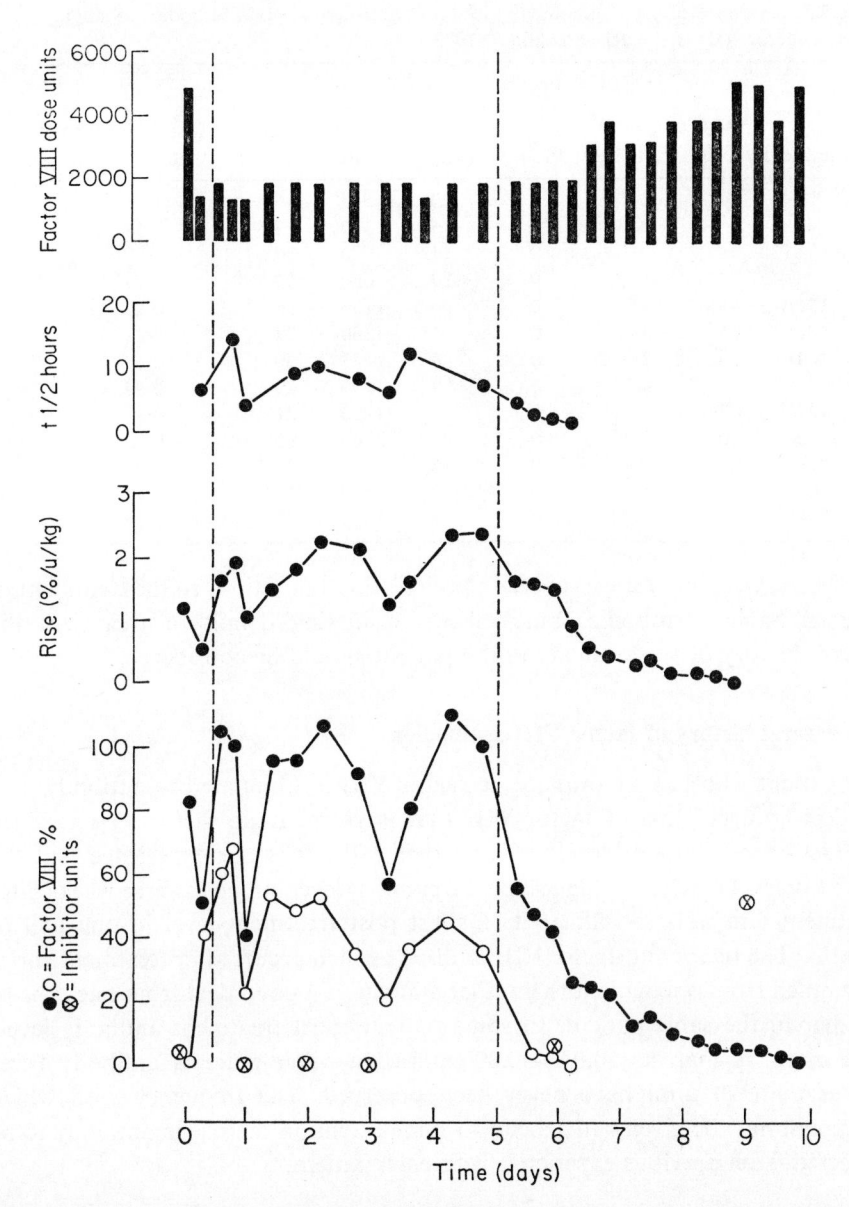

Figure 9.2. The record of results of laboratory tests on Case 203 having anti-factor VIII antibody who had an operation for invasive parotid tumour. The doses of factor VIII are related to the observed half-life of factor VIII and the rise in factor VIII level /u/kg. The observed factor VIII levels in the patient are shown below, the pre-infusion levels by open circles and the post infusion levels by solid circles. The levels of antifactor VIII antibody are shown ⊗. See text.

Table 9.5. Response of 9 patients having low titre anti-factor VIII antibodies to single doses of factor VIII (from Rizza & Biggs, 1973).

| | | | Factor VIII activities | | | | |
Patient	Wt. (kg)	Antibody	Pre	Post	Dose units	Dose (u/kg)	Rise in factor VIII %/u/kg
198	29	1·2	0	23	517	15	1·53
			0	6	370	17·5	0·48
			0	11	600	20	1·81
			0	20	690	23	1·15
181	43	3	0	6·5	1100	25	0·26
26	56	4	0	5	1360	24	0·21
64	56	2	0	6	1125	20	0·30
		4	0	3	1500	29	0·10
194	47·5	3	0	7	1000	21	0·33
200	40	1·25	0	43	3800	95	0·45
201	60	2·8	0	6	1600	27·5	0·21
197	27	1·6	0	8	450	17	0·47
202	51	2·2	0	8	1380	27	0·30

These experiences suggest certain policies and limitations to the treatment of patients having antibodies but before considering details of treatment the natural history of the antibody in the patient should be considered.

The natural history of factor VIII antibodies

The patient who has an antibody to factor VIII is stimulated to antibody production by each dose of factor VIII that is given. If no factor VIII is given production of antibody levels off and then falls. It is our experience that the antibody level reaches its highest post treatment level in one to three weeks after treatment and falls to half of its highest post treatment level in one to two months. The rise in anti-factor VIII antibody which occurs after treatment varies very much from one patient to another and varies a good deal from one time to another in the same patient. In some patients post treatment antibody levels have risen as high as 10,000–20,000 u/ml. In other patients antibody titres higher than 20 u/ml have never been observed. The frequency with which treatment may be given will depend to some extent on the rise in antibody to be expected from previous experience with each patient.

The circumstances which influence the decision to treat a patient having factor VIII antibody

In a study of 38 patients having factor VIII antibodies Rizza & Biggs (1973) treated about 40% of the lesions with which the patients presented at the clinic. Most frequently the treatment was required for haemarthroses or haematomata.

A patient who does not have anti-factor VIII antibody is always treated for incipient joint or muscle bleeds but a careful decision is taken about the patient who has antibody. The degree of pain and swelling is assessed, the amount of trauma that gave rise to the particular injury is taken into account. Much attention is given to rest, careful splinting and the avoidance of traumatic activities. Nevertheless many lesions are treated with great clinical benefit. When treatment is given antibody titre is measured and subsequent dose levels (if any) will depend on the antibody titre. In each case the dose level is judged according to the expected antibody titre and 2–4 times the usual dose is given. In time, experience and data about the treatment of individual cases accumulates and policy becomes more simply determinable.

If the patient has life endangering haemorrhage such as a cerebral haemorrhage, a fracture or other accidental injury or if the patient may require an operation then a very clear-cut decisive policy must be initiated. The patient should be seen by all doctors who could contribute to his treatment and at conference a policy decision must be reached at once before the first dose of factor VIII is administered. It must be remembered that a patient having factor VIII antibody cannot have more than 5 days of treatment before the antibody rises to dangerously high levels. Thus should surgery be required it must be done at once immediately after the first factor VIII dose. The most dangerous thing that can be done for such a patient is to give a moderate dose of factor VIII and then wait a day or two to see what may happen. Treatment should be at high dosage, immediate and continued and any surgical treatment done immediately.

If the patient comes to hospital with a high titre factor VIII antibody it is unwise to contemplate surgical intervention except in the event that death will certainly ensue if treatment is withheld. If the patient has a very severe haemarthrosis then a single very large dose of factor VIII will sometimes halt the bleeding even when no free factor VIII is detectable in the plasma after infusion.

THE USE OF BOVINE OR PORCINE FACTOR VIII FOR PATIENTS HAVING FACTOR VIII ANTIBODIES

In many patients antibody titre to human factor VIII may be higher than that to bovine or porcine factor VIII. In such patients the bovine or porcine factor VIII may have good clinical effect. However, with the high potency human factor VIII now available the need for animal factor VIII is less than it was in the past.

THE USE OF CYCLOCAPRON IN PATIENTS HAVING FACTOR VIII ANTIBODIES

For patients requiring dental extractions and who do not have factor VIII antibodies it has been found that fibrinolytic inhibitors such as EACA or

Cyclokapron treatment increases the effectiveness of factor VIII (Walsh *et al*, 1971). This conclusion has been discussed in Chapter 6. Probably the fibrinolytic inhibitor acts by preventing the lysis of intravascular clots which are formed as a result of the factor VIII treatment. It is very probable that Cyclokapron will increase the effectiveness of treatment for patients having factor VIII antibodies. Unless contra-indicated by recent or existing haematuria it is probably wise to use Cyclokapron in conjunction with factor VIII treatment for patients having factor VIII antibodies.

FACTOR IX AND THE TREATMENT OF PATIENTS
HAVING FACTOR VIII ANTIBODIES

Some batches of so called 'activated' preparations of factor IX concentrate caused thrombosis in some patients, such 'activated' factor IX preparations were used to treat patients having factor VIII antibodies (Sultan, Brouet & Debre, 1974; Ekert & McVeagh, 1975; Tishkoff, 1975; Kurczynski & Penner, 1974; Abildgaard, Britton & Roberts, 1974 etc.). It was supposed that the activated factors would bypass the factor VIII reaction and promote clotting by the introduction of activated factors IX, X or VII or even thrombin. In fact it is quite difficult to distinguish all of the so called activated factor IX preparations from ordinary factor IX preparations using any simple laboratory tests. It was observed by various authors that there was a shortening of the partial thromboplastin time in the plasma of patients who were treated with activated factor IX preparations. There was also the impression that some cases were clinically improved.

IMMUNOSUPPRESSIVE DRUGS AND THE TREATMENT OF
PATIENTS WHO HAVE FACTOR VIII ANTIBODIES

Patients who have anti-factor VIII antibodies and who have haemophilia do not in our experience benefit from treatment with corticosteroids, ACTH or immunosuppressive drugs such as Azathioprine. On the other hand when an anti-factor VIII antibody arises in a previously normal person immunosuppressive drugs may be beneficial (Rizza *et al*, 1972).

References

ABILDGAARD C.G., BRITTON M. & ROBERTS R. (1974) Prothrombin complex (Konyne) for patients with factor VIII inhibitors. *Blood*, **44**, 933.
BARKER L.F., SHULMAN N.R., MURRAY R., HIRSCHMAN R.J., RATNER F., DIEFENBACK W.C.L. & GELLER H.M. (1970) Transmission of serum hepatitis. *Journal of American Medical Association*, **211**, 1509.

BIGGS R. (1974) Jaundice and antibodies directed against factors VIII and IX in patients treated for haemophilia and Christmas disease in the United Kingdom. *British Journal of Haematology*, **26**, 313.

BIGGS R. & SPOONER R. (1977) Haemophilia treatment in the United Kingdom from 1969 to 1974. *British Journal of Haematology*, **35**, 483.

BLUMBERG B.S. (1964) Polymorphisms of the serum proteins and the development of isoprecipitins in transfused patients. *Bulletin New York Academy of Medicine*, **40**, 377.

BRINKHOUS K.M., ROBERTS H.R. & WEISS A.E. (1972) Prevalence of inhibitors in haemophilia A and B. Proceedings of the 2nd Conference held under the auspices of the International Society on Thrombosis and Haemostasis. *Thrombosis et Diathesis Haemorrhagica*, **51** (Supplement), 315.

DIKE A.E. (1970) Two cases of transfusion malaria. *Lancet*, **ii**, 72.

EDSON J.R. (1974) Prothrombin-complex concentrates and thromboses. *New England Journal of Medicine*, **296**, 403.

EKERT H. & McVEAGH P. (1975) Activated PPSB in the treatment of a patient with haemophilia and antibodies to factor VIII. *Medical Journal of Australia*, **2**, 675.

GAZZARD B.G., LEWIS M.L., ASH G., RIZZA C.R., BIDWELL E. & WILLIAMS R. (1974) Coagulation factor concentrate in the treatment of the haemorrhagic diathesis of fulminant hepatic failure. *Gut*, **15**, 993.

GIBSON B., MATTHEWS J. & RIZZA C.R. (1977) An operation on a patient having factor VIII antibody. In preparation.

GILES J.P. & KRUGMAN S. (1972) Viral hepatitis: differential diagnostic features between infections with type A and B viruses. *American Journal of Diseases of Childhood*, **123**, 281.

GOCKE D.J. (1970) The Australia antigen and blood transfusion. *Vox Sanguinis*, **19**, 327.

KASPAR C.K. (1973) Post-operative thromboses in haemophilia B. *New England Journal of Medicine*, **289**, 160.

KASPAR C.K. (1974) Prothrombin complex concentrates and thromboses. *New England Journal of Medicine*, **290**, 404.

KASPAR C.K. (1975) Thrombo-embolic complications of factor IX therapy. *Thrombosis et Diathesis Haemorrhagica*, **33**, 642.

KERNOFF P.B.A., DURRANT I.J., RIZZA C.R. & WRIGHT F.W. (1972) Severe allergic pulmonary oedema after plasma transfusion. *British Journal of Haematology*, **23**, 777.

KINGDON H.S., LUNDBLAD R.L., VELTKAMP J.J. & ARONSON D.L. (1975) Potentially thrombogenic materials in factor IX concentrate. *Thrombosis et Diathesis Haemorrhagica*, **33**, 617.

KRUGMAN S., GILES J.P. & HAMMOND J. (1971a) Viral hepatitis type B (MS-2 strain): prevention with specific hepatitis B immune globulin. *Journal of American Medical Association*, **218**, 1665.

KRUGMAN S., GILES J.P. & HAMMOND J. (1971b) Viral hepatitis B (MS-2 strain) studies on active immunization. *Journal of American Medical Association*, **217**, 41.

KRUGMAN S. & GILES J.P. (1970) Viral hepatitis: new light on an old disease. *Journal of American Medical Association*, **212**, 1019.

KURCZYNSKI E.M. & PENNER J.A. (1974) Activated prothrombin concentrate for patients with factor VIII inhibitors. *New England Journal of Medicine*, **291**, 164.

LANE J.L., RIZZA C.R. & SNAPE T.J. (1975) A five year experience of the use of factor IX type DE(1) concentrate for the treatment of Christmas disease at Oxford. *British Journal of Haematology*, **30**, 435.

MARCHESI S.L. & BURNEY R. (1974) Prothrombin complex concentrates and thromboses. *New England Journal of Medicine*, **290**, 404.

MAYCOCK W. d'A. (1972) Hepatitis in transfusion services. *British Medical Bulletin*, **28**, 163.

METSELAAR D., BLUMBERG B.S., MILLMAN I., PARKER A.M. & BAGSHAWE A.F. (1973) 'Hepatitis-B antigen in colony mosquitoes'. *Lancet*, **ii**, 758.

MOLLISON P. (1972) *Blood Transfusion in Clinical Medicine*. Blackwell Scientific Publications, Oxford.

MRC. Post transfusion hepatitis in a London hospital: results of a two year study (1974). *Journal of Hygiene*, **73**, 173.

MURRAY R. (1955) Viral hepatitis. *Bulletin of the New York Academy of Science*, **31**, 341.

PRINCE A.M., BROTMAN B., GRADY G.F., KRUHNS W.J., HAZZI C., LEVINE R.W. & MILLIAN S.J. (1974) Long incubation post-transfusion hepatitis without serology. *Lancet*, **ii**, 241.

RIZZA C.R., EDGCUMBE J.O.P., PITNEY W.R. & CHILD S.A. (1972) The treatment of patients having spontaneously occurring antibodies to anti-haemophilic factor (factor VIII). *Thrombosis et Diathesis Haemorrhagica*, **28**, 120.

RIZZA C.R. & BIGGS R. (1973) The treatment of patients who have factor VIII antibodies. *British Journal of Haematology*, **24**, 65.

ROBERTS H.R. & BLATT P.M. (1975) Post-transfusion hepatitis following the use of prothrombin complex concentrates. *Thrombosis et Diathesis Haemorrhagica*, **33**, 610.

ROSATI L.A., BARNES B., OBERMAN H.A. & PENNER J.A. (1970) Haemolytic anaemia due to anti-A in concentrated antihaemophilic factor preparations. *Transfusions*, **10**, 139.

SEELER R.A. (1972) Haemolysis due to anti-A of anti-B in factor VIII preparations. *Archives of Internal Medicine*, **130**, 101.

STEINBERG M.H. & BREILING B.J. (1973) Vascular lesions in haemophilia B. *New England Journal of Medicine*, **289**, 592.

SULTAN Y., BROUET J.C. & DEBRE P. (1974) The treatment of inhibitors to factor VIII with activated prothrombin concentrate. *New England Journal of Medicine*, **291**, 1087.

TAMAGNINI G.P., DORMANDY K.M., ELLIS D. & MAYCOCK W. d'A. (1975) Factor VIII concentrates in haemophilia. *Lancet*, **ii**, 188.

TISHKOFF G.H. (1975) Prothrombin complex to treat factor VIII inhibition. *New England Journal of Medicine*, **292**, 754.

VARTAN A. (1967) Transfusion malaria in a man with Christmas disease. *British Medical Journal*, **4**, 466.

WALSH P.N., RIZZA C.R., MATTHEWS J.M., EIPE J., KERNOFF P.B.A., COLES M.D., BLOOM A.L., KAUFMAN B.M., BECK P., HANAN C.M. & BIGGS R. (1971) Epsilon-aminocaproic acid therapy for dental extraction in haemophilia and Christmas disease: a double blind controlled trial. *British Journal of Haematology*, **20**, 463.

WESSLER S., REIMER S.M. & SHEEPS M.C. (1959) Biologic assay of a thrombosis inducing activity in human serum. *Journal of Applied Physiology*, **14**, 943.

WESSLER S. (1955) Studier in intravascular coagulation III. *Journal of Clinical Investigation*, **34**, 647.

Chapter 10. Organisation of Haemophilia Treatment

ROSEMARY BIGGS

Haemophilia and similar conditions are so rare that most doctors never encounter a single case in their entire working lives. In 1966 Trueta estimated that if haemophiliacs, most of whom had musculo-skeletal deformity at this time, were to attend the nearest orthopaedic specialist each specialist would see 1 or at the most 2 patients in their working lives. In the United States 95% of the doctors who treated haemophiliacs in the years 1970 and 1971 saw less than 10 different patients and only 11% of patients attended centres at which more than 50 patients were treated (NHLI, 1972).

There are dangers for haemophiliacs who attend centres where few such patients are seen. Many injuries or symptoms that would be trivial for a normal person portend disaster for the haemophiliac. Every problem that arises must be assessed against a background of knowledge about the patient's abnormal haemostatic mechanism. The situations that arise are so various that no set of rules can be applied which will forestall all of the mistakes that may be made. As in so many fields of medicine, nothing can replace experience and experience presupposes the gathering together of many patients under the care of one physician. This experience affects all departments of the medical services from the ambulance driver to the consultant surgeon. The difficulties of fitting patients into the usual pattern of medicine can be illustrated by considering the haemophilic patient against a background of medical organisation for the normal person.

A haemostatically normal person usually attends his general practitioner when he is ill. He may have to wait hours or even days for a convenient time. This waiting seldom injures the haemostatically normal patient but delay is usually disastrous for the haemophiliac. For this reason most patients with haemophilia are encouraged to go direct to hospital when they have a bleed.

The patient may telephone the hospital before leaving home. The interpretation of symptoms in telephone conversations is an art. Patients not infrequently misinterpret their own symptoms. Abdominal pain may be referred to as indigestion by the patient when it is caused by retroperitoneal haemorrhage. A headache may be of no significance in the chronic migraine sufferer but may be a very serious event for a small boy who has been out fighting. Small boys may in any case deny fighting when they have been forbidden to fight. The telephone conversation may seem to be about such trivial matters that a doctor who is not a haemophilia specialist may tell the patient to wait till the morning and see his own general practitioner.

Once on the way to hospital in the ambulance all difficulties may not be over. The ambulance driver may have definite instructions about the destination to which all patients must be taken and may be unwilling to make an exception for a haemophiliac. The patient may thus arrive at the wrong hospital.

When the right hospital is chosen the patient may come to the casualty department when a new doctor is on call and he may then not receive the correct treatment. The patient may even be admitted to a hospital under the care of a consultant who feels no need to ask advice from the Haemophilia Centre Director about treatment.

When the patient does arrive at hospital and is admitted to the correct ward under the care of the haemophilia specialist there may still be difficulties in centres where few patients are treated. The factor VIII for administration may be handled wrongly and even dangerously by laboratory technicians and nursing staff who seldom see a patient having haemophilia or a similar condition. In a surgical ward all patients may be expected to take part in more or less vigorous physiotherapy unsuitable for most haemophiliacs. Patients often receive aspirin for aches and pains in hospital but haemophilic patients should never receive this drug. The significance of the presence of antibodies to factor VIII may not be appreciated. Technical staff collecting blood samples may not be aware of the special care needed for venepuncture in haemophilic patients.

When the patient arrives in hospital he may need the care of a surgeon, paediatrician, orthopaedic or other specialist. These specialists may not be familiar with the special problems of haemophilic patients. The surgeon may wish to operate for appendicitis on all patients who have pain in the right iliac fossa, vomiting, pyrexia, constipation and a raised white cell count. In normal people 9 times out of 10 these symptoms and signs indicate appendicitis. For the haemophilic it is fair to say that on 9 occasions out of 10 the symptoms are caused by iliacus haematoma. Orthopaedic surgeons have been known to injure the damaged joints of haemophiliacs by methods of examination which would be harmless for normal people. For the ENT specialist, epistaxis in normal people may be a lesion easily cured by local cautery whereas in the haemophiliac epistaxis is often made worse by cautery. For the casualty officer many of the haemophilic lesions may seem too trivial to warrant a hospital visit much less admission to hospital or a consultation with the Haemophilia Centre Director.

A proportion of patients have a measurable amount of factor VIII or IX in their blood and are mildly affected. These patients do not have spontaneous bleeding and are seldom crippled. They usually appear so normal that doctors not experienced in this field of study may feel that they are not 'true bleeders' and need no special treatment. In fact these patients often bleed disastrously after injury. They need infusions of concentrate for trauma, dental extractions or operations.

These and other similar problems make it difficult to organise the treatment of haemophilic patients in centres where few such patients attend. Some general district hospitals do nevertheless provide an excellent service for the few patients who attend. This excellence usually stems from the devoted care of one doctor who has developed a good personal relationship with the patients and who has developed a good working relationship with a nearby Haemophilia Centre which caters for larger numbers of patients. Every effort should be made to promote co-operation between large Haemophilia Centres and hospitals or associate centres where few patients attend.

The Haemophilia Centre (historical)

The concept of treating patients at special Haemophilia Centres originated, in the United Kingdom, in 1950 when the Medical Research Council set up a committee to consider the social and medical problems of haemophilic patients. By 1954 the Committee had organised a list of Centres where special facilities for the study of haemophiliacs existed. At this time the main concern was to issue haemophilia identity cards to the patients and to establish diagnosis. Since little treatment was then available, skill and knowledge centred in haematology laboratories where specialist tests could be carried out. It is for this historical reason that the directors of many Haemophilia Centres are pathologists or laboratory haematologists.

In 1964 the introduction of cryoprecipitate greatly widened the possibility for treating haemophilic patients and by 1967 appreciable amounts of this product were available in the United Kingdom. In 1967 the first meeting of Haemophilia Centre Directors took place and a start was made to co-operate between the directors in the collection of statistics about treatment. Since then the directors have met annually to discuss problems of mutual interest. In 1964 the responsibility for the organisation of Centres was transferred to the Health Departments and in 1968 a memorandum (HM(68)8) on the care of haemophilic patients was issued. This memorandum defined the role of the Haemophilia Centres. In 1976 this memorandum was revised (FPN 105 HC (76) 4). The 1976 memorandum recognises 3 types of Centre with different responsibilities. The relevant part of this document is reproduced on the following pages.

Organisation of Haemophilia Centres

"Summary

1 This Notice advises general medical and general dental practitioners of the revised arrangements for the care of persons suffering from haemophilia and related conditions; the Appendix lists the centres at which treatment is available in the United Kingdom.

Background

2 The arrangements under which centres are designated for the diagnosis, treatment and registration of persons suffering from haemophilia and related conditions have been in existence since 1968. Following a review which was carried out in consultation with the Directors of the present Haemophilia Centres some alterations have been agreed; the new arrangements are described in the succeeding paragraphs.

Haemophilia Centres

3 The functions of these Centres are to provide:

(*i*) a laboratory service able:

(a) to carry out the tests, including the identification and assay of specific coagulation factors and anti-coagulants necessary for an exact diagnosis to be made.

(b) to monitor coagulation factors and anticoagulants during treatment.

(c) in collaboration with the appropriate Reference Centre (see paragraph 7 below) to investigate relatives of patients with haemophilia or related conditions.

(*ii*) a clinical service for the treatment of patients at short notice at any time of the day or night.

(*iii*) an advisory service to patients (and, in the case of child patients, to their parents) on matters of concern to them such as preventive medicine and dentistry, education, employment, genetic counselling and social medicine. Advice should also be given to general practitioners about the emergency treatment of haemophilic patients on their list and the procedure for securing these patients' admission to hospital when required including what the patient should do to obtain ambulance transport in an emergency.

4 A record of all patients to whom haemophilia cards are issued should be maintained at each Haemophilia Centre including at least the following information:

Name, address and telephone number of patient
Date of birth
Diagnosis
Mother's maiden name
Maternal grandmother's maiden name
Name, address and telephone number of general practitioner
Name of consultant in charge of the case.

Associate Haemophilia Centres

5 Centres which were designated in 1968 but which do not fully meet the new criteria laid down for designated Haemophilia Centres (see paragraph 3 above) may wish to continue to provide emergency treatment to haemophiliacs living or working nearby and registered with them. These centres will be known as Associate Haemophilia Centres. Each will be linked with a convenient designated Haemophilia Centre so that together they will be in a position to offer a full therapeutic, diagnostic and advisory service to haemophiliacs and their families.

Reference Centres

6 In 1968 the centres at Oxford, Manchester and Sheffield were designated at Special Treatment Centres where special skills were available to patients requiring major surgery. At that time management during and after surgery was the most difficult aspect of the treatment of haemophilia. This is no longer the case because the management of patients undergoing surgery has become easier as a range of therapeutic materials have become more widely available. Today the emphasis in the treatment of haemophilic patients is on the early day-to-day care on demand and this treatment must be provided at all centres.

7 However, although it is no longer necessary to designate centres for the specific purpose of carrying out surgical treatment there are administrative and other advantages to be gained in designating some centres to be Reference Centres, to which Haemophilia Centres can look for guidance and support. The centres currently so designated and the areas which they broadly cover are:

St Thomas's Hospital The Royal Free Hospital	London, The South East and East Anglia
The Churchill Hospital, Oxford	Oxford, Wessex, the South West, the Midlands and Northern Ireland
The Royal Infirmary, Manchester The Royal Infirmary with the Children's Hospital, Sheffield	The North West, North Wales, Trent and Yorkshire

Chapter 10

1 **Oxford**
West Midland RHA
Oxford RHA
Wessex RHA
South Western RHA
Northern Ireland RHA

2 **London**
East Anglia RHA
North West Thames RHA
South West Thames RHA
South East Thames RHA
North East Thames RHA

3 **Sheffield**
Trent RHA
Yorkshire RHA

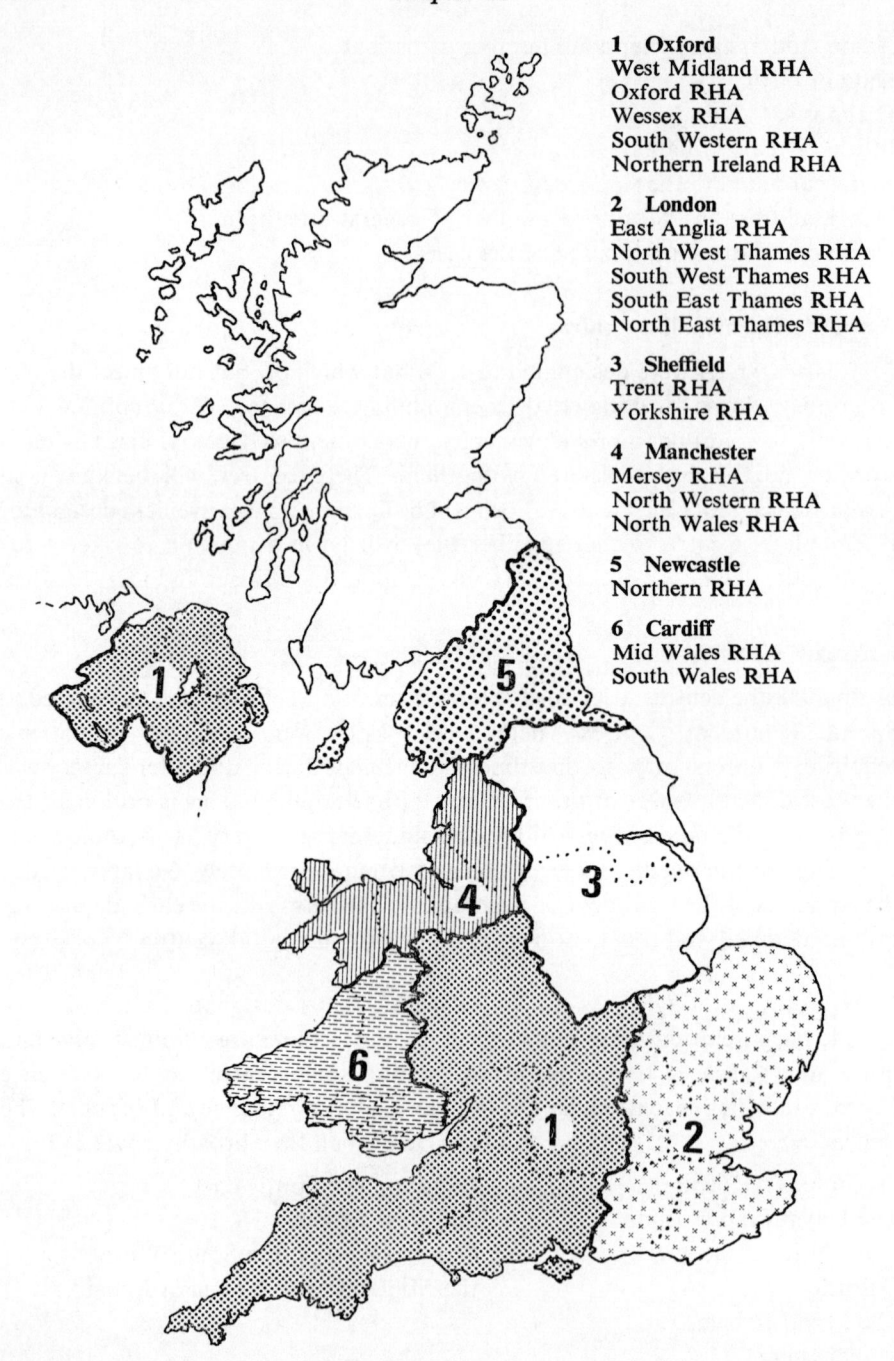

4 **Manchester**
Mersey RHA
North Western RHA
North Wales RHA

5 **Newcastle**
Northern RHA

6 **Cardiff**
Mid Wales RHA
South Wales RHA

Figure 10.1. Map of the United Kingdom showing the boundaries of the Haemophilia Reference Centre territories.

The Royal Victoria Infirmary, Newcastle } The North of England
University Hospital of Wales, Cardiff } South Wales
(See Figure 10.1)

8 The functions of these Reference Centres are:

(*i*) to provide a 24-hour telephone advisory service to Haemophilia Centres and Associate Haemophilia Centres and to support them particularly during holiday periods.

(*ii*) to provide a specialist consultant service for surgery and for orthopaedic, dental, paediatric and social care for those Haemophilia Centres and Associate Haemophilia Centres wishing to use such a service.

(*iii*) to advise on and organise when called upon home therapy and prophylactic therapy for haemophilia patients.

(*iv*) to provide a reference laboratory service for Haemophilia Centres and Associate Haemophilia Centres including the diagnosis of atypical cases, the assay of antibodies and the supply of assay standards and reagents.

(*v*) to provide education facilities for doctors, technicians, nurses and others as required in order to promote optimum care of patients and a comprehensive laboratory diagnostic service.

(*vi*) to ensure close co-operation between the Haemophilia Centres, Associate Haemophilia Centres and the Regional Centres of the Blood Transfusion Service.

(*vii*) to co-ordinate, as necessary, the allocation of available therapeutic materials to Haemophilia Centres and Associate Haemophilia Centres.

(*viii*) to co-ordinate statistics collected by Haemophilia Centres and Associate Haemophilia Centres.

(*ix*) to co-ordinate meetings and research programmes.

In the United Kingdom in 1976 few haemophilic patients are treated at hospitals which are not designated as Haemophilia Centres and the smaller centres now all have access to larger centres for advice and help when necessary. Despite the excellent progress that has been made in the United Kingdom some difficulties remain. One problem, referred to earlier, is that a number of Haemophilia Centres and Associate Centres cater for less than 10 different haemophilic patients each year. The second problem arises from the fact that the care of haemophilic patients is not easy to integrate into conventional hospital organisation. The visits by patients cannot be tidily disposed in out-patient clinics. Neither do most of today's patients need hospital admission. Patients need to be able to come to hospital and see an expert physician at any hour of the day or night. Without very special arrangements these irregular visits cannot easily be handled in a casualty department. In addition patients who need care from infancy to old age need to develop a much closer relationship with hospital staff than does a patient who has an illness of short duration. In the present chapter an attempt will be made to analyse the work generated by haemophilic patients at the Oxford Centre. It is hoped that this analysis may help those at other hospitals to plan the staff and services needed for the care of haemophilic patients and to arrange the organisation to ensure that patients feel safe and cared for when they enter the hospital."

The work of the Oxford Haemophilia Centre

The work carried out at the Oxford Haemophilia Centre can be considered according to the type of service involved:

1 Diagnosis and laboratory testing.
2 Treatment and general advice to patients.

The analysis considers only the work carried out directly by haemophilia centre personnel. On a consultative basis the centre relies very much on assistance and co-operation with nearly every other hospital speciality. In particular close co-operation is needed with orthopaedic specialists and physiotherapists. For special problems the haemophilic may need to consult hospital specialists in all other departments as do normal people who fall ill.

Diagnosis and laboratory testing

The number of laboratory tests carried out at the Oxford Centre from 1969 to 1975 has fluctuated between 5,500 and 7,700 annually with a mean of 6,304. The number of haemophilia A and B patients treated in each of these years has averaged 230. Thus an average of 27·4 tests has been carried out for every patient treated in one year. It is not very meaningful to relate the number of tests to the number of patients treated since a good many of the tests were carried out for diagnosis on patients who did not have any haemorrhagic state and thus were not treated. There is nevertheless likely to be some relationship, though not a precise one, between the general work load and number of patients who attend for treatment. It is to be expected that laboratories at Haemophilia Centres will give a general service to the Region in the diagnosis of cases with haemostatic defects. Many laboratories attached to Haemophilia Centres also carry out tests for disseminated intravascular clotting and are responsible for the laboratory control of oral anticoagulant therapy, heparin administration and thrombolytic therapy. At the smaller centres there is usually no special Haemophilia Centre or coagulation laboratory but one or two technicians in the General Haematology Laboratory carry out coagulation tests on a rotational system. In these small centres it is difficult to maintain expert technique. The number of staff required will vary according to the range of work undertaken. It is hoped that scientists in these small centres will avail themselves of the services of their Haemophilia Reference Centre.

The work in the laboratory in Oxford is carried out by 1 graduate scientist, 1 chief technician and 3 technicians. The work can also be considered in terms of tests per working day (assuming 5 working days per week). On average about 24 tests per day were carried out. In a general way it may be seen that at least 2 technical staff of whom one must be permanently employed on coagulation work and of senior status will be needed for centres with 100 patients and the number will need to be increased if routine anticoagulant control, the control of fibrinolytic therapy and general screening for haemostatic defects is undertaken.

Treatment and general advice to patients

The number of infusions given to patients gives some indication of the physical work involved in the treatment of haemophilic patients. The general trend in Oxford since 1962 is shown in Table 10.1. In 1975 just over 6,000 infusions were administered to 255 patients in Oxford, an average of 24·4 infusions per patient. The number of infusions can also be considered according to the number of infusions given per day. In 1974, for example, 14·3 infusions were given each day including weekends and holidays. Viewed over a long period of time about 15 to 20% of the infusions are given before 9.00 a.m. or after 5.00 p.m. The amount of work on Saturdays, Sundays and week day holidays is not much less than on a normal working day. The work in Oxford is currently carried out by 1 consultant physician, 1 medical assistant, 1 rotating registrar for about one quarter of the year, 2 senior house officers and 1 nursing sister.

The night work on weekdays during 4 months of 1973 was recorded and the results are shown in Table 10.2. It will be seen that on 15 nights in the 4 month period no patients came for treatment at night and that on other nights the number of patients attending varied from 1 to 6. The total number of calls experienced in the 88 nights observed was 214. In the last 2 columns of Table 10.2 are shown the terms of a Poisson series with a mean value of 2·43 calls per night which is the average observed number of calls for the 88 nights for which records were kept. It will be seen that the occasions on which different numbers of patients need treatment at night correspond fairly well with expectation based on the Poisson series with a mean value of 2·43. It is our opinion that the

Table 10.1. Number of doses of therapeutic material given to patients having haemophilia and Christmas disease in Oxford.

Year	Patients H	C	H+C	Doses H	C	H+C	Doses per patient per year H+C
1962	50	11	61	527	76	603	9·9
1963	77	17	94	589	59	648	6·9
1964	72	16	88	539	128	667	7·6
1965	104	23	127	1394	177	1571	12·4
1966	120	25	145	1318	252	1570	10·8
1967	147	27	174	1357	300	1657	9·5
1968	138	27	165	1622	279	1901	11·5
1969	190	38	228	1755	287	2042	8·9
1970	176	36	212	2036	200	2236	10·5
1971	198	25	223	2497	253	2750	12·3
1972	207	38	245	3383	536	3919*	16·0
1973	223	42	265	4227	462	4689*	17·7
1974	219	35	254	4778	434	5212*	20·5
1975	220	35	255	5540	689	6229*	24·4

* An increasing proportion of doses were given at home by patients to themselves or by relatives to patients.

Table 10.2. Number of night calls at the Oxford Haemophilia Centre during 4 months in 1973.

Numbers of calls per night	Observations Number of nights	Total number of calls	Theory Number of occasions	Total number of calls
0	15	0	7·744	0
1	12	12	18·818	18·818
2	17	34	22·864	45·728
3	22	66	18·520	55·560
4	11	44	11·251	45·004
5	8	40	5·467	27·335
6	3	18	2·214	13·284
7	0	0	0·769	5·380
8+	0	0	0·353	2·824
Totals	88	214	88	213·933

proportion of night calls has remained rather constant. These night calls are an important feature if an attempt is to be made to ensure that patients always see a doctor who is familiar with the treatment of haemophilia. With limited staff rather careful arrangements will have to be made to ensure the patient's safety during out of hours visits.

Table 10.3. The amounts of work generated by haemophilic patients measured in terms of infusions given at the Oxford Haemophilia Centre in 1974.

Number of different patients treated per year	Approximate number of treatments per day including night calls	Approximate number of calls at night	% of nights free of calls
254	14	2·1	12·2
100	5	0·75	47
50	2·5	0·375	69
20	1	0·15	86
10	0·5	0·075	93

From the observations made in Oxford it is reasonable to deduce, from the expectations of the Poisson series, the numbers of visits likely to occur during the day and at night at centres at which different numbers of patients are treated. To make the calculations it has been assumed that 15% of all visits by patients were made out of hours. The Oxford figures for 1974 have been used for comparison. The results of the calculations are set out in Table 10.3. In 1974, 254 patients were treated at the Oxford Haemophilia Centre and the approximate number of treatments given per day was 14. Of these treatments 2·1 treatments per day are assumed, on average and over a long time have been given at night and only about 12% of nights would be free of night calls. When 100 patients are seen in the year instead of 254 then about 5 treatments will be given each day and of these on average 0·75 will be given at night and nearly half of the nights will be free of night calls. At a centre where less than 50 patients are treated each year a substantial number of days will pass when no patients attend and night calls will become rare. For a centre where few patients are treated it would be unreasonable to appoint a medical consultant with no medical responsibilities other than the care of haemophiliacs. At 31 of the United Kingdom Haemophilia Centres less than 50 different patients were treated in the year 1974. For this reason the best method of combining the treatment of haemophilia with other responsibilities is most important and must be planned at each haemophilia centre.

These considerations suggest the conclusion that the organisation of a large centre such as that at Oxford is a quite different problem from the organisation of small centres. At Oxford full time staff are well occupied during the day and on night duty. An idea of the numbers of various kinds of staff required for centres which cater for different numbers of patients is shown in Table 10.4. The staff required for 250 patients seen every year is based on the Oxford experience. In the laboratory the number of staff will depend on the coagulation work that is done for patients other than those having haemophilia. It has been assumed that

Table 10.4. Staff required to carry out the work of a Haemophilia Centre.

Number of different patients attending for treatment annually	Probable* average number of visits by patients daily in working hours	Number of laboratory tests monthly	Medical	Nursing	Staff Technical and Scientific	Secretarial
250	12·5	500 (+250)	4	2	5–6	2
200	10	400 (+250)	3–4	1–2	4–6	1–2
150	7·5	300 (+250)	2–3	1	3–5	1
100	5	200 (+250)	2	1	3–5	1
50	2·5	100 (+250)	1–2	1	3–4	½
25	1	50 (+250)	1–2	1	2–3	½

The figures in brackets are extra tests which may be done if general coagulation tests for the control of anticoagulant therapy etc. are included in the work of the laboratory.
* It is assumed that a proportion of patients receive home therapy.

2 extra technicians will be required to do an estimate of 250 extra tests monthly if all the coagulation tests, including anticoagulant control and the diagnosis of DIC, etc, are carried out in the coagulation laboratory.

The medical staff must include one consultant who has responsibility for the organisation of haemophilia treatment. This consultant will supervise laboratory testing, interview new patients, arrange and plan treatment but will not normally expect to carry out infusions or to engage in out of hours work except on an emergency consultative basis. Night calls must be carried out by junior doctors and since these doctors often rotate from post to post at 3 monthly or even 6 weekly intervals it can be very difficult to maintain adequately trained junior staff. The junior staff engaged in haemophilia care should if possible have longer periods of duty in this work than 3 months. It is difficult for patients, and particularly difficult for child patients, if they see a different doctor every 2 or 3 months.

The nursing staff at the Haemophilia Centre are very important. A nursing sister permanently employed on Haemophilia Centre work will provide the continuity so essential for the care of these patients. The sister can carry out infusions, under medical supervision in the daytime, organise supplies of therapeutic materials, keep essential records and introduce the patients to the newly appointed doctors. It may be noted that the Haemophilia Centre cannot be thought of as a place for rotating nursing staff as are other hospital departments. A sister or staff nurse who is sent to do odd hours of duty at the Haemophilia Centre is not very useful. It is our feeling that all Haemophilia Centres which cater for 25 or more different patients a year should employ a full time nursing sister. At the smaller centres the sister can play a very useful role in the care of other patients who come to the laboratory or ward as out-patients.

The safety of patients at small centres might be improved by a number of organisational arrangements:

1   The centre may maintain a close relationship with its reference centre and arrange for patients to be registered at the Reference Centre and to be able to telephone the reference centre by arrangement in out of hours times and holidays.
2   As many severely affected patients as possible may be put onto home therapy.
3   Patients may be given very exact instructions about how to obtain out of hours treatment including such examples as:

(*a*) Cards to be shown to Ambulance drivers and Casualty Officers, etc.
(*b*) Patients may sometimes be given instructions about the whereabouts of a store of factor VIII or factor IX in the hospital. Bottles or packs of cryoprecipitate may be labelled with individual patients' names. The patient may be instructed to go to the store during out of hours times and extract a suitable dose of concentrate and take this to a specified ward or department where a doctor will administer the dose.
(*c*) Notices may be hung on Casualty Department walls to remind the hospital staff about the local arrangements for the care of haemophilic patients.
(*d*) Teach-in courses may be arranged for new doctors and staff nurses at which instruction about the arrangements for haemophilic patients is given.
(*e*) Specialised laboratory tests may be undertaken at the Haemophilia Reference Centre laboratory or uniform reagents may be distributed in the territory administered by the Reference Centre to all of the centres in that territory.

HOME THERAPY

Examination of the records at Oxford suggest that half of the infusions are given to one fifth of the patients. Thus of a total of about 250 patients who attend the centre every year, 50 patients use half of the material provided. The introduction of these 50 most severely affected patients to home therapy has lightened the load of infusion therapy at the centre. At present about one third of all infusions given to patients who attend the centre are given at home. The introduction of these particular patients to home therapy has not reduced the number of night calls substantially. The home therapy programme has enabled the staff to give a better overall service to patients. The institution of home therapy has not reduced the responsibility of Haemophilia Centre staff for the care of patients. However intelligent and well trained the patient may be he is not a doctor and he must have the continued support of his own general practitioner and hospital consultant. Organisational steps must be taken to ensure this support.

Arrangements may be made to hold follow-up clinics to which patients on home therapy come at regular intervals. It may be convenient for such follow-up clinics to have a social atmosphere with perhaps some period of time set aside for private consultations, some for conversation between parents and patients, some time for talks by doctors and nurses and some for general discussion between doctors and patients. Perhaps instead of formal out-patient appointments the centre might be 'at home' to patients on a certain day every month and patients who wish for a private interview should write for an appointment. Others may simply attend to hear of any new developments or to have reassurance from conversing with others who have similar problems. These sessions could of course be open to all patients registered at the centre and could encourage some to embark on home therapy who hesitate to take this step.

It seems possible that this sort of meeting could lead to a better organisation by clarifying the physician's concept of the patient's difficulties in attending hospital and putting forward, perhaps for the first time, the patient's expectations for a good centre.

In addition a close link should be kept between the Haemophilia Centre and the patient's general practitioner. If the general practitioner is aware that the patient is on home therapy then he (or she) can better support the patient. The general practitioner could also be asked to call on a patient who has not attended the centre for some time to discover any difficulties that may have arisen or if the patient has moved house without notifying the centre.

The Haemophilia Centre Director may also decide to hold a 'telephone clinic'. The patient may be informed of the physician's intention to telephone at a particular time and be asked to be at home for the call. This step initiated by the doctor may be very helpful for patients particularly in the early stages of home therapy.

These ideas presuppose a willingness and the availability of time for the Haemophilia Centre Director to organise such a programme. It may be difficult for the director of a small centre to set aside much time for specifically haemophilia centre activities and it may not be reasonable for such a doctor to undertake the responsibility of a home therapy programme. It may well be that home therapy should be organised from 20 to 25 larger centres in the United Kingdom where a member of staff could have special responsibility for the organisation of the home therapy programme. In some cases perhaps the training of patients and the more unorthodox clinics could be organised at the large centres and the therapeutic material distributed to the patients through the smaller local clinics.

CONSULTATION

The data about the work generated in the care of haemophiliacs concerns the carrying out of laboratory tests and the administration of doses. The physician-in-charge of the centre must of course organise and supervise all of this work. The physician-in-charge will talk to individual patients, if the need arises, either by appointment or on a more casual basis when patients come to hospital for diagnosis, treatment or to collect home therapy. The problems that may arise in these conversations have a wide range and include the choice of toys for children, the choice of schools and arrangements with head teachers to ensure safe schooling. Holidays and hobbies may also need planning and discussion. As the patient grows older many problems may arise with which the physician may help. These include the choice of occupation, marriage and genetic counselling (see Chapter 11). The detection of female carriers of haemophilia has been discussed in Chapter 3. The patient and his parents may well wish to discuss the implications which arise from the sex-linked type of inheritance and this discussion must start with the Haemophilia Centre Director even if ultimately it is taken up by a special genetic counsellor.

Conclusion

In most Regions of the United Kingdom the Haemophilia Centre is not a special clinic with its own staff. The centres cater for too few patients for this to be possible. The centre is more a concept which is effective because of the dedication of one particular doctor. If that doctor leaves and transfers to another hospital there is nothing to ensure that the new doctor will have the same interest in haemophilia. The director of the Haemophilia Centre may be a laboratory haematologist or a physician and in either case usually has many responsibilities other than the care of haemophiliacs. The organisation of out of hours cover in hospitals where house officers pass from one department to another and one hospital to another at 6 weekly to 3 monthly intervals presents almost insuperable difficulty. In the laboratory the Haemophilia Centre is usually represented by a bench with a waterbath and sometimes no more than 1 technician with experience in coagulation techniques.

It seems to us that there can be no general rules about the organisation of a Haemophilia Centre. Where 100 or more patients attend every year it should be possible to have staff whose sole responsibility is the care of haemophilic patients (see Table 10.4). When the centre is of this size it should be possible to organise both laboratory and clinical care of patients and to have safe arrangements for patients outside working hours. It may be that every patient should be seen at such a large centre at some time and registered at that large centre in case of need. The trouble about centres catering for many patients is that, except in very large cities, many patients will live a long way away from the Centre.

If it is to be general policy to introduce as many patients as possible to home therapy this implies training patients and their relatives to take more medical responsibility than is usual. A population of informed patients is a safeguard. Perhaps these trained patients and relatives should be issued with cards stating that they have received training at a particular centre and are able to carry out certain procedures such as infusions using particular apparatus and to make and apply splints. These trained patients or parents should be able to help doctors and nurses at hospitals where few haemophilic patients attend and should be in a position to safeguard themselves or their children. This concept presupposes a willingness of doctors to accept this sort of help. It is Utopian to suppose that every Haemophilia Centre will be a special clinic with a 24 hour service given at all times by specially trained doctors and nurses. Since this is true some compromise arrangements must be accepted.

It may be held that a little knowledge is a dangerous thing and that patients will do better always to rely on their medical advisors. In fact patients facing the future for the first time knowing that they have a haemophilic child are terrified and helpless. Suzanne Massie has described this desolation: 'we wept there, the three of us—Bob, my mother and I—clinging to each other, helpless and alone, without warning, as surely as if we had been abandoned on the bleak surface of the moon, our lives had changed'. A knowledge of simple procedures in case of emergency and a comprehensive knowledge of the services available and where these can be found will be reassuring. Very soon parents become well aware of their own limitations and equally well able to detect ignorance in others. Since they are advised always to telephone their own centre when in doubt, they may rightly expect medical practitioners who are not familiar with the treatment of haemophilia to take the same precaution.

References

DHSS Memorandum HC (76) 4. Health services development arrangements for the care of persons suffering from haemophilia and related conditions.

MASSIE R. & MASSIE S. (1975) *Journey*. Alfred Knopf, New York.

National Heart and Lung Institute report on Blood Resources.

TRUETA J. (1966) In: Biggs R. & Macfarlane R.G. *Treatment of Haemophilia and Other Coagulation Disorders*. Blackwell Scientific Publications, Oxford.

Chapter 11. Haemophilia, Medical Science and Society

ROSEMARY BIGGS & C. R. RIZZA

In this final chapter it is our intention to consider in a rather theoretical manner some different and unrelated problems that we have encountered and needed to think about while developing a treatment centre for the care of haemophilic patients. These topics are often discussed at the Oxford Centre and those discussions have contributed to the points of view expressed here.

Academic research and the treatment of patients

The first stage in the study of any inborn error of metabolism involves observations about clinical features by which the disease can be recognised. When the disease has been defined treatment cannot usually be devised until the abnormality in metabolism has also been identified. The academic studies which ultimately uncover the cause are usually diverse and unconnected but lead, at some stage, to a theory or series of theories about the nature of the abnormality. In favourable cases a theory can be tested by devising a form of treatment and observing the effects of the treatment. Usually the treatment has at least some disadvantages and a proportion of the experimental facts do not accord with the theory. There are thus nearly always further avenues to explore. All the same in medicine the reason for research is to discover cures. The academic studies and theories of causation are essential steps along the way but are not ends in themselves. As Medawar (1967) said:

'And so we make a special virtue of encouraging pure research in, say, cancer institutes or institutes devoted to the study of rheumatism or the allergies—always in the hope, of course, that the various lines of research, like lines of perspective, will converge somewhere upon a point. But there is nothing virtuous about it! We encourage pure research in these situations because we know no other way to go about it. If we knew of a direct pathway leading to the solution of the clinical problem of rheumatoid arthritis, can anyone seriously believe that we should not take it?'

In the study of haemophilia, the disease state was defined as sex-linked and recessive and various kinds of disastrous bleeding in haemophilic patients were described. Experiments showed that haemophilic blood had a long clotting time in glass tubes (Wright, 1893) and that the addition of normal to haemophilic plasma shortened the clotting time (Addis, 1910 and 1911). From 1910 to 1950, 40 years of studies concerning normal physiology of coagulation produced little further information about haemophilia. It was then shown that two disease states, haemophilia A and B were included in the original definition of haemophilia (Aggeler et al, 1952 and Biggs et al, 1952). It was found that each of these two diseases was associated with deficiency of an essential coagulation factor and that each of the two factors had a measurable effect on clotting as observed in glass tubes.

The experiments carried out between 1950 and 1960 provided important information about the reactions between clotting factors which occur before a clot can be formed (Biggs et al, 1953a, b, c; Margolis, 1957; Biggs et al, 1958). The clearer view of the complex interreactions of clotting factors made it possible to devise methods for measuring factors VIII and IX (Biggs & Douglas, 1953; Biggs et al, 1955; Biggs et al, 1961). The fractionation of human and animal plasma to provide therapeutic concentrates of clotting factors depends on the existence of methods for measuring the relevant factors. Thus in blood clotting, as in other studies, the background knowledge of theory led to the production of therapeutic substances (Bidwell, Dike & Snape, 1976 review the development of various fractionation methods). The concentrates of clotting factors that were made were used to treat patients and these were found to be highly effective whenever they were used. Experience in Oxford was presented by Biggs & Macfarlane in 1966. The success of methods of plasma fractionation and the success of treatment both add evidence to support the correctness of the theory on which this line of work was based. The theory was presented in a formal way by Macfarlane in 1964.

The present book was planned as a second edition of Biggs & Macfarlane (1966) but since 1966 the focus of interest has changed. The present book gives an established system of treatment which has been developed in Oxford in the past 20 years. The practical problems that have grown from the acknowledged success of treatment have occupied much of the time of scientists who might otherwise have been engaged in more academic studies. Since the aim of the academic studies in medicine is to discover effective treatment, we do not consider that time given to such practical issues was or is ill spent. There are, however, aspects of the more academic studies of haemophilia which have been somewhat neglected in recent years in the general enthusiasm over effective treatment.

Chemical studies of the structure of factor VIII

Perutz (1971) said: 'When I began the study of haemoglobin over 30 years ago, I thought that one could never find out how it worked without knowing its structure'. The same could be said of factor VIII. The unravelling of the structure and mode of action of haemoglobin has disclosed a small molecular machine with very special ability to combine with oxygen. Understanding the structure of a molecule gives the research worker an authentic sense of power. A similar sense of power may be felt by a skilled mechanic who understands the mechanism of a motor vehicle. The difference between the car mechanic and the scientist lies in the fact that the car mechanic has some hope of mending a vehicle which develops a defect whereas the scientist has at present little hope of mending a defective molecular machine.

To continue the analogy there are defects in cars which are so severe that the mechanic could reasonably advise the owner to use some other form of transport or to purchase a new car. Defects in the molecular machine may be slight in which case the machine may nevertheless serve. On the other hand if the defect is severe the molecular machine must be replaced or bypassed. In the case of factor VIII one may suppose that patients having a measurable level of factor VIII have a defective but still serviceable machine. The patients having no factor VIII have a machine which needs replacing.

There is very little that we know about the structure of factor VIII. Present knowledge has been summarised by Austen in Chapter 2. We do not really know the size of the factor VIII molecule; there are reasons to suppose that factor VIII circulates as an aggregate of smaller parts. We do not know if factor VIII is an enzyme or if it develops activity only in association with other constituents such as phospholipid and factor IX. We do not know in what sort of reaction factor VIII participates.

There are of course, degrees of understanding the mechanism of a molecule. Before the structure of haemoglobin was understood it was known that haemoglobin was a carrier of oxygen. Although we know very little about factor VIII we do know approximately how factor VIII fits into the clotting process. The outline general knowledge about haemoglobin suggested transfusion as a treatment for thalassaemia and so also our outline knowledge about factor VIII suggests replacement therapy. Had we waited until we understood the structure and mode of action of factor VIII in chemical terms before we started to consider treatment we should have waited a long time.

Practical aspects of treatment within existing knowledge are, of course, important but detailed knowledge of the structure and function of factor VIII is essential for many important advances that can be seen in outline for the future. These advances include the purification of animal factor VIII; the synthesis of a molecule with factor VIII activity; the bypassing of a reaction involving factor VIII or the identification of a faulty step in the pathway leading to factor VIII synthesis.

Why do haemophilic patients bleed in the way that they do?

The severely affected haemophiliac has no factor VIII clotting activity in his blood. When such a patient is injured predictably severe bleeding takes place from the site of injury and bleeding is predictably prevented by treatment with factor VIII. These severely affected patients also bleed 'spontaneously' into muscles or joints. The frequency of this spontaneous bleeding is very variable. In some patients episodes of bleeding occur in phases. Months may pass with no bleeding and then several episodes of bleeding may occur in one or two weeks. Some patients have a very constant pattern of frequent bleeding and some bleed very seldom. The individual pattern of spontaneous bleeding cannot be related to factor VIII levels since all of the patients being considered have no factor VIII.

INHIBITORS IN HAEMOPHILIA

The differences in clinical severity have been related to the presence of 'inhibitors' (other than anti-factor VIII antibodies) in haemophilic blood (Tocantins, 1942; Nour-Eldin, 1963). The observations of both of these authors consist of clearly described experiments which could be repeated by others. Some of the observations of Tocantins and Nour-Eldin have been confirmed but the interpretation of the results by other authors has not agreed with the conclusions of the original workers. In the case of Tocantins some of the observations purporting to demonstrate the removal of an inhibitor from haemophilic blood may have been caused by activation of factors XII and XI in the sample. In the case of Nour-Eldin some of the observed inhibitory effect could have been due to the citrate concentration of undiluted plasma or to other unexplained effects of whole plasma on certain test systems such as optimum requirements for phospholipid.

Observations on the inhibitory effect of abnormal variants of normal coagulation factors (Hemker *et al*, 1965) suggest a mechanism for inhibition in haemophilic blood. It seems likely that in haemophilic patients, a series of different abnormal proteins may replace the normal pro-coagulant factor VIII. In those patients who bleed most often their abnormal protein may act as a competitive inhibitor in the clotting process. It should be confessed that this superficially attractive idea has no foundation. The factor-VIII-related protein of haemophilic blood has shown no abnormality when tested by currently fashionable test systems.

ASPIRIN AND HAEMOPHILIA

Quick (1974) describes two brothers with haemophilia one aged 25 and the other 23. The elder brother was crippled from haemarthroses and muscle haematomata and the younger brother had very little permanent joint damage. Quick showed that the elder brother had a prolonged bleeding time after the administration of aspirin while the younger brother's bleeding time was normal after the same aspirin dose. Quick implies that intolerance to aspirin, expressed as a prolongation of bleeding time following a dose is yet another attribute of the von Willebrand protein or factor-VIII-related protein. Quick says that the abnormality of the factor-VIII-related protein which causes a long bleeding time after aspirin is very common in normal people, is dominantly inherited and causes no symptoms in the normal person. In 1966 Quick showed that the bleeding time was prolonged in 3 out of 10 normal subjects by a dose of 0·65 g aspirin and that a dose of 1·3 g prolonged the bleeding time of 8 out of 10 normals. A study of the effect of aspirin is made difficult by the technical variability inherent in the bleeding time test and by the fact that the effects of aspirin are dose related. No systematic studies of the effects of aspirin on the bleeding time of normal people or haemophiliacs have been made. It is nevertheless possible that there are features of the factor-VIII-related protein, other than its factor VIII activity, which may be abnormal in haemophilic patients.

HAEMOPHILIA AND VON WILLEBRAND'S DISEASE

It is difficult to imagine why deficiency of factor VIII in haemophilia A or factor IX in haemophilia B give rise to muscle and joint bleeding more frequently than bleeding into other sites. Explanations such as those of Tocantins (1947), Nour-Eldin (1963) and Quick (1974) could account for overall differences in severity of bleeding but not for the localisation of the site of bleeding. Patients having von Willebrand's disease lack factor VIII clotting activity and also lack factor-VIII-related protein. In these patients the bleeding is on the whole less severe than in haemophilia and the sites of bleeding are different. Haemarthroses are very uncommon in von Willebrand's disease; bleeding is usually from mucous surfaces giving rise to epistaxis, gastrointestinal haemorrhage and menorrhagia. It seems almost as if the possession of factor-VIII-related protein without clotting activity (as in haemophilia) is more damaging than the lack of both factors (as in von Willebrand's disease).

PLATELETS AND HAEMOPHILIA

Walsh *et al* (1973) studied a haemophilic patient who had no factor VIII but had been free of all spontaneous bleeding and was 12 years old when studied. This boy was found to have higher coagulant activity in his platelets than a haemophilic patient who had had much spontaneous bleeding. This finding prompted a study of 14 other haemophiliacs who were divided into 2 groups according to the recorded numbers of episodes of spontaneous bleeding per 100 days of observation, 0·5 to 5 in one group and 7·9 to 22·8 in the second. Without exception the boys with the most frequent bleeding had the least coagulant platelets. It is, of course, certain that the platelets contribute substantially to normal haemostasis and thus a particularly efficient platelet haemostatic system could compensate to some extent for a poor coagulation mechanism. These results have not been either confirmed or refuted and it must be admitted that the tests for platelet function devised by Walsh are not easy to carry out.

The limitation of haemophilia by genetic counselling

The effectiveness of genetic counselling for diseases controlled by recessive genes depends very much on particular features of the disease. Circumstances which favour success include:

1. THE CLINICAL SEVERITY OF THE DISEASE STATE

If the disease is always fatal in childhood and no treatment is available, then no parent would knowingly wish to give birth to an affected child and genetic counselling will tend to be heard and acted on.

2. THE POPULATION AFFECTED BY THE DISEASE

If the disease is limited to a reasonably circumscribed section of the population, then genetic counselling becomes more practicable. For example, Tay-Sachs disease, which is carried by an autosomal recessive gene, is 100 times more common in people of Eastern European Jewish ancestry than in other members of the population. Thus investigation limited to this section of the population is likely to have a relatively large effect.

3. THE DETECTION OF THE CARRIER STATE

If the carrier state can be identified with certainty then counselling is likely to be more helpful because normal family members can be reassured with certainty and because further supervision and counselling can concentrate on the known carriers and their families.

4. THE DETECTION OF AN ABNORMAL FOETUS

One method of reducing the incidence of a deleterious inherited disease is to arrange for the selective abortion of every abnormal foetus. Thus detection of abnormality in the foetus is important.

In Tay-Sachs disease all of these four favourable preconditions exist. In a study aimed towards the elimination of this disease (Kakack & Zeiger, 1973) it was calculated that 144,000 people of Eastern European Jewish origin lived in the USA. In this population the disease would occur in the offspring of marriage partners both of whom were heterozygous for the abnormal gene. In such a marriage one quarter of the children might be affected. In a marriage of two heterozygous people the examination of every pregnancy and selective abortion of every abnormal foetus would lead to the elimination of affected children. At the time of making the report Kakack & Zeiger (1973) had studied 4,000 couples and had identified 10 marriages in which both parents were heterozygous for Tay-Sachs disease. In these 10 marriages no abnormal foetus had been found. Thus even when all circumstances which favour genetic counselling exist the elimination of the disease is a gigantic task. It should also be noted that even if every case of Tay-Sachs disease were detected and eliminated before birth the disease would not die out. When an inherited disease caused by an autosomal recessive gene is maintained in the population despite the fact that affected persons die in childhood then it has been calculated that new genes arise by mutation at a rate equal to the incidence of the disease.

The difficulty in achieving positive results by genetic counselling in Tay-Sachs disease will highlight the problems that must arise in counselling haemophilic families. Haemophilia is a severely disabling disease but it is not fatal in childhood as is Tay-Sachs disease. Moreover, modern treatment has greatly improved the life-style of patients and the improvements already achieved raise hopes of an even brighter future in the minds of today's patients. Thus motivation for eliminating the disease is less than it was in the past.

Haemophilia is a very widely distributed disease and seems to occur with about the same frequency in all ethnic groups. Thus counselling cannot be limited to a particular group of people as in the case of Tay-Sachs disease.

In haemophilia the carrier state cannot be detected with absolute certainty by laboratory testing. Thus it is not possible to reassure normal women in haemophilic families. In families known to have haemophilia it is possible to predict that all of the daughters of haemophiliacs will carry the disease and that all the sons of a haemophiliac will be normal, thus limitation of the children of haemophiliacs to boys would reduce incidence of the disease. This limitation could be achieved by determining the sex of all children born to haemophilic fathers and selectively aborting all daughters. In a similar way the women who are known to be carriers in haemophilic families could be counselled to limit their children to daughters. Were such a counselling uniformly accepted and carried out the programme would exclude families where no knowledge of haemophilia exists prior to the birth of a haemophilic son (30–40% of all haemophilic families).

At present the effectiveness of genetic counselling in haemophilia is doubtful but the doctor has the responsibility to make sure that the patient understands the mode of inheritance as it may affect his or her particular situation and family.

Factor VIII and the Blood Transfusion Service

The United Kingdom Blood Transfusion Service was developed originally to supply whole blood for battle casualties and for patients who bled heavily after operations. The major effort of the transfusion service in the past has thus centred on the safe production of citrated whole blood. It is a relatively new idea that blood should be regarded as a primary resource from which large numbers of valuable derivatives can be made. As time has passed the idea of conserving a large number of blood derivatives as separate therapeutic materials has gained support and acceptance. The prominence of demand for coagulation factor concentrates to treat minority groups of patients arises from the fact that haemophilia and similar afflictions are life-long inherited diseases and that failure to treat the patients adequately has such distressingly unacceptable results. But coagulation factors are not the only or even the most important fractions of plasma now needed. Jeffrey (1976) has reviewed the demand for various blood components in relation to a population of 1 million people. He estimates that the product from 21,000 donors per million of the population is needed to provide red cells: plasma from 21,650 to 33,500 donors are needed to supply albumin and plasma from 10,000 donors to supply factor VIII for the 60 haemophiliacs likely to be encountered in a population of 1 million. Thus if the needs of patients for albumin are met there should be no difficulty in supplying factor VIII. The supply of plasma to make factor VIII should be seen in the general context of the urgent need for other valuable blood components.

The Regional Transfusion Centres in the United Kingdom were not designed to take part in large scale fractionation projects and many are ill equipped, under staffed and have no space for such projects. Indeed were they able to supply enough plasma it is doubtful if the present fractionation laboratories could cope with the increased work since the National Fractionation Laboratories were not planned with the aim of fractionating half or more of the blood collected in the United Kingdom.

The Regional Tranfusion Centres in the United Kingdom have developed each one with its own individual interests and its own relationship to the local community. From the point of view of donor recruitment this local orientation has its advantages. The Regional Transfusion Services are also paid for by money allocated for the general medical needs of each Region. Any new development in transfusion which involves the need for additional funds must be considered in relation to the other medical needs of each Region. There is thus difficulty in introducing changes in the transfusion service on a National scale. For example, the removal of fresh plasma from one third to one half of all donations would involve additional staff, space and apparatus in each Regional Transfusion Centre. Unless additional money is made available from central resources, the necessary restructuring must be planned locally and paid for from local funds which have already been allocated for other urgent medical needs.

The extraordinary success of commercial companies in fractionating plasma obtained by plasmaphoresis of paid donors must be seen against the difficulties which are encountered by the transfusion service in the United Kingdom. The success of commercial companies has been attributed by some to the payment of donors (Cooper & Culyer, 1973). It is concluded that unless the donors are paid it will never be possible to have enough plasma. In fact the whole question of remuneration or social recognition of the community service given by donors is a separate and important issue. The proportion of the population serving as voluntary blood donors in various regions of the United Kingdom has always varied widely (Titmuss, 1970) and there is no evidence that the average proportion could not be substantially increased. Moreover, the calculation of demand for blood is based on previous use of blood and this calculation regards the waste of red cells as a disgrace (Titmuss, 1970). In fact the use of red cells will never be exactly evenly distributed throughout the year and if peak requirements for red cells are met some red cells will always have to be discarded. If the demand for albumin fractions, as estimated by Jeffrey (1976), is met then there may be need to discard a third or more of all red cells collected. It is clearly important to have informed estimates of the future demand for all blood components and then approach the population to stimulate an adequate donor response.

The supply of plasma from volunteer blood donors also depends on the proportion of the blood collected that can be separated into components. It is claimed that for many purposes many doctors consider whole blood to be superior to concentrated red cell. In fact, in many parts of the United Kingdom and the world, it has been accepted that red cell concentrates are as satisfactory as whole blood in the treatment of haemorrhage and this view could almost certainly very readily be generally accepted. There should be little difficulty in arranging for at least half of the blood collected to be separated into components.

If the success of commercial companies in fractionation is not due to the ready supply of commercial plasma what is it due to? The commercial companies are organised to identify needs for medical products in society. Having identified the need their laboratories are equipped to study the product and its large scale manufacture. Having solved these problems the production of the substance is planned and financed and thereafter distribution and sale are promoted. The commercial firm has a highly organised team for the production and sale of new therapeutic materials. A new need that can be defined and met by the making of a new product is a welcome stimulus to a commercial firm. It portends increased scale of operation, increased profits and, for many of the personnel, a feeling of valuable service in supplying the needs of the community. The supply of blood is a relatively minor problem and most commercial companies would prefer to use blood collected from volunteer donors if a way could be found to arrange for the commercial companies to work with a National Transfusion Service.

In comparison to the commercial company the National Transfusion Service has quite different problems. The NHS in the United Kingdom has a very good system for identifying medical needs and for forecasting future demand. The Medical Research Council has Committees and working parties made up of specialists who are ideally qualified to provide information. When the DHSS needs advice the same experts are eager to help. A great gap exists between the identification of a need and the taking of any practical steps to satisfy that need. The identification of a need gives no stimulus to the DHSS as it does to the commercial company. This is because nearly all of the money allocated to the Health Service is given to the Regional Health Authorities and little is left over for National Schemes such as reorganisation of the Transfusion Service. In addition to lack of finance the DHSS has no co-ordinated team to promote a new product similar to that of the commercial firm. Both nationally and locally there is a built in conservatism in the NHS which tends to resist new developments.

It should perhaps be asked if the NHS has any business to be concerned with the manufacture of therapeutic substances. The NHS does not make drugs like aspirin and valium why should it make factor VIII? It is quite certain that if the the NHS has a real intention to make factor VIII and other plasma fractions on the scale required then a team of managers will be needed perhaps in the form of a National Transfusion Corporation and money will have to be made available to support the enterprise. In fact a number of drug companies are already supplying plasma fractions and seem to have solved many technical problems in the manufacturing process. The unsatisfactory aspect of the commercial companies concerns the source of their plasma. Perhaps the most economical development that could now take place would be to arrange integration on a National or Regional level between one or more drug companies and the Transfusion Service to produce factor VIII and other important plasma fractionation from blood collected by the Transfusion Service.

How much factor VIII is enough?

As the years pass the amount of factor VIII used per haemophilic patient has steadily increased. In 1974 the patients treated at Haemophilia Centres in the United Kingdom received on average 12,500 units per patient. In 1975 the average use was 14,800 units per patient per year. Present estimates suggest the need for 40,000,000 to 50,000,000 units to treat all patients. As discussed in Chapter 4 we believe it to be within our capacity to supply this amount of factor VIII from voluntary donations within the National Transfusion Service.

Until 1973 the use of factor VIII in the United Kingdom was 'rationed' to the amount that was made within the NHS. In 1973 the first commercial preparation became available and in 1976 there were 5 commercial suppliers of factor VIII and there was no longer a shortage of this material. Will there be a limit to the use of factor VIII and if so what will determine the limit? In the case of factor VIII the economic restraints of cost and restricted supply envisaged by Cooper (1975) do not now operate. The price of factor VIII is high but the patient does not have to pay the bill and no shortage of factor VIII exists. For the doctor, who has the welfare of his or her patients as a first priority, the use of factor VIII must now be adjusted to the needs of patients who are coming to have expectations to take part in more and more normal activities. The only obvious restraint in this situation is the limit when more treatment is judged to be harmful and this limit has not yet been reached. One may hope that some balance may be reached between available resources and the needs of patients. The practising physician who knows that there is no shortage of factor VIII who treats a patient (who knows that there is no shortage of factor VIII) cannot be expected to operate restraints. If there are to be restraints then they must be applied in some other way.

The treatment of haemophilic patients in society

The medical services of the United Kingdom, and in particular the hospital services, were developed with the main objective of caring for and if possible curing the sick. Sickness was thought of as a temporary lapse from health for which a cure was to be provided. Many of the diseases treated in hospitals during the nineteenth and early twentieth century are now curable in this sense. For example, antibiotics can now cure patients who have pneumonia, syphilis, tuberculosis and many other diseases that were previously treated in hospitals. Many other infections are virtually eliminated by immunisation. In addition whole categories of disease have disappeared as a result of good public health measures. Thus good drains, a safe water supply, good housing and adequate nutrition have eliminated typhoid, cholera, malaria, plague and rickets from our society.

These welcome advances have not reduced the amount of work carried out by the medical services; attention has simply been focused on other problems. Intensive care and coronary care units have been set up. Patients crippled with arthritis of the hip can have hip replacement operations. Spare part surgery has become a major laboratory and surgical speciality. Renal dialysis occupies large sections of most hospitals. There is no evidence that these medical developments are undesirable but some of them are fostered by the concept that large hospital institutions must be busy to be 'cost effective'.

In fact many modern causes of ill health are not easily cured by an intensive course of hospital treatment. In fact many diseases are not strictly speaking curable at all. Such diseases can be delayed in their onset and ameliorated by a much wider concept of medical care. Cardiovascular disease leading to cardiac infarction, for example, is accelerated by stress, smoking, high intake of animal fats, refined carbohydrate, overfeeding and inadequate exercise. The disease cannot be cured by a short course of treatment using anticoagulant therapy. In fact a 'European Organisation for the Control of Circulatory Diseases (EOCCD)' has been set up to consider the steps that should be taken to delay and ameliorate the effects of vascular disease. One of the suggestions for the care of patients with cardiovascular disease is the setting up of special Sanatoria or Health Farms where the patient may be weaned from addiction to cigarettes, introduced to a healthy diet, helped to reduce weight and given a sensible introduction to suitable exercise. In addition it is suggested that 'Coronary Clubs' for patients be set up and that frequent follow-up clinics be organised.

Twenty years ago haemophilic patients spent much time in hospital painfully recovering from acute haemorrhages and later they visited long-stay orthopaedic hospitals in the hope of ameliorating the late effects of bleeding. Now most haemophilic patients are safely treated at home or as out-patients. The haemophilic patients are not 'cured' by modern treatment but their whole mode of life can be improved with suitable medical support and they can live nearly normal lives with certain reasonable restrictions.

Hospital care has contributed substantially to the welfare of haemophiliacs in the past since without the haematology laboratories of large hospitals it is unlikely that research into haemophilia would have developed much momentum. Without the possibility of concentrating patients at hospitals designated as haemophilia centres the treatment for haemophilia would not have improved so fast. But the time may have come when conventional hospital care is no longer convenient or adequate for haemophilic patients.

The haemophilic patient cannot be 'processed' safely through the general hospital channels of out-patients, casualty and hospital ward with the inconstant staffing arrangement of these departments and the rigid formality of the system. The haemophilic patient needs a medico-social 'club' where the patients may receive treatment and be trained to carry out home therapy, where families may meet and talk to each other over a cup of tea, where nurse and doctor are available to discuss problems as they arise, where blood samples can be taken for regular follow-up studies, where physiotherapy and a visit to the social worker may be planned. This concept visualises at least some reasonably permanent staff and a place, however small, that could be called a Haemophilia Centre. The need for such special places and special organisations for the treatment of various diseases is now becoming obvious yet larger and larger District General Hospitals are built or under construction for which these needs have never been discussed.

How can the effectiveness of the medical services be judged?

As previously stated, the objectives of the NHS must be to preserve the health of citizens, to care for and cure those who fall ill and to ameliorate the condition of those with chronic or life-long conditions. It is difficult to know how to judge if this work is well or badly done or if the organisation as a whole functions well.

In a commercial company the criterion of success is profit or the production of good and useful objects. Increasing profit is achieved by large scale operation, automation, the elimination of time wasting procedures and good management and staffing organisation. The NHS can be thought of as producing health which might be assessed in terms such as infant mortality rates, average age at death or the lapse of time from the onset of illness to the restoration of full activity. These criteria are quite different and much less concrete than the simple objectives of the commercial company. The criteria are also unconnected with the individual relationship which develops between the patient and a health service worker. In the organisation to promote health very many different specialists are involved including nurses, physiotherapists, technicians, cleaning and catering staff, accountants, architects, planners, administrators and doctors. From the heterogeneity of the organisation has come the idea of 'team' work. In a sense these workers can be thought of as a team since the service needs all of these activities and unless the whole operates efficiently none of the parts will prosper.

The idea has grown up that the NHS is a big national organisation promoting health which should be judged by commercial type criteria such as cost effectiveness, bed occupancy times, and numbers of laboratory tests per technician. This concept obscures the real purpose of the NHS which is to care for and cure patients. There is of course nothing wrong with efficiency in the right place. For example certain laboratory procedures can be automated and thus made more reliable and cheaper to carry out. Less admirably, certain aspects of patient care can be handled in an organised manner. Tonsils, for example, can be removed from children on a more or less conveyor belt system and a similar routine can be developed for the safe hygienic delivery of babies. But even in these instances the process is not pleasant and is probably not desirable. A maternity clinic may be efficient if the mothers are displayed in rows awaiting the doctor who walks past, exchanges a few words with each patient, makes necessary observations and dictates notes to a recorder. The system is not very nice for the patient. The patient may wish to talk to the doctor in confidence and may have worries which may seem stupid to the doctor but which need to be discussed.

In fact the doctor–patient relationship has nothing to do with large scale organisation. The majority of patients come to hospital infrequently and see a different person on each occasion. Each episode is a distinct and usually unpleasant experience. The experience may be made less unpleasant by human personal relationships with hospital staff. The work of the NHS consists of millions of such personal encounters each of which is different. The concept that team work is involved in patient treatment arises from the attempt to draw analogies between the NHS and large industrial concerns.

The haemophilic patient is particularly unsuited to this team work idea though the concept of team work is often emphasised in relation to the treatment of haemophilia (e.g. Rosenthal, 1964). It is true that haemophilic patients cannot safely be treated in hospitals where the needs of the haemophiliac are not widely appreciated by all specialist departments. These specialists may need to consult with each other about the treatment of each episode of bleeding in some patients. This need for specialists to talk to each other is surely a basic need for the running of any hospital and for the care of all patients. For the haemophiliac the most certain need is that he shall have confidence in the doctors and nurses that he encounters on each visit and in the therapy that he receives.

The idea of team work in the care of patients and hospital organisation has another disadvantage. If there is a team then clearly its members must work together. Even a minor decision in one department cannot be taken without ludicrous multiplication of activity by team members. Suppose a junior technician leaves to take up other work and must be replaced. It might seem a simple matter to insert an advertisement by telephone in the local newspaper. But now that the team is operating, a form has to be filled in to justify the appointment.

The justification form must be considered by a committee most of whose members can have little idea of the work to be done by the technician. If the justification is approved the form passes to a department for framing advertisements and the applicants' replies are photo-copied and circulated before interviews are held. In other 'team work' it is often necessary for one department to carry out research in the work of another department in order to write reports for committee meetings. It might be more sensible in such cases for the specialist to be asked to speak.

One rather ludicrous aspect to the concept of team work in the hospital is the fact that hospital staff rotate from one job to another and from one department to another often after very short periods of work. The junior doctors change every 6 weeks or 3 months and similar rotation schemes affect nurses, physiotherapists and social workers. These rotation systems are designed to give staff training but are not in the interests of patient care and cannot be reconciled with a stable scheme for treating the same patients over a long period of time.

If certain myths about industrial organisation and team work are forgotten it is possible to begin to see how the effectiveness of treatment can be judged. Effectiveness can only be judged from an assessment of patient welfare on an individual basis. For the haemophiliac the main criterion is the ability to manage in a suitable sphere of activity as near to that of the normal person as possible. The child must attend regularly at a normal school and engage in the usual children's activities; his illness must not disrupt family life; as an adult he must feel able to cope and actually engage in useful work. Some of these healthy objectives such as school attendance and employment can be expressed quantitatively. The less measurable criteria concern the happiness and effectiveness of the family unit as a whole and this is well expressed in essays on the value of home therapy often written by patients in letters to their doctors (see Chapter 7).

Undoubtedly the most efficient treatment for haemophilic patients is provided by a well organised haemophilia centre. It seems to us that there may be a general lesson to be learnt from our study of haemophiliacs. This lesson is in the simple thought that more attention should be given to the care of individual patients with individual diseases and less to overall hospital organisation. More voices than ours have raised doubts about the value to modern patients of monolithic hospitals each costing hundreds of millions of pounds to build and each exceeding reasonably available revenue for day-to-day running. A disproportionate amount of time, energy and money is required to keep such institutions in running order yet the actual care of many patients must take place in more or less independent units within the general structure.

Conclusion

It takes a long time to make a specialist and to develop a satisfactory service for treating patients. The process of training really begins when all of the rotating from post to post and hospital to hospital comes to an end. The physician has then the time to learn by experience, to absorb the wisdom of others and to study the problems of a particular group of patients from every angle. At first this process of specialisation brings some sense of withdrawal from the main stream of medicine and fear that interests will become too narrowed. As time passes it is found that far from being narrow true specialization involves almost every field of human endeavour. In our own speciality, enzymology and chemistry were studied to consider the reactions of blood coagulation. Statistics were studied to consider populations of haemophilics and the setting up of laboratory techniques and standards. Our patients have suffered from diseases of every sort and description. The education of children has promoted a study of the educational system and the promotion of a special school for haemophiliacs. A sound knowledge of genetics is necessary for the study of inherited diseases. Plasma fractionation is a very important subject for the provision of therapeutic materials. Plasma fractionation cannot be carried out without the transfusion service. Finally expensive treatment is a political and social problem which requires central government finance.

We hope that this book reflects the development of a comprehensive service for patients at the Oxford Haemophilia Centre and that the subjects it discusses show the wide range of interests promoted by specialization.

References

ADDIS T. (1910) Hereditary haemophilia. Deficiency in the coagulability of the blood, the only immediate cause of the condition. *Quarterly Journal of Medicine*, **4,** 14.

ADDIS T. (1911) The pathogenesis of hereditary haemophilia. *Journal of Pathology and Badenology*, **15,** 427.

AGGELER A.M., WHITE S.G., GLENDENING M.B., PAGE E.W., LEAKE T.B. & BATES G. (1952) Plasma thromboplastin component (PTC) deficiency. A new disease resembling haemophilia. *Proceedings of the Society for Experimental Biology and Medicine*, **79,** 692.

ARONSTAM A., ARBLASTER P.G., RAINSFORD S.G., TURK P., SLATTERY M., ALDERSON M.R., HALL D.E. & KIRK P.J. (1976) Prophylaxis in haemophilia: a double-blind controlled trial. *British Journal of Haematology*, **33,** 81.

BIDWELL E., DIKE G.W.R. & SNAPE T.J. (1976) In: *Human Blood Coagulation, Haemostasis and Thrombosis.* Blackwell Scientific Publications, Oxford.

BIGGS R., BIDWELL E., HANDLEY D.A., MACFARLANE R.G., TRUETA J., ELLIOT-SMITH A., DIKE G.W.R. & ASH B.J. (1961) The preparation and assay of a Christmas factor (factor IX) concentrate and its use in the treatment of two patients. *British Journal of Haematology*, **7,** 349.

BIGGS R. & DOUGLAS A.S. (1953) The thromboplastin generation test. *Journal of Clinical Pathology*, **6**, 23.
BIGGS R., DOUGLAS A.S. & MACFARLANE R.G. (1953a) The formation of thromboplastin in human blood. *Journal of Physiology*, **119**, 89.
BIGGS R., DOUGLAS A.S. & MACFARLANE R.G. (1953b) The action of thromboplastic substances. *Journal of Physiology*, **122**, 554.
BIGGS R., DOUGLAS A.S. & MACFARLANE R.G. (1953c) The initial stages of blood coagulation. *Journal of Physiology*, **122**, 538.
BIGGS R., DOUGLAS A.S., MACFARLANE R.G., DACIE J.V., PITNEY W.R., MERSKEY C. & O'BRIEN J.R. (1952) Christmas disease—a condition previously mistaken for haemophilia. *British Medical Journal*, **2**, 1378.
BIGGS R., EVELING J. & RICHARDS G. (1955) The assay of antihaemophilic globulin activity. *British Journal of Haematology*, **1**, 20.
BIGGS R. & MACFARLANE R.G. (1966) *The treatment of Haemophilia and Other Coagulation Disorders*. Blackwell Scientific Publications, Oxford.
COOPER M.H. (1975) *Rationing Health Care*. Croom Helm, London.
COOPER M.H. & CULYER A.J. (1973) *The Economics of Giving and Selling Blood*. In the Economics of Charity published by the Institute of Economic Affairs.
HEMKER H.C., HEMKER P.W. & LOELIGER E.A. (1965) Kinetic aspects of the interaction of blood clotting enzymes. Derivation of basic formulas. *Thrombosis et Diathesis Haemorrhagica*, **13**, 155.
JEFFREY H.C. (1976) Blood transfusion and blood products. Problems of supply and demand. *Clinics in Haematology*. Volume 5. Number 1. W. B. Saunders.
KAKACK M.M. & ZEIGER R.S. (1973) Genetic counselling in Tays-Sachs disease. In: *Ethical Issues in Human Genetics*. Plenum Press. New York.
MACFARLANE R.G. (1964) An enzyme cascade in the blood clotting mechanism and its function as a biochemical amplifier. *Nature (London)*, **202**, 498.
MARGOLIS J. (1957) The initiation of blood coagulation by glass and related surfaces. *Journal of Physiology*, **137**, 95.
NOUR-ELDIN F. (1963) Bridge anticoagulant neutralising agent: properties and isolation. *Acta Haematologica*, **30**, 168.
Oxon Health (1976) Number 5. 'Where are we going?' Published by the Oxfordshire Area Health Authority (Teaching), Manor House, Headington, Oxford.
PERUTZ M. (1971) Haemoglobulin: the molecular lung. *New Scientist*, **50**, 676.
QUICK A.J. (1966) Salicylates and bleeding: the aspirin tolerance test. *American Journal of Medical Science*, **252**, 265.
QUICK A.J. (1974) *The Hemorrhagic diseases and the Pathology of Hemostasis*. Charles C. Thomas. U.S.A. p. 253.
ROSENTHAL M.C. (1964) Programmed care in haemophilia. In: *The Haemophilias*. North Carolina Press.
TITMUSS R.M. (1976) *The Gift Relationship. From Human Blood to Social Policy*. Allen and Unwin, London.
TOCANTINS L. (1942) Antithromboplastic activity of normal and haemophitic plasmas. *Federation Proceedings*, **1**, 85.
WALSH P.N., RAINSFORD S.G. & BIGGS R. (1973) Platelet coagulant activities and clinical severity in haemophilia. *Thrombosis et Diathesis Haemorrhagica*, **29**, 722.
WRIGHT A.E. (1893) On a method of determining the condition of blood coagulability for clinical and experimental purposes and the effect of the administration of calcium salts in haemophilia and actual or threatened haemorrhage. *British Medical Journal*, **2**, 223.

Index

ADP in platelet aggregation 9, 10
Adrenaline in platelet aggregation 10
Aluminium hydroxide in factor VIII
    purification 35, 41
Analgesics recommended 157
Antibodies
  to factor VIII 47–9
    absorption in haemophilia carriers
      80–2
    bovine or porcine factor VIII 199
    contraindicating home therapy 155
    cyclocapron 199–200
    decision to treat 198–9
    diagnosis 73–4
    in haemophilia carrier diagnosis 80–2
    and immunosuppressive drugs 200
    incidence 193–4
    interaction with factor VIII 74–77
      kinetics 74–7
      measurement 77–9
    natural history 198
    treatment 195–200
      low titre 195–8
      temporary disappearance 195–8
  to factor IX, incidence 194
Antifactor VIII antibodies 74–9
Antihaemophilic globulin, response to
    treatment 112
Aspirin
  contraindicated 157
  and haemophilia 223
Assay techniques
  factor VIII 66–70, 71
  factor IX 71–3
ATP, in platelet aggregation 9, 10

Bentonite in factor VIII purification 35, 41
Bleeding
  into intact skin or mucous membranes
    13
  into joints, clinical assessment 16, 60
    treatment 128–30
  von Willebrand's disease 173
  into mouth, treatment 130
  into muscle, treatment 13–18, 128–30, 131
  postoperative, clinical assessment 60
    case report 61–2
  reasons for 13–18, 222–4
  into scalp 130
  into soft tissues, muscles and joints
    13–18
    treatment 128–30
  into tongue, treatment 130
  after trauma, onset, clinical assessment
    60
    case reports 62, 63
Blood, amounts required to treat
    Haemophilia A & B 89–109
Blood coagulation defects
  clinical assessment 59–60
  genetic aspects 15
  and haemostatic failure 15–18
  incidence and effects 6–7
  inheritance 7
  due to inhibitor presence 86–7
  diagnosis, laboratory and clinical 58–88, 63–74
  to estimate treatment required, *table* 17
    mild or moderate 64–5
    severe 64
  laboratory tests, *table* 14
  mechanism, normal 2–9
    normal, factors 3–9
Blood donations
  amount of factor VIII required 104
  hepatitis transmission 181–2
    incidence 181
    infectivity 183
  voluntary service 105–6, 183, 227–8
Blood, surface contact 4–6
Blood Transfusion Service and amounts of
    factor VIII required 105–6, 226–9
Bronchospasm, reaction to infusion therapy
    189

236

Index

Bruising 59
  clinical assessment 60
    case reports 62, 63
  in von Willebrand's disease 173

Calcium citrate in factor VIII purification 35
Calcium phosphate in factor VIII purification 35
Capillary defects in von Willebrand's disease 174
Christmas disease
  antibodies to factor IX 194
  clinical features 25
  complications 181–200
    see also Hepatitis: Antibodies, Bronchospasm; Malaria; Pyrogenic; Pulmonary Congestion; Urticaria; Haemolytic reactions; Pyrexia; Rigor; Thrombosis
  dental care 135–141
    extraction 138–9
    regime 139–41
  diagnosis, laboratory 64
  distinction from haemophilia A 26
  factor IX, dose, calculation 124–5
    estimate of treatment required 17
  home therapy 134–5
    see also Home therapy
  incidence 26
  response to factor IX 115, 120, 124
    following surgery 146–51
      response 147–50
  treatment 106–7
    half-life 115–20
    prophylactic 134–5, 157
Clotting factors, see Factors
Clotting time, in severe coagulation defect diagnosis 64
Coagulation, see Blood coagulation defects
Commercial
  fractionation 227–9
  human factor VIII, activity 100, 103, 105
    characteristics 121
    response of haemophiliacs 123
Counter electrophoresis, virus detection 182
Cryoprecipitate
  characteristics 121
  and factor VIII activity 109, 101–2, 105
  and hepatitis transmission 183
  response of haemophiliacs 122
Cryoprecipitation in factor VIII purification 35–6
Cyclokapron 140, 141
  in factor VIII antibodies 199–200

Dental care 135–41

Dental extraction 135–41
  acrylic plate during healing 138
  bleeding, clinical assessment 60
    case reports 61, 62
  cautions 141
  and haematuria 141
  regime 139–41
  in von Willebrand's disease 178–9
Donation, blood, see Blood donations

EACA, see Epsilon amino caproic acid
Ehlers Danlos syndrome, haemostatic failure 18
Emergency treatment, awareness of patient's needs 58
Epistaxis
  clinical assessment 60
    case report 61
  treatment 132
  in von Willebrand's disease 173
    management 178
Epsilon amino caproic acid (EACA) with factor VIII treatment 136–7
  side effects 141

Factors
  cascade theory 7–8
  diagram 11–12
  first named 4
  nomenclature and common synonyms 5
  in normal clotting 3–4
  as proenzymes 7–8
Factor I (fibrinogen)
  deficiency, diagnosis 85
  estimate of treatment required 17
Factor II (prothrombin) deficiency
  diagnosis 85–6
  estimate of treatment required 17
Factor V defect
  estimate of treatment required 17
  diagnosis 86
Factor VII deficiency
  diagnosis 86
  estimate of treatment required 17
Factor VIII 29–57
  active, molecular weights 41–5
    segregation 41–5
    sub-units 41–5
  activity in haemophilia A 31–3
    identification 49–51
    in von Willebrand's disease 33
  administration 132–4
Factor VIII, amounts required 89–106, 229
  annually 104
  average units per infusion 98
  blood donations 104

Factor VIII, amounts required (*contd.*)
    and blood transfusion service 105–6
    individual 93–4
        yearly dosage, Oxford 94–8
    home therapy, proportion used 163–5
animal 37–9
    activity 100, 103
    causing platelet aggregation 39
    causing thrombocytopenia 38, 39
    in haemophilia A treatment 123–4
    as therapeutic material 38
    therapeutic resistance 38–9
antibodies, *see* Antibodies
assay 64, 65–71
    one-stage 65–7
        clotting time assessments and errors 66–7, 70
    two-stage 67–70
        errors 70
and Blood Transfusion Service 226–9
body levels 34
buffers 37
chemical factors 49–51
commercial human, activity 100, 103, 105
    characteristics 121
defect, estimate of treatment required 17
deficiency, genetic aspects 34
    in von Willebrand's disease 174
in dental extraction 135–8
    see also Dental
dosage in haemophilia, calculation 124
    home therapy 159
freeze dried, response of haemophiliacs 122
gel filtration chromatography 42–5
half-life, in factor VIII deficiency 115–20
intermediate purity NHS, properties and clinical use 100, 102–3, 105
levels in diagnosis of haemophilia carriers 79–80
    following surgery 145–6
measurement 30–1
molecular weight, in polyacrylamide gels 46–7
NHS, characteristics 121
nomenclature 29–30
number of infusions 132–3
purification 34–6, 99–100
reaggregation 47
related antigen, after gel filtration chromatography of factor VIII 43, 45–6
    activity in haemophilia A 32–3
    in haemophilia carrier detection 82–4
    identification 49–51
    nomenclature 29–30
    sub-units 45–6, 50

and von Willebrand's disease 27, 29–30, 175
    levels 31–3
relation to defective haemostasis 16
response, to treatment 100–6, 112–15
    in von Willebrand's disease 172, 173
    transfusion studies 175
in spontaneous bleeding 130–2
source, concentrated preparations from human plasma 121–3
stability 36–7
standards of normality 70–1
structure, chemical studies 39–41, 221
synthesis *in vivo* 33–4
as therapeutic material, best form 104–5
and thrombosis 190–3
treatment, haemophilia A, pre-operative 145
    following surgery 143–6
    von Willebrand's disease 179
whole blood or plasma as sources 120–1
yield 99
Factor IX
administration 132–4
antibodies, *see* Antibodies
assay 69, 71–3
    one-stage 71
    two-stage 71–3
deficiency, *see* Christmas disease
in dental extraction 135, 138–9
    see also Dental
dosage, home therapy 159
    calculation 124–5
half-life, in Christmas disease 115–20
and thrombosis 190–3
treatment of Christmas disease following surgery 146–51
    see also Christmas disease
whole blood or plasma as sources 120–1
Factor X
deficiency, diagnosis 86
estimate of treatment required 17
Factor XI
clotting, contact phase defects, diagnosis 86
deficiency diagnosis 84–5
estimate of treatment required 17
Factor XII
clotting, contact phase defects, diagnosis 86
estimate of treatment required 17
Factor XIII deficiency
diagnosis 86
estimate of treatment required 17
review 18
Fibrinogen
characteristics 3
separation in factor VIII purification 35
Foetus, abnormal, detection 225–6

Index

Fractionation, national or commercial 226–9
Freeze dried factor VIII, response of haemophiliacs 122
Fresh frozen plasma, definition, action and use 100–1, 105

Gastrointestinal bleeding
  clinical assessment 60
    case report 61
  treatment 132
  in von Willebrand's disease 173
Gel filtration chromatography, factor VIII
  normal, activity after 42–5
  purification 36

Haemarthroses 60
  clinical assessment 60
  treatment 128–30
  von Willebrand's disease 173
Haematomata
  into mouth 130
  muscle, treatment 131
  scalp 130
  tongue, treatment 130
Haematuria
  clinical assessment 60
  and dental extraction 141
  in haemophilia 23
  treatment 132
Haemolytic reaction to infusion therapy 189
Haemophilia (*see also* Haemophilia A)
  academic research and treatment 219–20
  admittance to hospital 204–5
  antibodies, to factor VIII, see Antibodies
  and aspirin 223
  carriers, diagnosis 79–84, 224–5
    diagnosis, antibody absorption of factor VIII 80–2
    factor VIII level 79–80
    factor VIII related antigen 82–4
  control of haemostasis 127–52
    see also Haemostasis
  dangers, and small centres 203–4
  delayed visits to hospital 133–4
    dangers 203
  diagnosis, laboratory 64–74
  disruption and insecurity caused by 133–4
  genetic aspects 19–20, 60, 92, 93
    counselling 224–6
  incidence 20–1, 203
    in various populations 91
Haemophilia A
  age distribution 128
  bleeding, into abdomen 22
    into joints 22
    into nervous system 22–3

overt 23–4
reasons 222–4
into tissues, blood cyst formation 22
  continual 24
bruising 21–2
clinical picture 19–25
complications 181–200
  see also Hepatitis; Antibodies: Malaria;
    Pyrogenic: Urticaria, Bronchospasm;
    Pulmonary congestion, Pyrexia;
    Haemolytic reactions; Rigor;
    Thrombosis
dental care 135–41
  extraction 135–7
  regime 139–41
diagnosis, laboratory 64–74
distinction from Christmas disease 26
factor VIII activity 33
  related antigen activity 32–3
  synthesis 33–4
  see also Factor VIII
first manifestations 21
gastrointestinal bleeding 23
genetic data 92, 93, 19–20
  counselling 224–6
home therapy, *see* Home therapy
incidence 20–1, 203
inhibitors 222
latent period 24
life expectancy 25
mildly-affected patient 60
  and surgery 143
overt bleeding 23–4
platelets 223–4
prevalence 90–3
requirements, individual, of factor VIII 93–4
types of therapeutic material 98–103
treatment, estimate 17
  factor VIII 25, 123–4
    dose, calculation 124
    half-life 115–20
    plasma dose and response 120
    response to commercial human factor VIII 123
    response to cryoprecipitate 122
    to freeze dried factor VIII 122
    following surgery 143–6
  inadequate, too late 23
  local 24
  prophylactic 134–5
  organisation 208–18
  response 112–15
    case report 116–20
  and von Willebrand's disease, relation 223
  yearly dosage, Oxford 94–8
Haemophilia Centres 58
  associate 207

Index

Haemophilia Centres (*contd.*)
   consultation 216–17
   functions 206–7
   history 205
   organisation 206–10
   patients treated 91–2
   records 206–7
   References Centres 207–9
     functions 209–10
     boundaries 208
     problems 209–10
   staff required 214–5
   Oxford, *see* Oxford Haemophilia Centre
Haemophiliacs
   children born to 92
   in society, care, welfare 229–31
Haemophilia B, *see* Christmas disease
Haemorrhage
   and haemostatic failure 13–15
     see also Haemostasis
   following major surgery, control 142–51
   see also Bleeding
Haemostasis
   control in haemophilia 127–52
   defects, clinical assessment 59–63
     inheritance 19–20, 60, 92, 93, 224–6
       mildly affected patient 60
   failure, consequences 12–18
   home therapy 134–5
   and major surgery 142–51
   mechanism, in injury, factors 11–12
   normal 1–2
   plug at wounds 10
   vascular and tissue function 10–11
Hemophil (commercial human Factor VIII)
   activity 100, 103, 105
Hepatitis complicating treatment 181–8
   cryoprecipitate and concentrate studies 183
   diagnosis 183–4
   HB$_s$Ag 182, 186, 187–8
     in diagnosis 184
   prevention 187
   risk and choice of treatment 185–7
   source 187–8
   susceptibility 184–7
   transmission in transfusion 182–3
   virus A (infective) 181–2
   virus B (serum) 181, 182
Home therapy 134–5, 153–71
   assessment 167–71
   Christmas disease 165–6
     factor IX dosage 159
   comments of patients and parents 169–71
   complications 166
   criteria 154–6
   G.P.'s cooperation 156
   haemophilia A, factor VIII dosage 159
   observations 159–61
   one year's record of schoolboy 167–9
   Oxford Haemophilia Centre 215–6
   reasons for giving doses 160–1
   special occasions 166
   therapeutic material, amounts and types 162–5
   training 156–7, 158
5-hydroxytryptamine in platelet aggregation 10

Immunisation procedures 158–9
Immunosuppressive drugs and factor VIII antibodies 200
Inhibitors of blood coagulation 86–7
Intermediate purity NHS factor VIII, properties and clinical use 102–3, 100, 105
International Standard Unit, plasma 71

Jaundice, complicating home therapy 166
   see also Hepatitis complicating treatment
Joints, bleeding into
   treatment 128–30
   hip 130
   knee 129–30
   swelling in von Willebrand's disease 173

Kaolin Cephalin Clotting Time (KCCT)
   in factor VIII assay 65
   in mild or moderate coagulation defect 64–5
   in severe coagulation defect diagnosis 64

Laboratory diagnosis
   coagulation defects 63–74
   at Oxford Haemophilia Centre 210–11
Lord Mayor Treloar College
   average dosage 97
   treatment used 129

Malaria complicating treatment 188–9
Menorrhagia
   clinical assessment 60
     case reports 62
   in von Willebrand's disease 173
   management 179
Mildly-affected patient
   and surgery 143
   symptoms 60
   von Willebrand's disease 177
Mouth, bleeding into 130
Muscles
   bleeding into, treatment 128–30
   deep, haematomata, treatment 131

Index

National Health Service
  efficiency, and humanity 231–5
  fractionation 226–9
  teamwork 231–3
  training of staff 233
NHS high purity factor VIII, characteristics 121
Night calls at Oxford Haemophilia Centre 212

Oxford Haemophilia Centre
  diagnosis and laboratory testing 210–11
  home therapy 215–16
  treatment and general advice 211–15
  treatment statistics 211–15
  work 210–17

Penicillin in dental extraction 140
Plasma
  characteristics 121
  concentrated preparations as source of factor VIII and factor IX 110–26
  dose, and response to factors VIII and IX 120
  volume, and response to treatment 110–12
  see also Fresh frozen plasma
Platelet
  adhesion in von Willebrand's disease 174
  aggregation and adhesion 9–10
    caused by animal factor VIII 39
  in von Willebrand's disease 174
  and haemophilia 223–4
Precipitation
  factor VIII, animal 38
  in factor VIII purification 35
Prothrombin
  consumption test, in mild or moderate blood coagulation defect 64–5
  factors concerned with activation 6
  time 3–4
    one-stage in severe coagulation defect 64
Pulmonary congestion, reaction to plasma infusion 189
Pyrexia, reaction to plasma infusion 189
Pyrogenic reactions to plasma infusions 189

Radio immuno assay, virus detection 182
Registration of patients with haemorrhagic states 58
Rigor, reactions to plasma infusion 189
Risocetin co-factor
  function 29-30
  after gel filtration chromatography of factor VIII 43

identification 49
sub-units 45–6
in von Willebrand's disease 174

Scalp, haematomata 130
Soft tissues, bleeding into, treatment 128–30
Staff required, Haemophilia Centre 214–15
Statistics, treatment, visits, staff, calls; Oxford 211–15
Surface contact, blood 4–6
Surgery, major
  haemorrhage following, control 142–51
  in von Willebrand's disease 179

Tannic acid in factor VIII purification 35
Tay-Sachs disease, genetic counselling 224, 225
Teamwork 231–3
Telangiectasia
  genetic aspects 16, 18
  as haemostatic failure 16–18
Thrombocytopenia
  caused by animal factor VIII 38, 39
  severe, due to haemostatic failure 13–15
Thrombocytopenic purpura, bleeding 13–15
Thromboplastin generation test 5
  in factor VIII assay 67–9
  in mild or moderate blood coagulation defects 64–5
Thromboplastin, tissue, action 4–5
Thrombosis, and administration of clotting factor concentrates 190–3
Tissues, function at haemostasis 10
  see also Bleeding
Tongue, bleeding into, treatment 130
Training of staff 233
Transfusions
  hepatitis transmission, diagnosis 183–4
    HB$_s$Ag 182
    susceptibility 184–7
  studies in von Willebrand's disease 175–6
Treloar College, see Lord Mayor Treloar College

Ulcer, gastric or duodenal, bleeding, management 132
Urticaria, reaction to plasma infusions 189

Vascular function in haemostasis 10–11
Venepuncture
  difficulties 166
  home therapy 156, 157, 158

von Willebrand's disease 172–80
  bleeding time 173
  capillary defects 174
  clinical features 26–7, 172–3
  defects 173–6
  dental extraction 178
  diagnosis 59–61, 176–7
    differential 26
    laboratory 64, 84
  epistaxis 173
    management 179
  estimate of treatment required 17
  'factors' missing 175–6
  factor VIII deficiency 174
  factor-VIII-related antigen 27, 175
    levels 31–3
  factor VIII response 172, 173
    transfusion studies 175
    synthesis 33–34
  genetic aspects 173
  and haemophilia, relation 223
  management 178–9
  menorrhagia 173
    management 179
  mildly affected patient 177
  platelets, adhesion 174
    aggregation 174
    defects 174
  sites of haemorrhage 27
  surgery 179
  transfusion studies 175–6

Weight and response to factors VIII and
    IX, and plasma dose 120
  and response to treatment 110–12
Wound areas, platelet aggregation and
    adhesion 9–10